I

S

CANCER - THE LIFE-EXTENSION & CONTROL OF AGEING APPROACH ©

CHADD EVERONE - PRINCIPAL INVESTIGATOR & GOVERNING TRUSTEE
CHADD ALEXANDER EVERONE, II - PROOFING & COMPOSITION

THE CLAIM IS MADE THAT THERE IS ONE AND, REALLY, ONLY ONE PRACTICAL AND RATIONAL APPROACH TO CANCER, AS IS EXPLAINED IN THIS BOOK. WITHIN ABOUT 30 MINUTES, USING THE EASY TO FOLLOW ROUTINES HERE, YOU CAN OBTAIN THE STATE-OF-THE-ART PROTOCOLS FOR THE DIAGNOSIS AND TREATMENT OF ANY TYPE OF CANCER.

THEN, ADVANCE TO THE INFORMATION ON ALTERNATIVE AND SUPPORTIVE CARE AND HOW EXPERIMENTAL TRIALS AND "PHASE I" LIFE-EXTENSION APPLICATIONS MIGHT APPLY TO YOUR INTERESTS.

THE CONVENTIONAL APPROACH TO CANCER IS NOT REALLY WORKING; AND WE ARE IN A RAPID TRANSITION TO A NEW ORDER OF MEDICAL SCIENCE. HOWEVER, IT WILL REQUIRE THE INVOLVEMENT OF A LARGE NUMBER OF PEOPLE TO ADVANCE IT. AND THE EVENTUAL CONQUEST OF CANCER REQUIRES A FUNDAMENTALLY DIFFERENT DIRECTION - ONE WHICH WE CALL THE "LIFE-EXTENSION & CONTROL OF AGEING APPROACH".

THIS BOOK IS RELEVANT AT ANY STAGE (I.E., NEWLY DIAGNOSED, IN TREATMENT, IN REMISSION, OR RECURRENT) AS WELL AS FOR PREVENTION. IF YOU ARE DEALING WITH CANCER - THIS BOOK IS AN ESSENTIAL TOOL.

THE BOOK IS UP-DATED ROUTINELY AND CHANGES ARE INCORPORATED. PLEASE NOTE THE VERSION DATE ON THE FRONT COVER; AND IF THIS COPY IS MORE THAN 6 MONTHS, THEN CHECK FOR THE MOST RECENT VERSION FROM THE SITE BELOW. ALSO, WE ENCOURAGE YOU TO REGISTER FOR SUPPORTING INFORMATION AND SERVICES: **http://www.doctorinternet.com/cancer** PLEASE REPORT ANY ERRORS AND OMISSIONS AND SUGGESTED IMPROVEMENTS USING THE ABOVE LINK.

BY PROVIDING THIS INFORMATION, WE ARE NOT ENGAGING IN THE PRACTICE OF MEDICINE; THAT IS THE RESPONSIBILITY OF THE ATTENDING PHYSICIAN(S). OUR ROLE IS TO PROVIDE SUPPORTING INFORMATION AND SERVICES TO THE PATIENT, FACILITATOR, AND PHYSICIAN TOWARD OBTAINING THE BEST POSSIBLE CARE. THANK YOU FOR YOUR INVOLVEMENT.

FOUNDATION FOR INFINITE SURVIVAL (Est. 1972)
(*science and philosophy in a unified system of thought*)
LIFE-EXTENSION & CONTROL OF AGEING PROGRAM
DOCTORINTERNET.COM
BERKELEY, CALIFORNIA
© COPYRIGHT 2015

Synopsis

The approach to cancer which is presented here (what we call the Life-Extension & Control of Ageing Approach to Cancer) represents a substantially different way of dealing with this disease. (The British spelling of "ageing" is used rather than the American, "aging" because the former is phonetically accurate). The claim is made that there is one, and really only one, approach to dealing with cancer, and that is explained in this book. This will appear to be a bold claim; but the approach is realistic and straight-forward. It is integrative and practical - focusing on the immediate situation within a longer-range perspective. First, any person who is presented with this situation needs to know how to obtain the most appropriate, state-of-the-art, conventional medicine; and this is done, here, in a step-by-step fashion that most people can easily understand. If you do nothing more than the procedures in Chapter 1, then you will have done a significant service for the Patient. Beyond that, greater improvements can be achieved. Concurrent with the Curative Medicine aspect of the Life-Extension Approach there are other aspects which are called "Phase I - Life-Extension Modalities" and which work to improve the general physical and psychological condition in support of the therapy. Further, instructions are given on how to research experimental treatments. And, most fundamentally, this work brings to the fore-front the understanding that unless the underlying disease of biological ageing, itself, is cured, then cancer will never be prevented nor successfully cured.

To expand on these different aspects of the book, when dealing with any type of cancer, the first consideration is to understand what the current, conventional, medical treatments have to offer. This is the subject of the first several chapters of the book; and we will show you how to obtain the state-of-the-art, diagnostic and treatment protocols. Keep in mind that Conventional Medicine changes in tandem with advances in bio-medical science and technology, which is now in a stage of rapid evolution. Also, consider that the side-effects of conventional medicine are a major concern and a "cost/benefit" type of assessment needs to be made regarding the likelihood of a cure and the extension of quality survival *versus* the detrimental effects of therapy. Concurrent with medical treatment, a program of diet and nutritional support, physical exercise, meditation techniques, detoxification, and other adjuvant practices is advised to boost biological vitality during and after treatment. A rational and well-informed approach to Curative Medicine along with Adjuvant Health Practices are, what we call, "Phase I - Life-Extension Modalities"; and this aspect is the main theme in the book. In addition, one is encouraged to investigate the participation in experimental therapies and become versed in the research literature. More fundamentally, the control of biological ageing is paramount. In terms of the eventual eradication of cancer, this is the most fundamental aspect but one which is completely over-looked; and I will encourage you to become involved in advancing this approach.

Beyond the medicine and the science, there are philosophical and psychological aspects that play an important role in dealing with cancer.

The Life-Extension & Control of Ageing Approach to Cancer is relevant whether one is newly diagnosed, in treatment, in remission, or the cancer has recurred. The central plan is to do what is appropriate with available technology and practices in order to extend functional life-span, while staying in touch with medical advances so that one can take advantage of them as soon as they are ready to be employed. Survival is a dynamic strategy. We are in a kind of relay race for truly effective treatments in which incremental scientific advances are "passing on the baton", so to speak, toward the final goal of curing and preventing this disease. If your interest is to obtain the most appropriate treatment and to stay abreast of the most current, state-of-the-art information on any type of cancer, then this book will be of great benefit. Only by having such information can one be equipped to make the best, informed decisions and participate in advancing the science.

The dynamics of change needs to be emphasized. The genetic and molecular mechanisms of cancer are now reasonably well understood, and entirely new methods of diagnosis and treatment are emerging. Our approach is, in large measure, about staying current on and managing this changing technology, as it becomes relevant to a particular person. The procedures in this book should enable one to accomplish that. Please consider that, if the version of the book is more than 6 months from the date on the Cover, it is best to check with us to see if a more recent edition has been issued. Also, we publish separate research reports on individual cases; and you might want to have access to one of those. See the support site: http://www.doctorinternet.com/cancer

Historically, the procedures in this book are an aspect of our work in the Life-Extension & Control of Ageing Program, established in the 1970's. When a participant in that Program encounters a medical condition, particularly cancer, we routinely do a comprehensive report which organizes the current best-practices and research as a basis for helping the various parties who are involved (the Patient, Facilitator, and Physicians) to plan and employ a dynamic strategy. Again, these procedures are useful at any stage, whether the Patient is newly diagnosed, already in treatment, or in remission and, particularly, if the cancer has recurred. As the Principle of the Program and the author this book, I have done hundreds of such individualized reports; and they are always of benefit and well received - not only by the Patient and Facilitator by also by treating Physicians. The reports and other services are explained on the DoctorInternet.com site at the above link. We welcome you to our expanding network of people who are dedicated to conquering this disease.

Synopsis

TABLE OF CONTENTS

Research

"Phase I Life-Extension" - Improving General Health

"Phase II Life-Extension" - Biological Regeneration

Forward

On a recent airplane flight to a conference, I happened to sit next to an executive of a large, high-tech company that makes an advanced radiation system, using a proton beam technology, for the treatment of cancer.

He was interested in talking about the company's latest developments. He said that their newest system is able to treat 5 patients concurrently within a 15 minute period of time. The system costs $100 million for the machine and another $100 million for the special building; and that does not include their income from the software and income from maintenance and support. In his words, these systems were "cash cows" for the radiologists and they were selling like "hot cakes". He was definitely enthusiastic but spoke nothing about rates of cure.

Then, he added that he would "never be in need of a job", to which I replied: "True, that is until you get *your* cancer and have to use one of *your* own machines." He paused and gave a knowing shrug. Nothing more needed to be said on that point, so we went on with discussing the details of the technology and the history of radiation therapy for cancer which originated with the work at Berkeley of John Lawrence (who was the younger brother of famous nuclear scientist, Ernest Lawrence, who, among many things, over-saw the invention of the atomic bomb). I explained how radiation research of the 1950's set much of the foundation for my own work in ageing research, (i.e., radiation accelerates ageing) and how the solution to cancer and ageing are inter-related. He was not aware of that correlation nor about this history of his technology.

The point of this story is that conventional technologies for cancer are big business, but they will not get us much in terms of curing cancer, regardless of how elaborate and profitable those treatments may be. If we are going to solve the problem, a more fundamental approach is required.

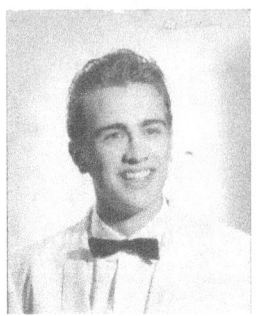

Author at age 17

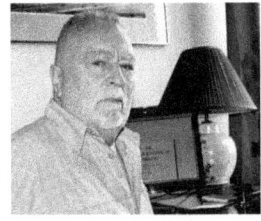

Author at age 73

The difference in form and function is biological ageing - i.e., the decline in vitality due to the decline in cell number, rate of cell functioning, and quality of cell structure. At the level of optimal biological vitality (age 20 ± 5), the incidence of cancer and other chronic diseases is almost zero. As the system ages, control mechanisms deteriorate and the incidence of cancer escalates.

The control of ageing and the cure of cancer are inter-linked. We are all in this together.

Introduction

It is understood that most readers are dealing with a present, medical problem and want to get started as soon as possible with the information that is relevant to one's situation. So, this Introduction will be brief with further background information given throughout the various sections of the book. In fact, you can skip this section and go directly to the procedures in Chapter 1, coming back to this at a later date. However, I do want to bracket the procedural details with some further comments about what is the "Life-Extension & Control of Ageing Approach to Cancer" and to whom this work is directed.

This book is an outgrowth of work which began in the early 1970's, when the author (Chadd Everone) together with a small group of like-minded people (scientists, medical doctors, and creative thinkers) were engaged in developing the Life-Extension & Control of Ageing Program. That initial work was published in two position papers, [1] and there has been no change in the basic strategy since that date - the sole exception being a shift in the basic research strategy from an emphasis on gerontology to regeneration biology as the solution to ageing. This Program constitutes a fundamentally new approach to medicine and health, one which is based on the emerging, life-extension sciences, with a focus on biological regeneration. The central idea is as follows: unless and until biological ageing is controlled (meaning reversed and prevented), our current efforts in disease prevention and curative medicine will never amount to much; and indeed, without the control of ageing, we are headed into a social catastrophe because intermediate improvements in preventive and curative medicine will only result in virtually the entire population surviving into advanced senility and a geriatric condition. Cancer and the other chronic diseases can be said to be caused by ageing, which will be explained more fully in Chapter 11. And unless we cure ageing, cancer will be an inevitable prospect for virtually all of us. This is a harsh but indisputable truth, and it must be confronted explicitly if the problem is ever to the solved. The concept of ageing being the fundamental disease with the consequences becoming a geriatric society, if not cured, was first observed by demographers and social planners in the 1950's. However, the medical profession, scientific community, political leaders, and the general public remain either unaware or in denial of this obvious fact. To get to a human condition that is free of cancer and chronic diseases, we must deal with the problem at its most fundamental level - molecular and cellular wear and tear of the ageing process(es). We know where that science stands today; and we have a good

---

[1] Everone CA, 1977; A Systematic Approach To Life-Extension And Control Of Ageing; Journal of Applied Nutrition, 29(3&4) p.32-47, 1977.

Everone CA, 1978; A Uniform System For The Delivery Of Life-Extension Applications And The Advancement Of Ageing Research; Presented at XIth International Congress of Gerontology, Tokyo, Japan, August 1978.

idea about where the research needs to go. The challenge is to get from where we are to where we need to be as expediently as possible. This book, although dealing specifically with cancer, works in that direction.

Our approach to life-extension and control of ageing entails three components: 1) a specialized, clinical program for, what we call "Phase I" and "Phase II" life-extension applications, as explained below; 2) a research strategy that focuses on the control of ageing *via* regeneration biology; and 3) a specialized animal colony for the verification of therapies to be applied in the clinical program. This is fairly straight-forward approach to technological invention and transfer.

Life-Extension Science can be divided into two categories. *a*) Phase I Applications include those practices that are presently available and are scientifically established to be useful in optimizing health and the prevention and treatment of disease and which will help to extend healthy life-expectancy within the normal, genetically determined, life-span. This could yield a functional life-span of about 80-90 years. *b*) Phase II Applications would employ incremental advances in Life-Extension Science that improve health by slowing ageing. There will be intermediate technologies which slow ageing; but the main one will be the regeneration of biological structures back to an optimum condition and, thereby, maintaining health and function, preventing disease, and extending the healthy life-span well beyond the genetically determined maximum. Phase II applications are still in the experimental, research stage of development. Thus, the main practical efforts in the Life-Extension Program are, currently, in Phase I.

Phase I Applications include certain practices in Nutrition, Physical Conditioning, Toxicology, Preventive Medicine, Psychological Practices, and Curative Medicine which have been established to have some benefit in helping to maintain biological vitality, prevent disease, and to support therapy if a medical condition arises. In addition, there is an important role which philosophy plays - indeed, it can be argued that the major barrier to making progress in the science is our existing world-view or philosophy and personal self-image.

Specifically, the treatment of Cancer is part of the Curative Medicine component of Phase I Life-Extension Science, with the other components playing an important, supportive role in treatment.

When these Phase I Applications are put together in a programmatic way and tailored to each particular person's situation, most people can achieve a reasonably functional and

3

Introduction

healthy, normal life-span with the practices and technologies that are currently available. As Life-Extension Science progresses by advancements in Phase II Applications, such improvements in medical treatment and health maintenance will yield increases in biological vitality and increments in life-extension, with the ultimate objective being, as said, regeneration.

Although the emphasis in our program is on health maintenance and disease prevention, serious medical problems do arise, in which case the challenge becomes one of designing the most appropriate approach to Curative Medicine for the particular individual, given the current state of medical treatment. In this situation, we recommend that one follow the set of procedures that are explained in the book. This we call the Life-Extension Approach to Medicine, of which the approach to Cancer is a specialized sub-set. Over the course of several decades, the author has done hundreds of formal medical reports for clients on a wide array of diseases within this frame-work of life-extension science. Many of those reports have been on cancers; and this book will take the reader through the procedures which are used for that disease.

The Life-Extension & Control of Ageing Approach to Cancer involves the following.

1 - Diagnosis. The staging of the disease and the cellular classification is central to any strategy for therapy, particularly if newer treatments such as "biological response modifiers" are to be considered. The proper diagnosis applies not only at the on-set of the disease but also re-diagnosis during the course of management.

2 - Watchful Waiting. In some cancers, it is advisable to simply monitor the progression of the cancer while, at the same time, implementing Phase I applications before initiating aggressive treatments. Phase I applications are relevant in both newly diagnosed cases and during the course of therapy.

3 - Phase I Life-Extension Applications. The objective is to improve the patient's physical and psychological condition and general health. Optimizing nutrition and physical exercise, reducing exposure to toxins, close monitoring of any disease processes, and working on one's personal psychology are all supportive of medical therapy and can be therapies in themselves, some times. If no medical therapy is warranted, then these procedures are even more important in an effort to maintain well-being, while exploring experimental treatments.

4 - Conventional Medical Therapy. The first issue in the Life-Extension Approach to Cancer is an assessment about the efficacy of the available "conventional" medical treatments. Whether a patient is newly diagnosed, or is already in the course of treatment, or is in remission, or has had recurrence, it is essential to evaluate what Conventional Medicine has to offer the Patient. The questions are these: What is the current "state-of-the-art" therapy for the particular type of cancer? What are the potential benefits versus adverse effects of various treatments? A decision needs to be made whether or not conventional modalities are appropriate and, if so, how to treat. Then, what is the state of research in the area, and is some kind of experimental method appropriate? One should stay in touch with the changing treatment protocols, re-checking this information every 3 to 6 months, because therapies are evolving. Further, how does the program of nutrition, physical conditioning, and other Phase I life-extension applications both support and augment medical treatment? All of this needs to be bracketed by the person's religious and philosophical values and what each individual person wants to achieve with one's life. Thus, evaluating the "state-of-the-art" medical protocols is the first set of procedures, and how to do that is covered in the initial Chapters of the book. Again, staying in touch with progress in conventional protocols is relevant at any stage of the cancer.

5 - Adjuvant Medicine. "Adjuvant" refers to treatments that are in support of the primary care. In addition to the other Phase I life-extension modalities, this includes other medical approaches such as: Supportive and Palliative care, Complementary and Alternative Medicine, and, in general, an Integrative, holistic approach to Medicine. One might consider using some of these modalities as part of a treatment program. Or, if the decision is to not employ Conventional Medicine or to postpone it, then one would consider these various modalities as primary treatments.

6 - Experimental Treatments. If conventional treatments have been exhausted or seem unlikely to be effective or there are too many adverse effects, then experimental approaches should be investigated. This is applicable for newly diagnosed cases as well as during or after the course of therapy. These are called "Clinical Trials" and researching these takes a fair amount of erudition on the part of all parties: Patients, Facilitators, and the Physicians. We will provide some guidance in that regard.

7 - Basic Research. We encourage one to survey and become familiar with the basic research on one's topics of interest. This entails learning how to use the MEDLINE database, which, like the experimental treatments, requires a fair amount of erudition on the part of all parties. Again, we will provide basic routines and guidance.

8 - Advancement of Basic Research. Research on the Conventional Medical approaches to cancer treatment (i.e., surgery, chemotherapy, and radiation) is already well funded by government agencies, foundations, and commercial entities. In truth, that effort has not yielded much progress; and it will ultimately fail because unless and until the technology for biological regeneration is developed and ageing is cured, cancer can never be preventable or curable. Further (and this is the most striking fact), even if very advanced treatments were devised to prevent or cure all cancers, as a specific disease, it would only increase the average life-expectancy by about 3 years because other chronic diseases would ensue and conventional cancer treatments probably accelerate their likelihood. Indeed, if all the particular causes of death were eliminated, the life-expectancy would be increased by only about 12 years, and then everyone would end up in the geriatric ward to die of chronic senescence. A dismal prospect, indeed! But this will be discussed in more detail, later in the closing chapters of this book. For the moment, we are concerned about obtaining the best possible and most appropriated and currently available treatment for the cancer of a particular individual.

The book is directed to three audiences - the Patient, the Facilitator, and the Physician; and a few words about each is warranted here.

The Patient is, obviously, the person with the cancer and in whom this effort counts. Many Patients are in denial and traumatized and will be relying on a Facilitator and, ultimately, on one's Physician(s). Still, increasingly, Patients want to be more involved in decision making, and the better informed the Patient is, the better one is in a position to ask relevant questions and make judgments that are appropriate.

The Facilitators are, in the broadest sense, the community which supports the Patient. In particular, a Facilitator is a person who is helping the Patient to obtain the most appropriate medical treatment. This can be a relative or friend, or it can be a trained counselor. The Facilitator can be in a better position to be more objective, understand the facts of the particular situation, and to help the Patient judge what is most appropriate. The Facilitator also can serve as an intermediary between the Patient and the Physician, helping the latter to give effective care of the former.

The Physician and Health Professionals are the ones who implement the medical treatments; and many of the procedures in this book will help them to stay on top of the rapidly evolving treatment of cancer. To the extent that the Physician wants an informed Patient, one can refer the Patient and Facilitator to some of the procedures in this book, thus serving professional due diligence and informed consent.

Almost everyone who is dealing with cancer will come to rely on the conventional medical professions and the diagnostic and treatment practices which they offer - as imperfect as they may be. **R**egardless of how much a person might be disaffected by the "Establishment" and be a rebel in other aspects of one's life, we almost certainly will acquiesce to the established way of doing things when it comes to medicine. **W**e are compelled to this by the inertial force of convention, the emotional need for authority in a situation of fear and uncertainty, the opinion of others, and the economics of the matter. **T**herefore, it is appropriate to start with how to get the most appropriate treatment from conventional medicine. **S**o, with this brief Introduction, let's move into those recommended procedures; and in the course of doing so, additional explanatory information will be provided.

Introduction

CHAPTER 1

PDQ - PHYSICIAN DATA QUERY - INTRODUCTION

The first step in dealing with any serious, medical problem is to evaluate what "conventional medicine" has to offer in terms of cure or amelioration or management of the problem.

In regard to cancer, the starting point is to use the database, known as Physician Data Query (PDQ).

Regardless of the stage in the progression of the cancer (i.e., newly diagnosed but not in treatment, already in treatment, in remission, or recurrent), the first thing to do is to obtain a current understanding of the conventional, state-of-the-art protocol for the particular type of cancer of concern. This is done by using the Physician Data Query or PDQ database. (Later, we will elaborate on and critique what "conventional medicine" actually is.)

PDQ (Physician Data Query) is the primary source of information for the most current, scientifically authoritative, state-of-the-art treatment protocols for any type of cancer. The database is generated and maintained by National Cancer Institute (NCI). The NCI was created in 1937 by Congress and President Roosevelt, and the Institute is the world's largest organization that is dedicated solely to cancer research. It is one component of the National Institutes of Health. The budget for 2013 for those institutes is about $29 billion, of which about $5 billion is for the National Cancer Institute.

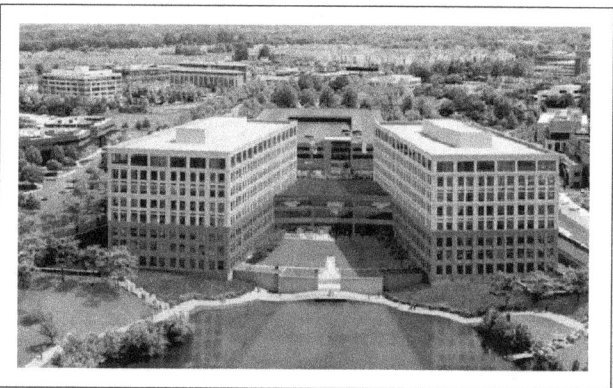

Rendering of the new research headquarters for the National Cancer Institute at Shady Grove Life Sciences Center in Rockville, Maryland.

The PDQ database is a comprehensive, cancer database, which contains a wide-range of information. Of particular use, at this point in our mission, is the "Cancer Information Summaries" section of PDQ. These are formal, peer-reviewed, evidence-based protocols

8

for the diagnosis and treatment of over 70 types of cancer. There is no better source of this kind of information than PDQ. The reports are in a version for the Patient and a version for the Health Professional or treating Physician.

* The Patient version for each type of cancer is written in lay language and includes links to the NCI Dictionary of Cancer Terms. Many Patient Summaries also include illustrations. It is for the general orientation of the Patient and Facilitator; and the Physician may want to give a copy of this version to the Patient as part of medical informed consent and due diligence.

* The Health Professional or Physician version of the PDQ provides more detailed information and is written in technical language. It is fully referenced with links to PubMed (MEDLINE), research reports. Further, there are summaries for Supportive and Palliative care, for Screening and Prevention, for Complementary and Alternative Medicine summary, and for Experimental treatments that are in clinical trials. Also, the Patient and Facilitator can use this independently and in conjunction with the treating Physician(s).

Again, the main focus, at this point, is on the "Cancer Information Summaries". The PDQ Cancer Information Summaries are produced, maintained, and updated regularly by six PDQ Editorial Boards that are comprised of oncology specialists in fields including medical oncology (chemotherapy), surgical oncology, and radiation oncology; epidemiology; psychology; genetics; and complementary and alternative medicine. Each Editorial Board reviews published research findings on a monthly basis and meets several times a year to review and discuss updates to their summaries. The six Editorial Boards are the following:

- Adult Treatment Editorial Board - 18 members
- Pediatric Treatment Editorial Board - 22 members
- Supportive and Palliative Care Editorial Board -16 members
- Screening and Prevention Editorial Board - 19 members
- Cancer Genetics Editorial Board - 30 members
- Cancer Complementary and Alternative Medicine Editorial Board - 19 members

Further, the PDQ Editorial Boards are supported by Advisory Boards, each of which is similarly comprised of experts in cancer and related specialties. These boards include a broad range of experts from the following:

- President's Cancer Panel,
- National Cancer Advisory Board,
- Board of Scientific Advisors,
- Board of Scientific Counselors - Basic Sciences,
- Board of Scientific Counselors - Clinical Sciences and Epidemiology,
- Clinical Trials & Translational Research Advisory Committee,
- Director's Consumer Liaison Group,
- NCI Frederick Advisory Committee
- NCI Initial Review Groups,
- Special Emphasis Panel, and
- Office of Federal Advisory Committee Policy.

By publishing these PDQ protocols for particular types of cancer, the NCI's objective is to bring the clinical, medical practice, that is "out in the field", more in line with what is held to be state-of-the-art, best practices. It needs to be emphasized that these protocols are not a policy for the NCI nor should they be seen as over-ruling the judgment of the treating physician. But they do give a good set of guidelines and a "second opinion", so that the Patient and Facilitator can evaluate the treatment of the physician, and the protocols give the treating Physician a consensus reference for judging one's treatment strategy.

For the most part, these protocols represent "conventional medicine". Some consideration is given to what is called "alternative" and "complimentary" types of medicine. But those modes of therapy are not well studied within a scientific frame-work. This is because research is not well funded in those modalities. Because these are not patentable, there is little economic incentive to advance them.

In the following sections, I will walk you through the procedures for retrieving the protocols from the PDQ databases - first for the Patient and, then, for the Health Professional. Simply follow the procedures, as described, to retrieve the information; and download the report. Use it as suggested and however it may be appropriate to your situation.

Once you have used a particular database, the procedures will be pretty intuitive; and after that, you may not need the detailed instructions which follow. Accordingly, in the prolog of each Chapter, we have provided "Expert Summaries" of the procedures for acquiring the data for quick reference.

Because the PDQ Summaries are revised on a routine basis, it is worthwhile to retrieve a new report periodically and to note any significant changes.

PDQ - PATIENT PROTOCOLS

The Patient Summary of the PDQ report is designed for the Patient and for the Facilitator. It explains the nature of the particular cancer, the various stages, and treatment options. It usually contains a glossary of medical terms that are relevant. The Patient/Facilitator should have the Physician go over the report and identify which sections are relevant to the particular case. Make notes on your printed copy.

Below is an "Expert Summary", which many people will be able to use.

Expert Summary

- *Go to:* http://www.cancer.gov/cancertopics/pdq

- *Select:* **"PDQ Cancer Information Summaries"**. Then select either: **"Adult Treatment Summaries"** or **"Pediatric Treatment Summaries"**.

- *Find:* The type of cancer desired and select "**[patient]**".

- *Select:* In upper right-hand section of the page, there are 3 icons – one for viewing the document, the other for printing it, and the third for sending it as an e-mail. Select your desired option.

- *Use:* Your desired print option in your browser.

If you were able to use this Expert Summary, congratulations! You have just completed, in a couple of minutes, an extremely complex retrieval of the most current, state-of-the-art, conventional medical protocols for the cancer of your interest - something which has required hundreds of millions of dollars to create and maintain and the dedication of a large number of professionals over many decades - all of which is due to public funding and costs you virtually nothing. If you do no more than this single routine, present the report to your physician, and use it as a basis to better understand your situation, then you will have done for yourself a very tangible service.

If this Expert Summary worked for you, then you can skip over the next couple of pages and go directly to the **Discussion** section of this Chapter. If the above Summary did not work for you, then the following instructions repeat the above steps and guide you through the same procedures with more detailed instructions and graphic representations.

To retrieve the report for the **PDQ - Patient**, connect to the Internet and go to:

http://www.cancer.gov/cancertopics/pdq

You will see this page.

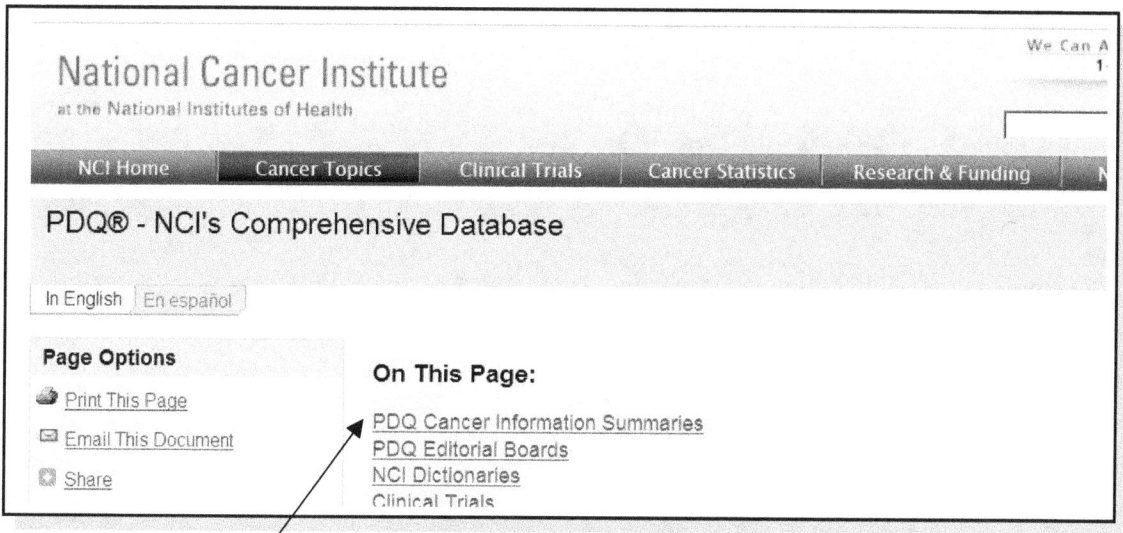

Select the link "**PDQ Cancer Information Summaries**", which takes you to:

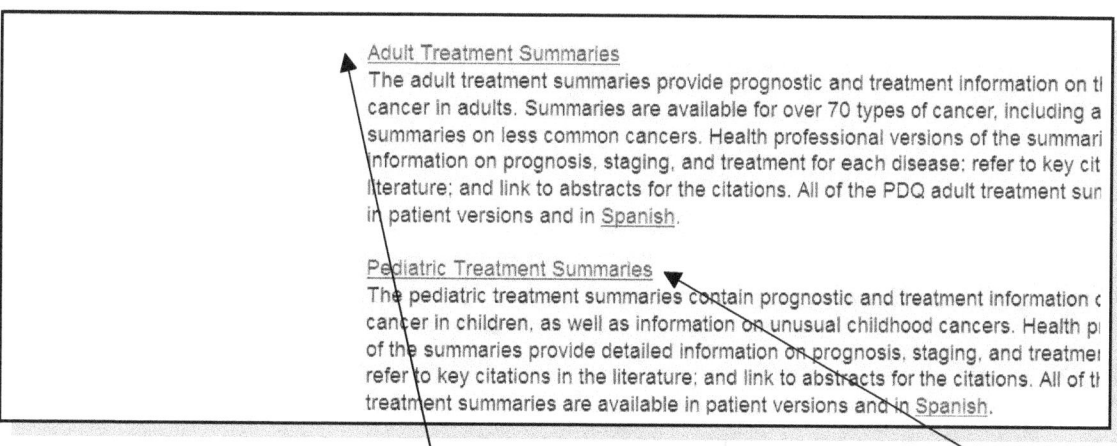

Select the appropriate link "**Adult Treatment Summaries**" or, for children, "**Pediatric Treatment Summaries**". Note that there are other links on this page which go to different databases; but do not diverge at this point because we will come back to some of those, later.

This will lead you to the page, which lists the various cancer reports that are available.

There are various ways to find the cancer of interest to you.
Scroll down the **List** or by using the **Index** .

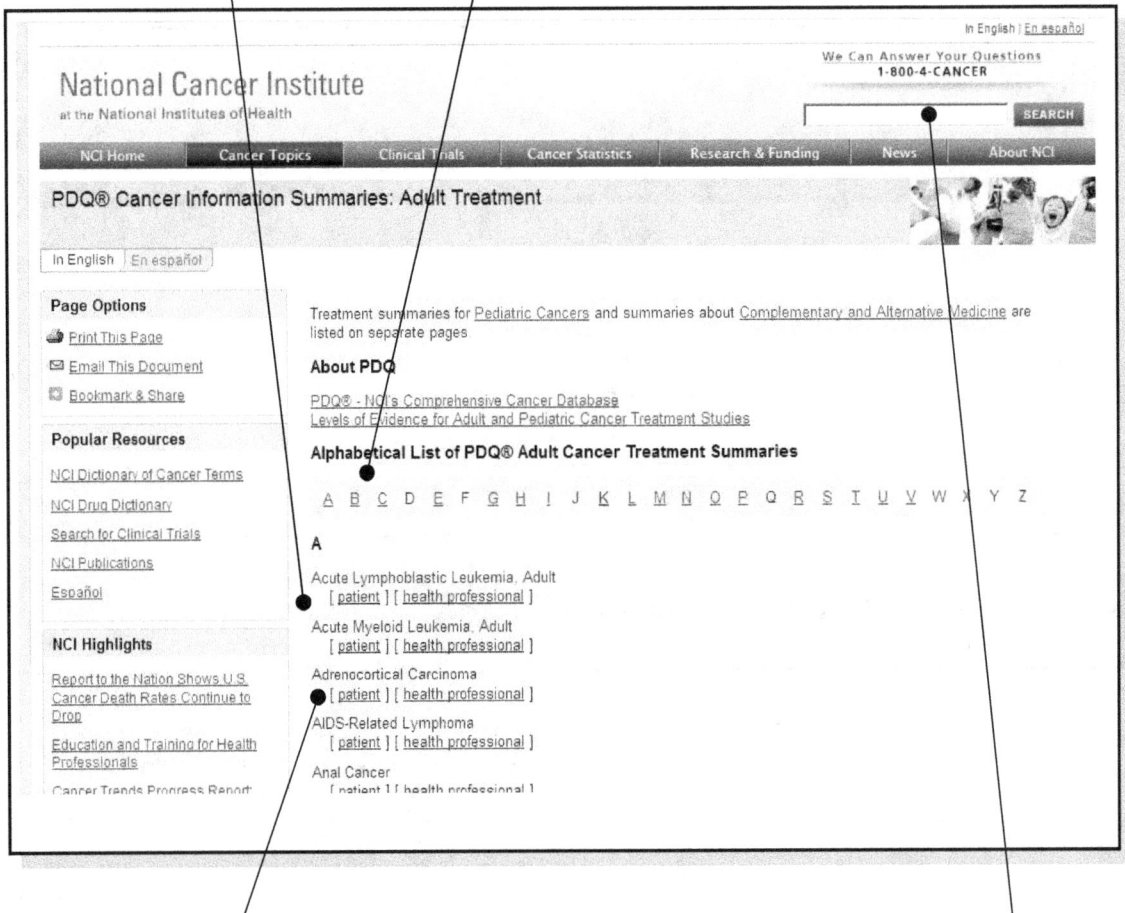

Select the link ["**Patient**"] when you find the proper type.
If you cannot find the particular cancer or want expanded information, use the **Search Box** and type in the term.

Before doing this procedure, it is best to make sure that you have the proper diagnostic term of the type of cancer from your physician. Also, from your physician, obtain the cell type and stage, as emphasized at the beginning of this chapter. Include this report and all other information in your clinical records portfolio, as will be discussed in Chapter 3.

13

Using "**Acute Lymphoblastic leukemia**", as an example for our purposes here, this will lead you to the first page of the desired report as represented below.

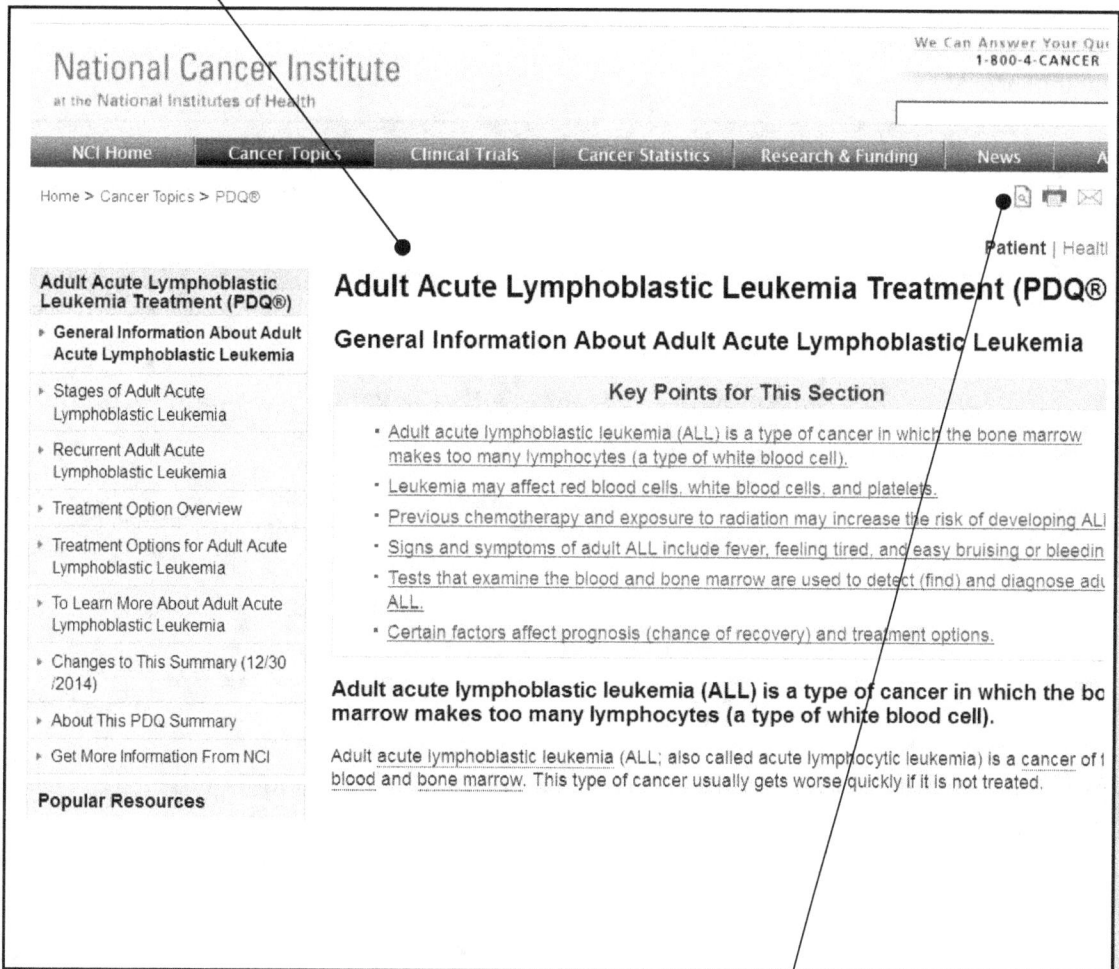

You can read this on-line and page through the report using the "**Next Section >**" at the bottom of the page. **B**ut it is best to retrieve the entire report and either print or download and store it on your disk. **N**ote the View Entire Document **icon**.

14

That will display the full report; and then, you can review the document on the screen, or you can use the **"Print"** function. Note, this only displays the document on your screen in a printer friendly format and does not actually send it to your printer. You must use your browser functions to do that. Also, you can **Email** the report, or forward it on various social media systems.

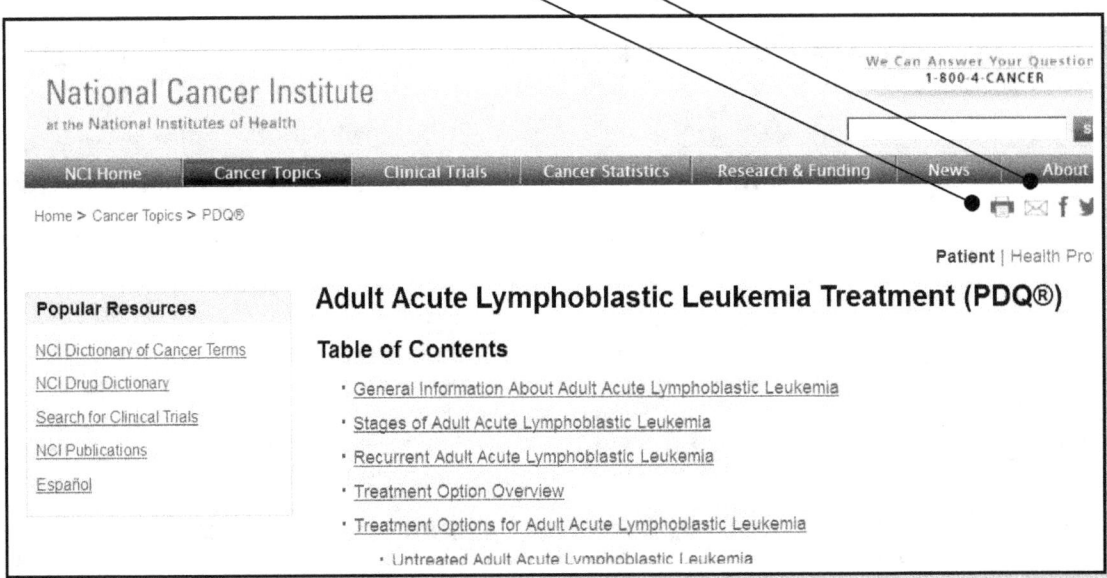

For the date of the most recent revision of this report, see, at the bottom of the page, when it was last **Updated**.

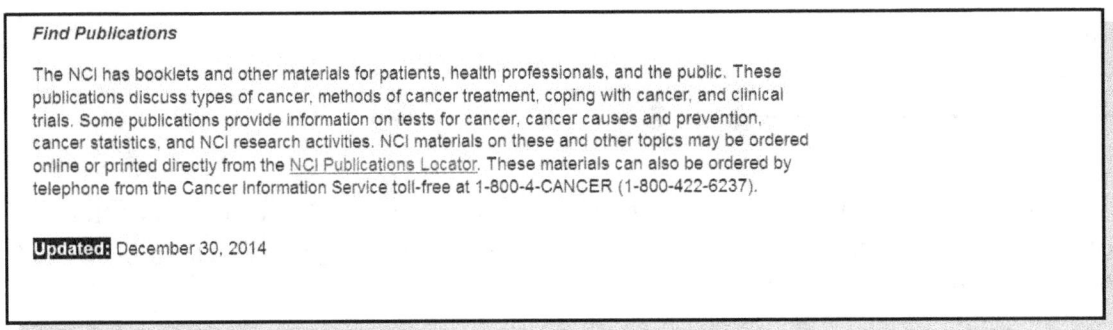

Discussion

Having done the above, you (even if someone who is naïve to this type of research) have retrieved the most current, state-of-the-art protocol on the cancer of interest; and you have done so within in very short period of time. If you were to do nothing more than this, you would have accomplished a great deal. Even a professional researcher could not have done any better - at least up to this initial point. And any professional researcher would have to start with this procedure. (Again, take into consideration that you have just been the beneficiary of hundreds of millions of dollars of public funding and millions of hours of expert work - a cumulative effort of over half a century. We should be grateful!)

Now, your study begins. Here are some general suggestions for how to approach this information.

> **To The Patient.** If you are the Patient, you can simply print out the full report, bind it in some fashion, make a copy for yourself and for the others involved, and provide your physician with a copy. Have the physician go over the report and point out which sections apply to you, in particular. If you did nothing more than this, you would be doing for yourself a considerable service, as well as making the job easier for your physician(s).
>
> However, you are encouraged to study the report, make notes, and use the basic information to proceed further in your research. Again, the objective is to do what you can to obtain the state-of-the-art diagnosis and the most appropriate treatment for your particular situation. Get a clear and objective idea about the stage of the cancer and the cellular type of the cancer. Usually, the stage will be some variation of the extent of migration from the original site. Tumors start as one localized cell that proliferates into a cluster that is "encapsulated" - Stage I. Then, if it progresses, it invades the surrounding tissue - Stage II. And finally, it can spread (metastasize) to other organs - Stage III. However, different tumors are staged differently. The aggressiveness and type of treatment (or no treatment) will relate to this "staging". Note the date of the PDQ report - at the top of the report, entitled "Last Modified:". Where a particular field is advancing rapidly, the report will be revised more frequently. Some revisions are minor; some are major; so go back and get a fresh report periodically. Get a clear idea about the efficacy and adverse effects of the

available types of treatment - surgery, radiation and/or chemotherapy, and biologic response modifiers (i.e., stimulating the body's natural defense against cancer). Much of the treatment strategy is a judgment call and relative to personal and social factors in addition to the medical assessment. The Patient's decisions are integral to that judgment; and the better informed one is, the better the judgment. Again, provide a copy of the Patient Summary to the Facilitator and the Physician(s). Do not be intimidated about giving information to your doctor and asking pointed questions - it is your body and you should understand what is happening. You should make the judgment calls even if it is to defer completely to the recommendations of your physician(s). And do be patient about studying the report - it takes some time and effort and repetition. To the extent that you become well informed, you can participate in a peer-network and can help others with the same problem

To The Facilitator. The Facilitator is one who is helping the Patient obtain the most appropriate care - dealing personally with both the Patient and the Physician. The Facilitator can be a relative or friend, a counselor, or other type of professional. This is one of the most important roles in cancer therapy. Patients can be frightened and not in an emotional state to make objective decisions. Knowing the Patient's personality, circumstances, and philosophical beliefs (including religious) are critical in the treatment strategy; and the Facilitator should not be reticent about being engaged in the interactions between the Patient and the Physician, assuming that the Patient gives permission.

To The Physician. It can be useful to you to provided one of these PDQ - Patient Summaries to your Patient to aid in your communications. It can also serve as part of the "informed consent" process. Also, having a copy of the more technical PDQ - Health Professional report could be useful in determining your therapeutic options; and the instructions for retrieving that more specialized report is in the next Section.

Again, the PDQ database is focused mostly on Convention Medicine; however, there are sections for Alternative Therapies and for Supporting Care; and there is a listing for Clinical Trials (experimental therapies) as well as other functions. All of those will be discussed later; but the single most important issue, at this point, is to get you to down-load the Patient Summary for the particular cancer of concern, to study it, and give a copy to the various parties, who are involved.

17

PDQ - PHYSICIAN PROTOCOLS
(PHYSICIAN & HEALTH PROFESSIONALS)

The protocols in the PDQ for Physicians and Health Professionals are more technical versions of the Patient reports. One feature is that references to the scientific literature are linked to PubMed (MEDLINE) database and from there related articles are available. That research information will be discussed separately in the "Chapter 8 - PubMed Search Engine and the MEDLINE Database".

Although designed for professionals, these Summaries are accessible to Patients and Facilitators who want a more technical understanding; and they are advised to download this report and provide a copy to the Physician(s).

Expert Summary

☉ *Go to:* http://www.cancer.gov/cancertopics/pdq

☉ *Select:* **"PDQ Cancer Information Summaries"**. Then select either: **"Adult Treatment Summaries"** or **"Pediatric Treatment Summaries"**.

☉ *Find:* The type of cancer desired and select "**[health professional]**".

☉ *Select:* In upper right-hand section of the page, there are 3 icons – one for viewing the document, the other for printing it, and the third for sending it as an e-mail. Select your desired option.

Use: Your desired print option in your browser.

As before, many people will find the above Expert Summary sufficient to retrieve the desired report. However, if that is not the case, then the following instructions will guide you through these procedures with their graphic representations.

To retrieve the report for the **PDQ - Health Professional** (Physician) **Summary**, go to:

http://www.cancer.gov/cancertopics/pdq

You will see this page.

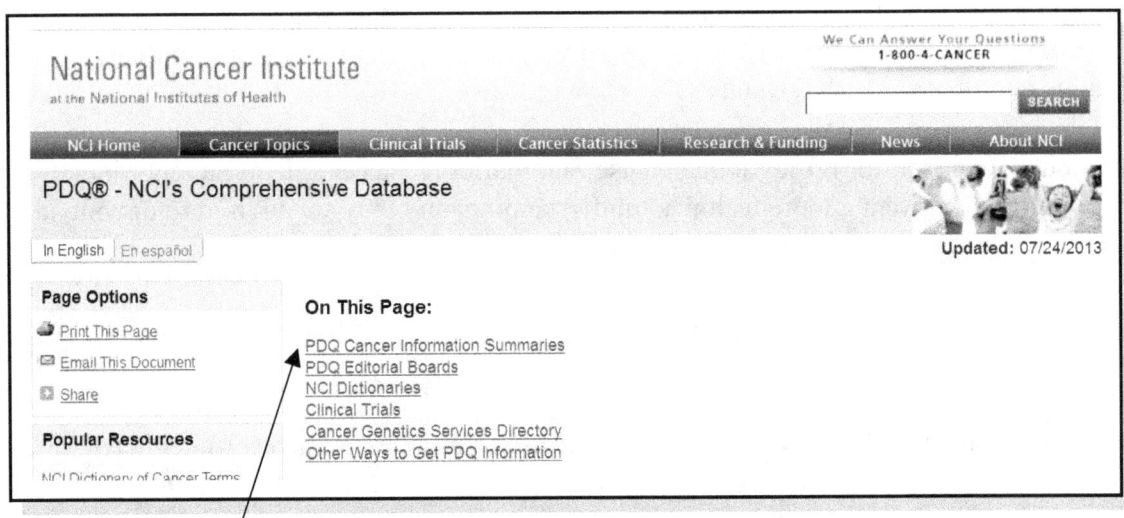

Select the link "**PDQ® Cancer Information Summaries**", which takes you to:

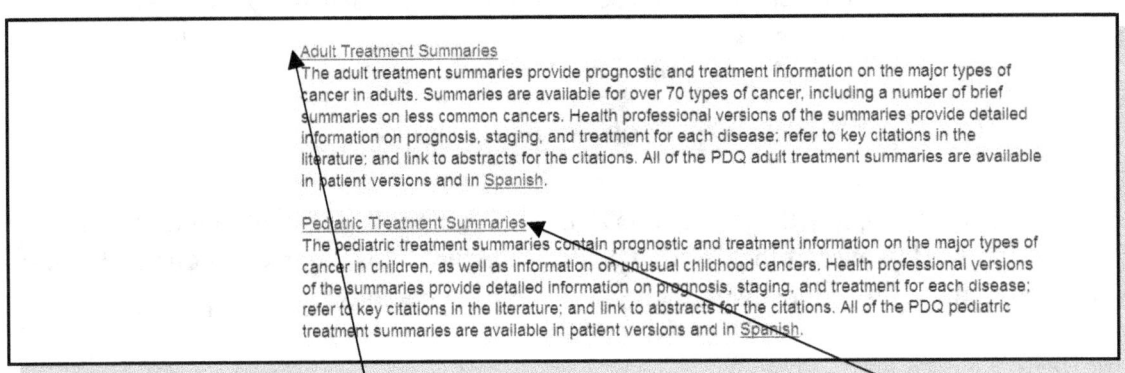

Select the appropriate link "**Adult Treatment Summaries**" or, for children, "**Pediatric Treatment Summaries**". Note that there are other links on this page which go to different databases; but do not diverge at this point because we will come back to some of those, later.

This will lead you to the page which lists the various cancer reports that are available.

Find the particular type of cancer of interest by scrolling down the **List** or by using the **Index** .

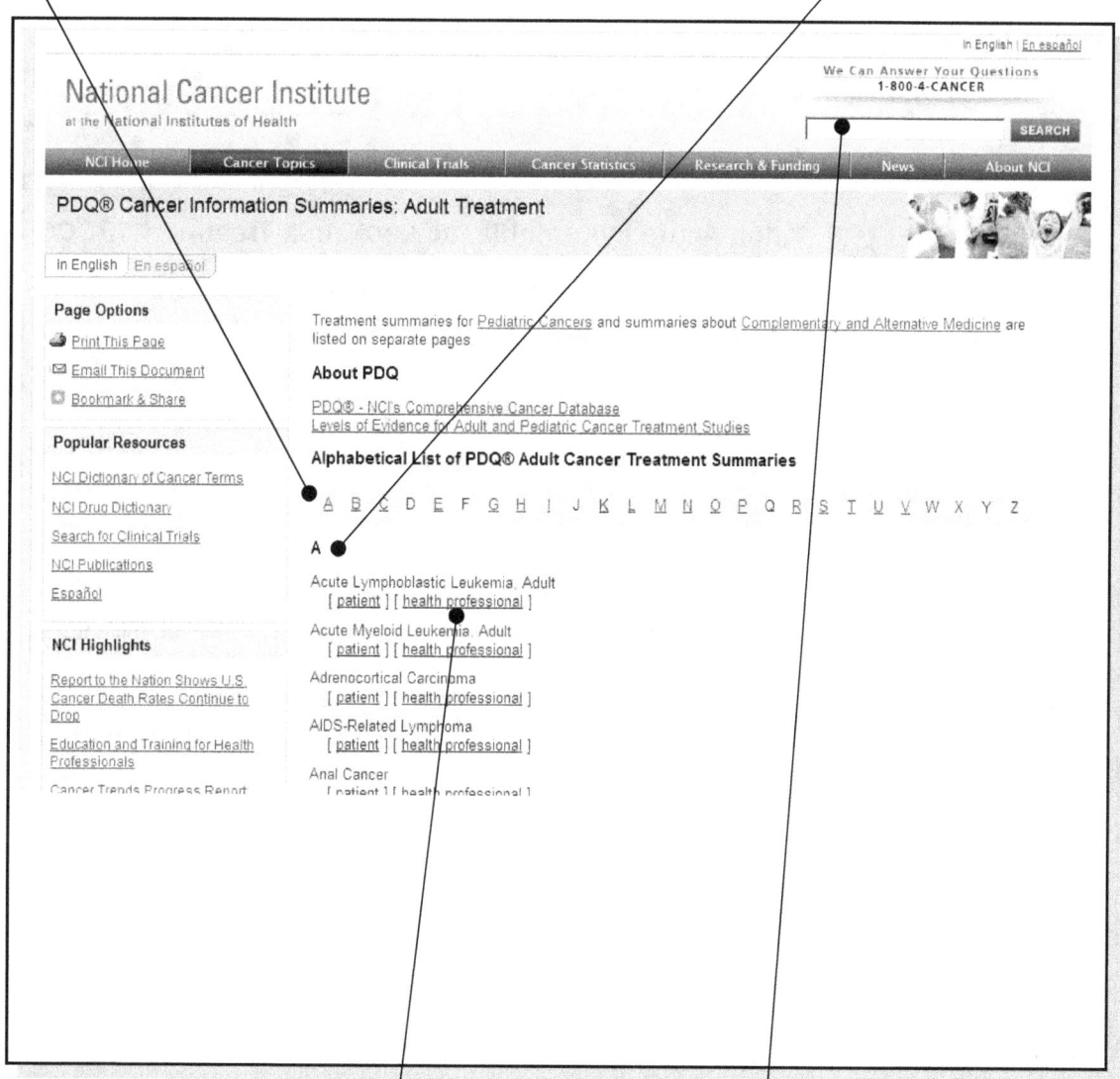

Then, Select the link ["**health professional**"]. Use the **Search Box**, if you cannot find the particular cancer or want more extensive information.

Using "**Acute Lymphoblastic Leukemia**" as an example, this will lead you to the first page of the desired report.

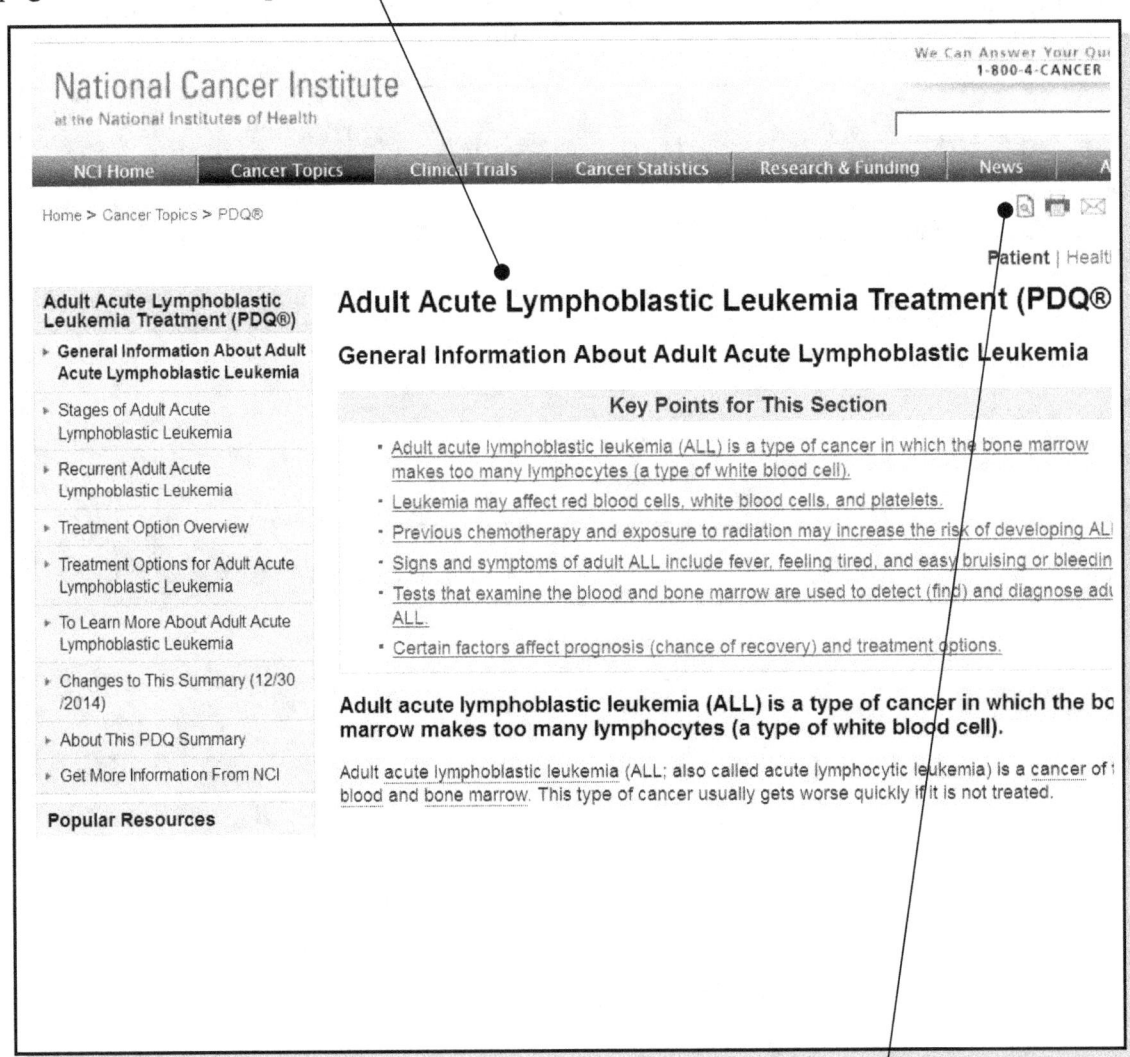

You can read this on-line and page through the report using the "**Next Section >**" at the bottom of the page. **B**ut it is best to retrieve the entire report and either print or download and store it on your disk. **T**o do that use the View Entire Document **icon**.

That will display the full report; and then, you can review the document on the screen or you can use the "**Print**" function. Note this print function only displays the document on your screen in a printer friendly format and does not actually send it to your printer. You must use the browser functions to do that. Also, you can "**Email**" the report or forward it on various social media systems.

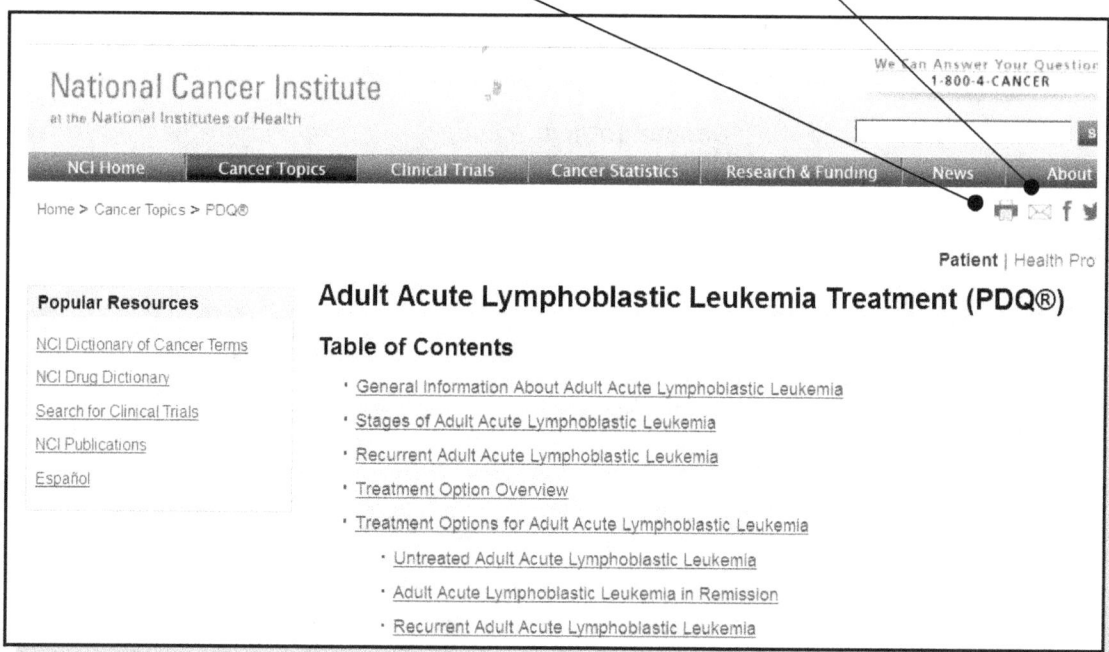

The date of the most recent revision is at the bottom of the page - **Update**.

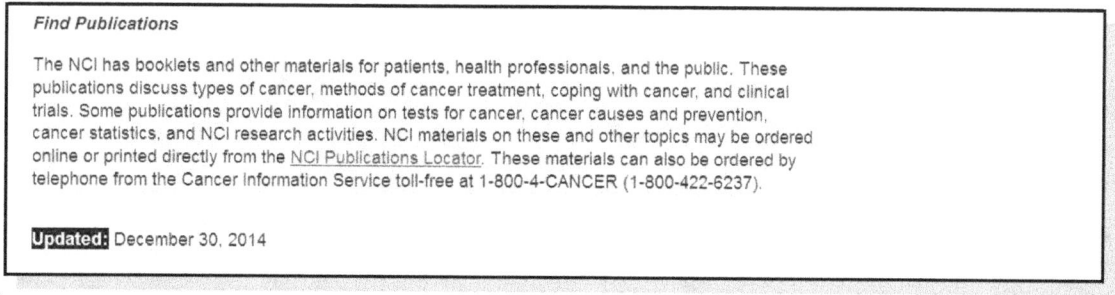

If you are the treating Physician, this is a state-of-the-art diagnostic and treatment protocol that is peer-reviewed, consensus, and evidence-based. **O**bviously, it is up to you to evaluate its applicability for a particular patient, and you will want to download these reports frequently to see what changes might have been made. **A**lso, the links to the PubMed database research reports might be interesting and helpful. **Y**ou might want to give a copy to a particular Patient or a Facilitator as part of your due diligence and informed consent.

22

Cancer Topics

The web-site of the National Cancer Institute has many sections. One of the more helpful is Cancer Topics. Go to: http://www.cancer.gov/cancertopics

Of particular interest in this section is "**Treatment**". Select that link.

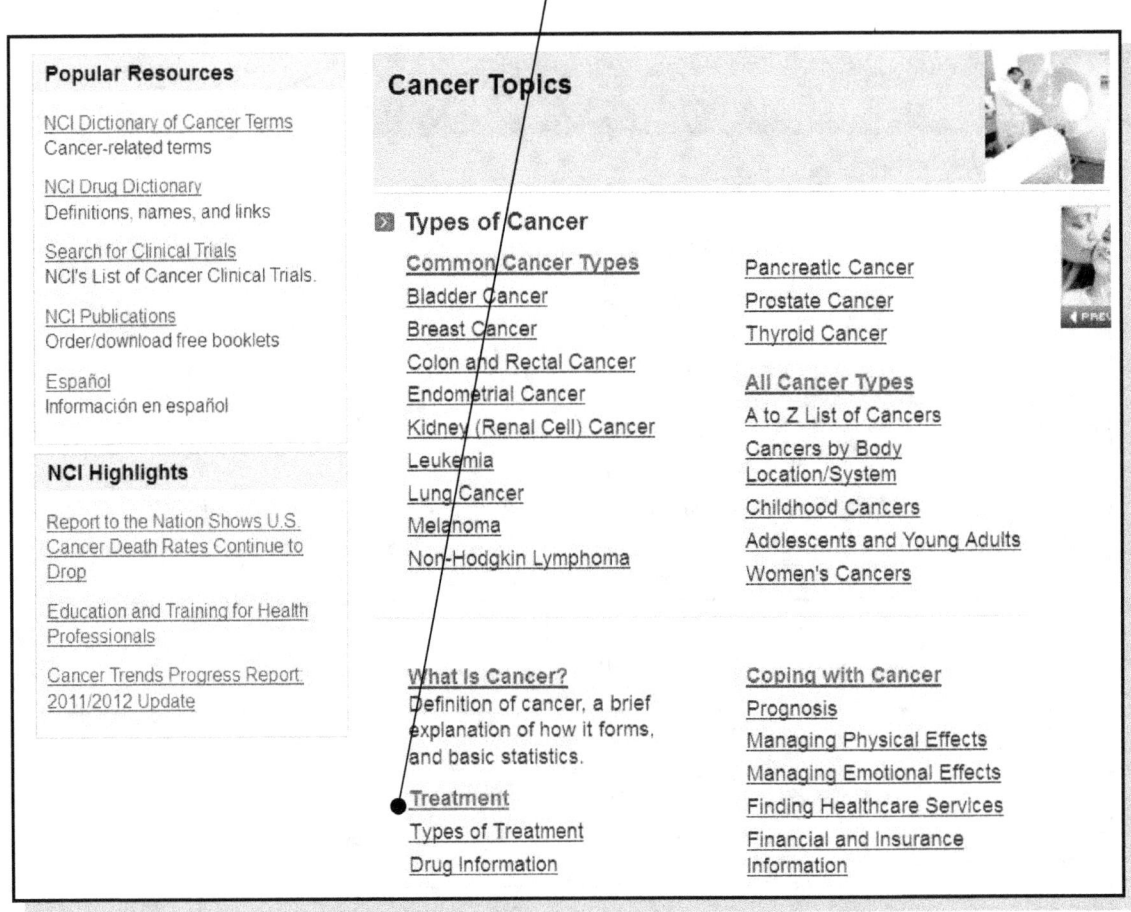

CHAPTER 2 - COMMENTS

After retrieving and reviewing the PDQ Patient and Physician reports, it is appropriated to make some incidental comments regarding:

1) "Conventional" Medicine;

2) A History of Medicine In General; and

3) Cancer - What Is It?

Being mindful that the reader is probably most interested in dealing with a particular medical problem, then one may want to stay with that pursuit, at present, and defer this Chapter. If so, then go on to the procedures in Chapter 3 and beyond; and come back to this background discussion at some other time. The PDQ reports are stated to be the most current, state-of-the-art information on specific types of cancer; and that is true. However, this section will give some perspective on how to interpret the validity of those protocols.

Conventional Medicine

The practice of medicine, today, is substantially different than it was 25 years ago and certainly different from what it was 50 or 100 years ago. Surely, it will be substantially different in 25 years hence, being that it is changing at a ever increasing rate. The PDQ protocols in Chapter 1, deal with, for the most part, what is called "Conventional Medicine", and this needs to be explained because Conventional Medicine is contingent on relative circumstances; it adapts over time; and it is behind where experimental science actually is. Given the current treatment options, this element of transformation or evolution of therapy is worthwhile to keep in mind when considering the most appropriate treatment strategy.

"Conventional" means whatever is the convention or accepted practice for a particular society at a particular time. It can vary from society to society, and, again, it changes over time. It is what the medical profession within a particular society generally agrees is acceptable medical practice; and this is determined by the social values, and the type of physician training, degree of patient education, the state of scientific understanding, and the available technology. Further, and most importantly, because the modern, conventional practice of medicine has become so elaborate and expensive, what is practiced, now, is determined mostly by what insurance agencies (government or private companies) are willing or able

24

to pay. If each patient had to personally pay for one's own medical treatment with today's Conventional Medicine, most of modern medicine would not be practiced even if it were extremely effective.

While, here in the U.S., we are bombarded by public relations and advertising hyperbole from the medical industry about how advanced our medicine is, what great progress is being made in research, and how our conventional medicine provides "the best health care in the world", there is considerable reason to be skeptical about all of that. Indeed, it simply is not true. Medical costs in the U.S. now consume 17.6% of the entire annual economy (Gross Domestic Product) with that representing over $8,000 per person per year, which is 2.5 times what is spent in the European Union, where they achieve substantially better life-expectancy and medical results for less than half the cost. For example, over the last 50 years, the average life-expectancy in the U.S. increased by 8.8 years, whereas in Europe it increased by 12.1 years. In Japan, life-expectancy increased by 14.9 years. [1] And those increases are due largely to improvements in standard of living and health practices rather than improvements in medicine

The situation is further distorted by the fact that, in the U.S., the elderly (65 years of age and older) consume more than 33% of the entire medical care spending with their medical expenses being substantially higher in the last year of life. In other words, a lot of medical over-treating is being done on people who are at the end-stage of life and obviously have no prospect of recovery. [2]

Keep in mind that medicine is no longer a calling with a high degree of philan-thropy and humanitarian motives, as it used to be some 50 to 100 years ago. Rather, now, it is mostly a business - a big and profitable business. Diseases have become "markets" that are, for the most part, socialized - i.e., the Providers (doctors, hospitals, supporting staff, manufactures of pharmaceuticals and thera-peutic devices, etc.) perform their services for Customers (Patients) and, then, third party Payors (government and insurance companies) pay the bill. If medicine were

---

[1]   See European Union (Organisation for Economic Co-operation and Development) - Health profile. Use the "Compare ... with" boxes. This is difficult to read, at first; but scroll over the various bars and points on the graphic line, and you will see the data. Note on the bar graph for current life- expectancies, the U.S. is 9th lowest among the 35 cited, with Switzerland being the highest. http://www.oecd-berlin.de/charts/health/

[2]   Medical Expenditures during the Last Year of Life. http://www.ncbi.nlm.nih.gov/pmc/articles/PMC1464043/

Chapter 2 - Comments - Conventional Medicine - History of Medicine - What is Cancer?

a "free market" economy (like computer technology), it could be expected that competition would improve quality and drive costs down; but medicine is a "regulated market" not a "free market" economy, being highly controlled by its guilds and governments. Particularly in regulated markets, there is strong inertia to stay in place and a resistance to disruptive change which might diminish position and profitability; and this is particularly strong in the market of medicine. The more medicine that is done, the more money is earned by the Providers, and being that the Customers do not pay directly for the charges, they welcome as much service as they can get. In the past, Patients paid, out-of-pocket, for their own services and the relationship was between the Patient and the Physician. Now, the third party Payor is the intermediary between Physician and Patient and thereby determines, in larger measure, what is to be done. In terms of traditional medical ethics, this situation is, technically, unethical because the Physician's client is, in effect, the insurance provider rather than the Patient, *per se*.

Present day Conventional Medicine is in a state of turmoil. And in practical terms, it is not certain how long the current *modus operendi* can be sustained. This aspect will be discussed later in the following history section.

Another confounding trend is the transformation of the medical profession from one of highly trained and experienced Experts, who have had decades of professional, hands-on practice, to what is called "Best Practices" treatment protocols in which the guidelines are established by committees, and then the treating physicians and support staff can be inter-changeable "administrators" of the protocol. This is an extension of the industrialization of medicine, using technicians as inter-changeable parts. It is thought to be more cost effective but not, necessarily, more effective in terms of patient care and out-comes. It also has a dampening effect on individualized patient management and innovative personalized treatment.

Many people are in the process of re-evaluating some of fundamental premises of the current, Conventional Medicine. One such premise is that diseases must be treated as soon as diagnosed, when in fact many times a disease does not need to be treated immediately or ever; and "Watchful Waiting" may be the proper strategy in certain cases. "Watchful Waiting" is a clinical management approach wherein immediate therapy is not provided, but there is a period of life-style modification and close diagnostic observation, during which the patient is periodically tested and the progression of the pathology is monitored to better determine if and how a problem needs to be approached for the particular individual. This will be discussed later.

26

For example, in a recent paper entitled "Overdiagnosis and Overtreatment in Cancer - An Opportunity for Improvement" [3], the authors comment:

> "Over the past 30 years, awareness and screening have led to an emphasis on early diagnosis of cancer. Although the goals of these efforts were to reduce the rate of late-stage disease and decrease cancer mortality, secular trends and clinical trials suggest that these goals have not been met; national data demonstrate significant increases in early-stage disease, without a proportional decline in later-stage disease. What has emerged has been an appreciation of the complexity of the pathologic condition called cancer. The word "cancer" often invokes the specter of an inexorably lethal process; however, cancers are heterogeneous and can follow multiple paths, not all of which progress to metastases and death, and include indolent disease that causes no harm during the patient's lifetime .... *Physicians, patients, and the general public must recognize that over diagnosis is common and occurs more frequently with cancer screening.*"

The authors of the report recommend to the National Cancer Institute a change in conventional medical thinking - one that moves away from general screening and early diagnosis and early treatment of certain cancers to "... better characterize the biology of the disease detected and to use disease dynamics (behavior over time) and molecular diagnostics that determine whether cancer will be aggressive or indolent to avoid overtreatment." And they go on to observe that the emphasis on early screening for example of breast, prostate, other types of cancer appears to detect cancers that are potentially insignificant, while the early screening and treatment for colon and cervical cancer are, in fact, effective in reducing incidence and late-stage disease.

In another recent article "A Decade of Reversal: An Analysis of 146 Contradicted Medical Practices" [4] a group of medical investigators reviewed 1,344 original articles concerning particular conventional medical practices, as published in a major medical journal over a decade (2001 to 2010). They conclude that 40% of conventional practices were found to be ineffective and were reversed over that period of time.

---

3   Overdiagnosis and Overtreatment in Cancer - An Opportunity for Improvement; Esserman, Laura J., *et alia*; Journal of the American Medical Association, July 29, 2013)

4   A Decade of Reversal: An Analysis of 146 Contradicted Medical Practices; Vinay Prasad, *et alia*; Mayo Clinic Proceedings; August 2013, Vol. 88 #8, 790-798).

Chapter 2 - Comments - Conventional Medicine - History of Medicine - What is Cancer?

"Of these, 981 articles (73.0%) examined a new medical practice, whereas 363 (27.0%) tested an established practice. A total of 947 studies (70.5%) had positive findings, whereas 397 (29.5%) reached a negative conclusion. A total of 756 articles addressing a medical practice constituted replacement. 165 were back to the drawing board, 146 were medical reversals, 138 were reaffirmations, and 139 were inconclusive. Of the 363 articles testing standard of care, 146 (40.2%) reversed that practice, whereas 138 (38.0%) reaffirmed it. **Conclusion**: The reversal of established medical practice is common and occurs across all classes of medical practice. This investigation sheds light on low value practices and patterns of medical research."

As presently configured, Conventional Medicine (certainly in the United States) seems to be caught in a maelstrom of conflicting vested interests. Amid complex government regulations about what constitutes "evidence-based medicine", the oversight of Community Medical Societies and State Medical Boards, insurance agencies (private and governmental) who are continuously faced with the affordability of medical coverage and a decline in the number of subscribers, the "medical industrial complex" which is constantly pressing for more revenue, and a research community that seems to be more interested in chasing grants than in translating new findings into applied therapeutics that provide tangible, improved benefits, one wonders about where the proper care for the Patient, *per se*, is in this vortex.

Obviously, the reader should not interpret the above to be a categorical condemnation of Conventional Medicine. Rather, it is a suggestion for caution and circumspection. And many dedicated people are attempting to work through the various entanglements toward a better medical paradigm. However, the popular image of medicine as being a pure science, ethically above reproach, and strictly interested in the betterment of humanity does need to be taken down a couple of notches until we really see a substantial improvement in outcomes. Medical progress is, after all, judged by improved outcomes and the improvement of patient well-being - not by increasingly fancy technologies many of which do not improve out-comes and, indeed, can decrease the quality of survival. This theme will be elaborated in the following discussion about A History of Medicine.

In addition to Conventional Medicine, one must also consider the status of Conventional Research. The term "scientists" is also imbued with an aura of sacredness - a person dedicated to the pursuit of truth and the perfection of humanity. There can be some truth to that; but like medicine, Conventional Research has

Chapter 2 - Comments - Conventional Medicine - History of Medicine - What is Cancer?

become, since the end of World War II, a big business relying most on government grants through universities. Much of the research is directed by people who have a vested interest in established knowledge - so there is a resistance to radically new approaches. And there is a long lag-time from the actual laboratory science to publication and then from publication into the collective consciousness of the scientific community and from there into practical applications by the industry (physicians and associated businesses). One can easily say that by the time scientific finding are made in the lab, it can take decades for it to get into application - from both the inertia of transmission and from barriers to acceptance. There are some rudimentary efforts being made on how to shorten the time from discovery to application in the fields of "Translational Research" and "Translational Medicine". We have further comments in Chapter 11 - Cancer and the Control of Ageing, discussing also how the readers of this book might play a role in that important aspect of cancer research.

A History of Medicine In General

Humanity's perennial pursuit has always been a life without deprivation, pain, suffering, disease, and death. Those are the absence of negative conditions. In the affirmative, the pursuit has been for "life, liberty, and the pursuit of happiness". Obviously, over-coming the negatives is necessary for achieving the affirmatives; and great advances have, indeed, been made in this regard, particularly over the last century. However, contrary to popular belief, rather than medicine, most of the improvements in health have come, thus far, from increases in standard of living and public health programs, all of which have had the effect of preventing disease and death, mostly, during early development - thus enabling people to naturally live close to the maximum, human, genetically programmed life-span. Paradoxically, however, we have become victims of our own success because most of us will now survive into advanced old age and suffer from the chronic diseases (including cancer) and varying degrees of senescence. Medicine has played a role in our progress; but it has been relatively minor, particularly with respect to what it will have to play if we are to make further gains in the future, because we have exhausted the potential gains from improving our circumstances. Let's take a panoramic sketch of the history of medicine to give a perspective not only of where we are today but also were we need to go in the future.

The first thing to consider is that the history of medicine is deeply intertwined with religion. From the earliest of times, priests were physicians, tending to the sick and dying; and *vice versa*, being a physician involved elements of being a priest, particularly when there was not much that could be done to cure the sick. The interplay between physician and priest is, in subliminal ways, still operative in today's medicine.

Going back to origins, the fossil records demonstrate and modern anthropology holds that we, humans, evolved from an original cluster of some 12, in-bred, mutant primates in East Africa, beginning about 200,000 years ago. (The reason they say "12" is because that number is thought to be the minimum which would be necessary to establish a new specie). Over those hundreds of thousands of years of evolution, only the last 5,000 years can be said to be in a civilized state of existence. Advanced, technological civilization begins only about 100 years ago. And, as one example, it has only been since the year 2000 that the molecular and cellular mechanisms of cancer have been scientifically understood - i.e., that cancer arises, in stages, from a single cell with damaged DNA and deterioration of the cellular micro-environment. In other words, scientific medicine is just beginning.

Our primitive ancestors migrated first throughout Africa, then over the Sinai land bridge, and out to the other continents - naked and barefooted for most of our evolution. These Stone Age people, living in "nature, red in tooth and claw", as Hobbes (1642) characterized the early human condition, had a maximum life-span of not more than about 30 years - similar to the other wild mammals. The causes of their death were mostly in child birth and diseases during early infancy, preda-tors, famine, accidents, warfare, and various causes which were held to be mysteri-ous such as fever and infection. Burial mounds of these people indicate that about 50% of their populations died before 5 years of age. Deeply imbedded in the natural environment, they originally worshiped and sought the advice of their ancestors, who lived in the after-life; and they understood the world around them as being inhabited by many tumultuous spirits (both benevolent and malevolent) which governed human fate and which are embodied in the entities and forces of nature (e.g., fire, wind, water, earth, burning bushes, animals, sacred stones, and the like) - recall that Moses talked to his God, who spoke as a burning bush. With the advent of agriculture and the progressive conquest of Nature, those Nature gods became replaced by gods who lived in the Sky, who were anthropomorphic projec-tions such as the Greek pantheon of an immortal super race called the Titans and who later were over-thrown by a descendant group of gods - Zeus and the Olympi-ans. Then, as Nature came increasingly under human control and societies became more integrated and complex, those tribal Sky Gods became superseded by the current theological conception of a single, abstract, all-mighty God - the creator

30

Chapter 2 - Comments - Conventional Medicine - History of Medicine - What is Cancer?

and ruler of everything. (Hindu philosophy had that idea long before it developed in the West.)

While people always did attempt to cure disease with natural substances and practices (herbs, waters, smoke, amulets, dance, saunas, sacrifice, exorcism, and other techniques of sympathetic magic), for the most part, it was believed that disease and death were caused by gods or evil spirits and pretty much beyond human control. Disease, it was thought, was an out-come of some kind of wrong doing by or a defect in the person who was afflicted. Indeed, this superstitious notion still carries forward today; and I recall as a young boy, when my mother bent down and whispered a secret into my ear: "Aunt Mini has cancer but do not say anything about it to anyone". It was as if Aunt Minnie had committed something morally wrong - something which should not be discussed openly. And there is still an aura of guilt and taboo that is associated with any disease - particularly cancer.

Western civilization, from its adoption of Christianity in the 4th Century to the present, inherited some of its fundamental philosophical values from the more ancient Hebrew traditions as codified in the Old Testament or Torah. The early Hebrews must have taken stock of the human condition and come to the conclusion that the reason life was so nasty, dirty, brutish, and laden with suffering was because our original ancestors must have greatly offended God who, then, expelled them out of paradise to wander the world and endure their suffering - passing the curse along to us, their descendants. It is a quirk of the mind that once we believe that a condition becomes sanctified as being the will of God, then any attempt to change it becomes forbidden - i.e., interference with divine will is a major sin. The reference here is to the Biblical story called The Fall of Man (Genesis III), wherein Eve and Adam violate God's prohibition against eating the fruit from the Tree of Knowledge. Because of that, God feared that they would make an attempt on the second tree, the Tree of Life, and become immortal like himself. As a preemptive strike, God expels the two from paradise giving punitive sanctions on them both. On Eve, the woman, he places a curse: "I will intensify the pangs of your child-bearing; in pain shall you bring forth children." This divine execration on women was taken so literally by religious conservatives that people were persecuted over the centuries for attempting to mitigate pain and suffering during child-birth. For example, as late as 1591 (some 4,000+ years after the writing of the Old Testament), King James VI of Scotland had a midwife (a gentlewoman of high rank by the name of Euphanie Macalyane) burned at the stake for the crime of using a remedy to relieve a woman's pain in child-birth - to him and the intellectuals of his

31

Chapter 2 - Comments - Conventional Medicine - History of Medicine - What is Cancer?

time, this was a clear and literal violation of God's mandate. And still into the 19ᵗʰ Century, for the same reason, a leading Scottish obstetrician (James Young Simpson) was strongly rebuked by his physician colleagues for his use of chloroform as anesthesia in child-birth. He was only saved from being ostracized from the medical profession, when Queen Victoria commanded that he administer his chloroform to her in the birth of her sixth child. That exonerated him from persecution and broke the taboo against relieving pain in birth. To this day, physicians seem to retain a phobia about administering pain relieving medication even to dying patients; and the Catholic Church continues to have a similar reluctance to pain relief for terminal patients, due to the belief that it might interfere with the last rites and the transmigration of the soul.

Given the idea that disease is caused or allowed by God, sacrifices and prayers were the only available method to invoke Divine intervention for healing; and these devices are still widely practiced today, with prayer for the sick still being, probably, the single most widely used "therapy" by patients and people who are associated with them, even though there is, regrettably, no empirical evidence to show that it works. In fact, some scientifically controlled studies have been done in an attempt to prove the efficacy of prayer, and they have not shown any beneficial results.[5]

History records that the first person to investigate health and disease from the perspective of natural causes, without reference to Gods, was the Greek physician, Hippocrates (460 - 370 BCE); and he is considered to be the founder of Western (i.e., modern) Medicine. A generation after Hippocrates, Aristotle (382 - 322 BCE) initiated the scientific study of biology; and since then, the study of biology and medicine have advanced in tandem with each other, with biology leading the way. From a realistic perspective, it can be said that the Hippocratic approach to medicine was a cult which gradually gained some acceptance on into the Roman era; but because the knowledge of biology and the techniques for intervention were so crude at the time, the main, prevailing mode of treating illness continued to be temples that were dedicated to the Gods of healing, where people would visit and make offerings - giving their donations and receiving special waters, unction, prayers, and such. The naturalistic approach to medicine (correlating physical conditions with physical causes) was carried forward into the Roman era, with such works as the anatomy of Galen (129-216). However, when Christianity took hold

---

5   See research on Faith Healing and Treatment Outcomes.
     http://www.ncbi.nlm.nih.gov/pubmed?term=("Faith+Healing"[Mesh])+AND+"Treatment+Outcome"[Mesh]

Chapter 2 - Comments - Conventional Medicine - History of Medicine - What is Cancer?

of the Roman Empire and theology became the dominant power, scripture and belief came to be what mattered most rather than the pursuit of knowledge about nature. The science of the Greeks and early Romans became persecuted - stagnating and receding into an underground of quackery from which it did not start to recover until some 1,200 later with the re-discovery of classic culture during the Renaissance in the 1500's and from there into the Enlightenment. A similar history happened to the Arab or Islamic civilization, which, as the Roman civilization was collapsing, became the safe haven for much of Greek and Roman knowledge until eventually it too gave way to the dominance of belief over the pursuit of knowledge. For over a millennium, a shroud settled over Civilization where belief in Scripture and Authority stifled the advancement of practical knowledge. (A 1,000+ years is a great loss of time that could have been spent doing the hard work on physically improving the human condition.)

The idea of "Progress" is that the world and the human condition can become increasingly better through science, technology, modernization, liberty, democracy, quality of life, etc.. Curiously, this idea did not exist as a social value until very recent history - i.e., a couple of hundred years ago during the "Age of Enlightenment/Reason" in the 17th and 18th Centuries. People simply did not have the idea that current conditions could be improved by intelligent, collaborative effort.

One of the main drivers of historical change is the invention of new technologies. Technologies change conditions, the change in conditions causes people to behave and think differently, and that forces the modification of social organization, which then is amplifies by the inventions of new technologies, as so forth. For example, historians believe that the stirrup, as a device for securing the rider in the saddle of a horse, enabled warfare to be conducted by mounted cavalry which radically changed the nature of war and thereby the political and social organization of civilization; the iron plow enabled the cultivation of previously non-arable land, causing population explosions; the steam engine made feasible long-distance travel for masses of people; our entire modern society rests on, more than anything, capturing the energy of fossil fuel; and so on with a myriad of inventions at a rate of increasing acceleration. In the future, one of the main driving forces of history will be medical inventions, which do not exist, yet. For a highly informative and entertaining over-view of technological change, see "The Ascent of Man" by J. Bronowski and "Connections" by James Burke are both documentary television essays on human history. [6]

---

6   See Wikipedia:
    "Connections" J. Burke: http://en.wikipedia.org/wiki/Connections_%28TV_series%29

Chapter 2 - Comments - Conventional Medicine - History of Medicine - What is Cancer?

The single, greatest, land-mark event in the history of scientific medicine was the invention of the microscope (Leeuwenhoek, 1660's) which revealed an entirely new universe of invisible life-forms, including the sub-structure of the human body. That invention led to: the discovery of cells as the basic unit of life (Hooke, 1673); to the discovery of microscopic life-forms as a cause of some of the major diseases (Pasteur, 1862); and to antibiotics, the single most significant tool against disease (Fleming, 1928). Once it was understood that cells formed the basic unit of life which then formed tissues that constructed organs which were integrated to form the whole body, it was a logical deduction that disease was caused, most fundamentally, by loss or malfunction of cells. The study of cells eventually leads to the investigation of their molecular construction (19th Century to the present) and which has now lead to the understanding of the genetic mechanisms which regulates the constructions of cells (mid 20th Century to the present).

Medicine can be divided into two approaches - 1) techniques which destroy pathologic cells/tissue and 2) methods which facilitated the healing of cells/tissues. The two are reciprocal - destroying pathologic tissue allows for natural healing to recover, and facilitating natural healing can over-come pathology. Almost all current medical practices can trace their roots to some traditional or ancient observation or practice; but it was not until the 18th Century and hence to the present that the stochastic, empirical knowledge of tradition became elucidated by rational and formal scientific methodology and then translated into wide-spread application by the medical profession.

Although there are numerous kinds of therapeutics, the main-stay of medicine is surgery and pharmacology. With respect to destroying or correcting pathologic tissue, surgery is the most direct approach. Although surgery has been practiced since ancient times; it was only until the invention of antiseptic techniques, anesthesia, and antibiotics that it became a practical procedure - i.e., Semmelweis (1846) and washing of hands; Long (1849) with the discovery of ether for anesthesia; Pasteur (1862) the germ theory; Lister (1865) with the use of carbolic acid as an antiseptic during surgery; and Fleming (1928) antibiotics. Without antiseptic techniques to prevent infection, anesthesia to inhibit pain and shock, and antibiotics to treat infection, surgery would not be practical due to shock and infection.

Like surgery, pharmacology has an ancient tradition, with Paracelsus (1493 - 1541) being consider the pioneer in the use of chemicals and minerals in medicine. The

"The Ascent of Man" Jacob Bronowski: http://en.wikipedia.org/wiki/The_Ascent_of_Man
Check YouTube http://www.YouTube.com to see if the videos are posted.

Chapter 2 - Comments - Conventional Medicine - History of Medicine - What is Cancer?

beginning of modern therapeutics is credited to Withering (1758) for the discovery of Digitalis, from the foxglove plant, for cardiac conditions. And, of all of the drugs used in today's medicine, perhaps 70% are derived from natural botanicals. It is not surprising that biologically active molecules would be discovered in other life-forms, given the great molecular variations that have resulted from some 4.5 billion years of evolution by trial and error. And specific therapeutic modalities will be carried to a new paradigm as we make progress in genomic medicine. To illustrate the effect of general progress, of which medicine has played a role, consider the historic shift in survival as illustrated in the graphs on the following page.

Chapter 2 - Comments - Conventional Medicine - History of Medicine - What is Cancer?

In the adjacent graph, the percent surviving for a given population of humans, on the Vertical axis, is plotted against chronological age categories on the Horizontal axis. All groups begin with 100% surviving and end with 0% surviving. The survival curve **"A"** is for Stone Age people, as evaluated from their burial mounds. These were hunters and gathers. At age "0", 100% of the population is surviving, but almost 50% are dead by the age of 5 years and virtually all are dead by the age of 45. Effectively, ageing

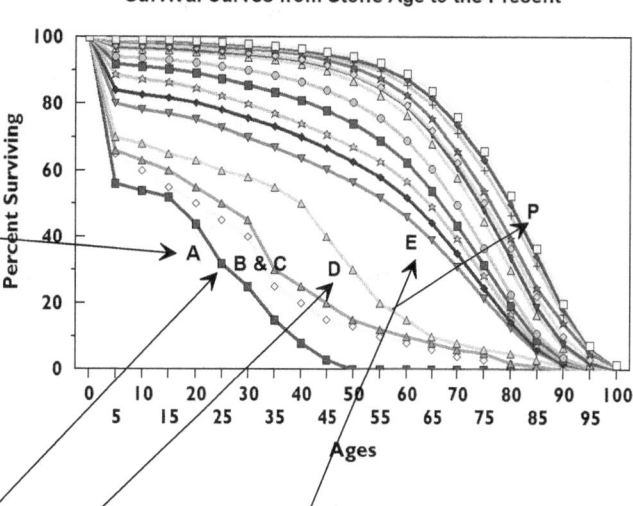

Survival Curves from Stone Age to the Present

did not afflict Stone Age people. The environment was so harsh that people did not survive long enough to age. The adults were sturdy and functional until they were killed or died early of natural causes.

The survival curves **"B" and "C"** are for the classical Greek (300 BCE) and Roman periods (50 CE). Here again, about 50% of these groups were dead early in life - by the age of about 25. However, more people did survive into their 50's and a few rare ones survived to 80. These populations represent farming or agrarian cultures - still harsh but improving. Curve **"D"** represents the 1800's in England or early industrial civilization. Still there is a high mortality in infancy and early adulthood, but the survival begins to increase during the middle years. Curves **"E" through "P"** range from 1900 - 2012 and are accurate, coming from census data. What is demonstrated here is that, as industrialism advanced with the food supply being more constant, improvements in hygiene, heating, and people living off the dirt, clean water, then immunizations, and conventional medicine particularly during child birth and through early development, more and more people have survived into old age, such that death during the early ages goes to almost zero and almost all of the population now survives into advanced age. 50% of the population is now living beyond 80 years, which is well into the period of senescence. Note that the maximum life-span of about 95 has not changed over the millennia, which, because there are still no effective treatments for biological ageing, has yet to be affected.

One amazing fact is that the life-expectancy, for those people who have reached the age of 65, has changed very little of the last 100 years. For those who were 65 years of age in 1900, the life-expectancy was 11.86 years; while today, in 2010, it is 19.10 years - for a difference of only 7.24 years improvement over a period of a century. And most of that

Chapter 2 - Comments - Conventional Medicine - History of Medicine - What is Cancer?

has been achieved not by medicine but by improvements in standard of living and personal hygiene and a healthier life-style. Given that in 1900 there was essentially no effective medicine and today we have this massive amount of sophisticated and high-tech medicine, it is amazing that there is only an increase of 7.24 years - again most of which was achieved not by medicine. The comparative life-expectances are recorded in the table below. [7]

Comparative life-expectancy at 65 years of age from 1900 to 2010 - all races and sexes		
Decade	Life-expectancy years	Living to age
1900	11.86	76.86
1910	11.60	76.60
1920	12.47	77.47
1930	12.23	77.23
1940	12.80	77.80
1950	13.83	78.83
1960	14.39	79.39
1970	15.00	80.00
1980	16.51	81.51
1990	17.28	82.28
2000	17.77	82.77
2010	19.10	84.10

How medicine is practiced is another element that has radically changed. Until recent history, there was no medicine except folk medicine for the common people (95% of the population). Sturdy people survived, and those who got injured or sick either recovered by themselves or they died. The medicine that was available for the wealthy could be provided by a doctor, making a house call, or by the person traveling to some healing center such as a temple (in ancient times) or a health-spa-type of facility such as Lourdes, France, which receives patients to this today. Neither the common people (without medicine) nor the wealthy (with medicine) had much difference in survival rate. As we approached the modern era, most medicine was practiced as a cottage industry with the physician having one's clinic in his house, seeing local people in that setting or making

---

7   Table 21. Life expectancy by age, race, and sex; Death-registration states, 1900-1902 to 1919-1921, and United States, 1929-1931 to 2008, Page 52.
     http://www.cdc.gov/nchs/data/nvsr/nvsr61/nvsr61_03.pdf

house calls to the patient. Local churches provided rudimentary hospital facilities where nuns would administer palliative procedures to the sick and a local physician might provide some over-sight. The main hospital treatment was kindness and patience as palliative care during the natural course of a disease; and that must have been the origin of the term "patient" or the endurance of suffering when referring to someone under medical care. In a modified form, this model lasted into the 1950's when most doctors were general practitioners, having an individual office and privileges to admit one's patients to a local hospital which usually was owned by the community or a religious or philanthropic order. The general practitioner would frequently be the physician to multiple generations of a particular family (the family doctor) and would do surgery, obstetrics, immunizations, and virtually all types of medicine, except more specialized surgery, in which, even then, the family physician might assist in the operating room. In terms of payments, the physician would charge the patient directly and work out the payment of fees; and a common practice was for the more wealthy patients to pay a higher fee, which would compensate for the *pro bono* services which the doctor would provide to his lower income patients.

It is commonly admitted that, scientifically speaking before the 20th Century, medicine was, in large measure, quackery. Common practices included: blood letting by incision or leaches; acupuncture and moxibustion or cupping; restraint and trauma; electro-magnet generators for the relief of pain; metallic tractors; purgatives (Rush's revenge); medicines using mostly opium and cocaine; Mesmerism; unregulated concoctions containing mercurials, quinine, powders, arsenic; and an infinite variety of other nostrums and placebos. As stated previously, surgery was not really a practical modality until after the invention of antiseptic procedures, anesthesia, antibiotics, and, more recently, artificial life-support technologies. Beginning in the early 20th Century and in a effort to purge the profession of quackery and such mal-practices, an effort began to organize medicine in a more professional manner with the formation of local and national medical societies, the government licensing of physicians, accreditation of medical schools, and formal protocols for licensing drugs and devices for which safety and efficacy needed to be proven. The more traditional methods of healing such as herbs and nutrition, massage, and the use of cocaine, opium and such naturopathic medicine did continue on, but in a more underground manner outside the medical profession; and indeed, they are probably used by more people today than the practices of Conventional Medicine.

As knowledge in biology, physiology, and medicine started to increase exponentially, doctors were forced to become more and more specialized, such that today the traditional, general practice doctor is almost extinct. Also, as the professional reforms took hold, physicians began to form group practices and medical insurance became a viable method for paying for services. At first, individuals contracted with insurance carriers; physicians provided services to patients; and then patients paid the bill and submitted it to the insurance carrier for re-imbursement. But that soon gave way to physicians billing insurance carriers directly. Thus began the "billing wars" between insurance provides and physicians. Physicians held fast to the privilege that only they had the right to determine what was the proper practice of medicine and what the fees should be. Insurance providers were obligated by contract to pay for the medicine which was provided to the subscribing patients. Thus, the two parties (the Provider and the Payor) became locked in an adversarial position - the Provider kept increasing fees and doing unnecessary services that forced the Payor to increase insurance premiums, which resulted in negative feed-back loop - forcing subscribers to drop out of the system, which then required a further increase in premiums.

Different responses to this situation emerged called "health maintenance organizations" or "pre-paid health plans"; and somehow, the term "medicine" got changed to "health", probably for advertising purposes. Various configurations have evolved; and thus far, the model which has seemed to be most successful in terms of member satisfaction and cost containment is the one created by a pugnacious industrialist by the name of Henry Kaiser, who was well accustomed to confronting vested interests and willing to oppose the medical establishment. He organized Kaiser Permanente in 1945 to provide medical care for his construction employees, and then subsequently it was expanded to open enrollment. The company has three interlocking entities: 1) Kaiser Foundation Health Plan is a non-profit organization which manages the patient membership and performs essentially the functions of the insurance company; 2) The Permanente Medical Group is a for profit organization of physicians, nurses, and clinical staff who work only for the members of the Kaiser Foundation Health Plan; and 3) the Kaiser Foundation Hospitals, a non-profit organization, which runs the hospitals for the physicians. There are other competing plans, but Kaiser is the largest in the U.S. which, as of their 2013 report, has some 9 million member/patients, 37 hospitals, 611 medical offices, 17,157 physicians, and 175,668 supporting employees.

Still, these "pre-paid health plans" are economically unstable because the cost of medicine keeps increasing which causes individuals and employers to drop out of the system, thus forcing an increase in premiums and thus resulting in a negative feed-back loop, as mentioned above. In the U.S., the effort to shore up the economics of the system has, most recently, been the enactment in 2010 of the "Quality, Affordable Health Care For All Americans" (Public Law 111-148), which effectively forces all people to become part of such a health plan or to purchase insurance - increasing the patient base by some 30 million people who were previously uninsured. While publicly speaking, most of the medical profession was opposed to this law, it effectively puts a governmentally subsidized cushion under the medical profession; but the cost controls and oversight of quality

39

Chapter 2 - Comments - Conventional Medicine - History of Medicine - What is Cancer?

remain weak; and therefore, the same problem continues - escalating medical costs without improved outcomes. It will be some time before one can judge if this is a sustainable economic model and if it improves the quality of medicine.

European countries took a somewhat different path to providing medicine to their citizens. After the devastation of World War II and as a way of thwarting the possibility of Communist take-overs, the governments created a social policy of full-employment and socialized medicine, among other government sponsored programs. With full-employment, everyone had an income from which earnings could be extracted to pay for government regulated medicine; and that controlled costs as well as provided good care. However, with the European Union (EU) now experiencing high unemployment, there are not the earnings from which to extract the costs of medicine; and the EU is facing somewhat the same problem as in the U.S.

It is all very complex and in a state of dis-equilibrium - particularly with a revolution about to take place in medical technology. From the current "industrialized" model for providing medicine to the emerging high-tech, genomic-based, personalized medicine, it is unclear what will become the *modus operendi* of future medicine. This will be discussed further in Chapter 11 - Cancer and the Control of Ageing.

To finalize this section on the History of Medicine, you might get a feel for the interplay between medicine and science by glancing down the table, below, which lists the Nobel Prizes for the joint fields of medicine or physiology from 1901 to the present. Take note that the prize is usually given many years after the discovery. Again, keep in mind that, even with all of these achievements of the 100 year span of time, for those over 65 years of age, there has been only an increase of about 7 years in average life-span, most of which did not come from medical progress.

Nobel Prize in Physiology or Medicine [8]		
Date	To	For the
1901	Emil Adolf von Behring	work on serum therapy, especially its application against diphtheria, by which he has opened a new road in the domain of medical science and thereby placed in the hands of the physician a victorious weapon against illness and deaths
1902	Ronald Ross	work on malaria, by which he has shown how it enters the

---

8   "All Nobel Prizes in Physiology or Medicine". Nobelprize.org. Nobel Media AB 2013. Web. 24 Aug 2013. http://www.nobelprize.org/nobel_prizes/medicine/laureates/

Nobel Prize in Physiology or Medicine [8]		
Date	To	For the
		organism and thereby has laid the foundation for successful research on this disease and methods of combating it
1903	Niels Ryberg Finsen	contribution to the treatment of diseases, especially lupus vulgaris, with concentrated light radiation, whereby he has opened a new avenue for medical science
1904	Ivan Petrovich Pavlov	work on the physiology of digestion, through which knowledge on vital aspects of the subject has been transformed and enlarged
1905	Robert Koch	investigations and discoveries in relation to tuberculosis
1906	Camillo Golgi and Santiago Ramón y Cajal	work on the structure of the nervous system
1907	Charles Louis Alphonse Laveran	work on the role played by protozoa in causing diseases
1908	Ilya Ilyich Mechnikov and Paul Ehrlich	work on immunity
1909	Emil Theodor Kocher	work on the physiology, pathology and surgery of the thyroid gland
1910	Albrecht Kossel	contributions to our knowledge of cell chemistry made through his work on proteins, including the nucleic substances
1911	Allvar Gullstrand	work on the dioptrics of the eye
1912	Alexis Carrel	work on vascular suture and the transplantation of blood vessels and organs
1913	Charles Robert Richet	work on anaphylaxis
1914	Robert Bárány	work on the physiology and pathology of the vestibular apparatus
1915	No Nobel Prize this year.	
1916	No Nobel Prize this year.	
1917	No Nobel Prize this year.	
1918	No Nobel Prize this year.	
1919	Jules Bordet	discoveries relating to immunity
1920	Schack August Steenberg Krogh	discovery of the capillary motor regulating mechanism
1921	No Nobel Prize was awarded this year.	
1922	Archibald Vivian Hill	discovery relating to the production of heat in the muscle
1922	Otto Fritz Meyerhof	discovery of the fixed relationship between the consumption of oxygen and the metabolism of lactic acid in the muscle
1923	Frederick Grant Banting	discovery of insulin

Chapter 2 - Comments - Conventional Medicine - History of Medicine - What is Cancer?

Nobel Prize in Physiology or Medicine [8]		
Date	To	For the
	and John James Rickard Macleod	
1924	Willem Einthoven	discovery of the mechanism of the electrocardiogram
1925	No Nobel Prize this year.	
1926	Johannes Andreas Grib Fibiger	discovery of the Spiroptera carcinoma
1927	Julius Wagner-Jauregg	discovery of the therapeutic value of malaria inoculation in the treatment of dementia paralytica
1928	Charles Jules Henri Nicolle	work on typhus
1929	Christiaan Eijkman	discovery of the antineuritic vitamin
1929	Sir Frederick Gowland Hopkins	discovery of the growth-stimulating vitamins
1930	Karl Landsteiner	discovery of human blood groups
1931	Otto Heinrich Warburg	discovery of the nature and mode of action of the respiratory enzyme
1932	Sir Charles Scott Sherrington and Edgar Douglas Adrian	discoveries regarding the functions of neurons
1933	Thomas Hunt Morgan	discoveries concerning the role played by the chromosome in heredity
1934	George Hoyt Whipple, George Richards Minot and William Parry Murphy	discoveries concerning liver therapy in cases of anaemia
1935	Hans Spemann	discovery of the organizer effect in embryonic development
1936	Sir Henry Hallett Dale and Otto Loewi	discoveries relating to chemical transmission of nerve impulses
1937	Albert von Szent-Györgyi Nagyrápolt	discoveries in connection with the biological combustion processes, with special reference to vitamin C and the catalysis of fumaric acid
1938	Corneille Jean François Heymans	discovery of the role played by the sinus and aortic mechanisms in the regulation of respiration
1939	Gerhard Domagk	discovery of the antibacterial effects of prontosil
1940	No Nobel Prize was awarded this year.	
1941	No Nobel Prize was awarded this year.	
1942	No Nobel Prize was awarded this year.	
1943	Henrik Carl Peter Dam	discovery of vitamin K
1943	Edward Adelbert Doisy	discovery of the chemical nature of vitamin K

Nobel Prize in Physiology or Medicine [8]		
Date	To	For the
1944	Joseph Erlanger and Herbert Spencer Gasser	discoveries relating to the highly differentiated functions of single nerve fibres
1945	Sir Alexander Fleming, Ernst Boris Chain and Sir Howard Walter Florey	discovery of penicillin and its curative effect in various infectious diseases
1946	Hermann Joseph Muller	discovery of the production of mutations by means of X-ray irradiation
1947	Carl Ferdinand Cori and Gerty Theresa Cori, née Radnitz	discovery of the course of the catalytic conversion of glycogen
1947	Bernardo Alberto Houssay	discovery of the part played by the hormone of the anterior pituitary lobe in the metabolism of sugar
1948	Paul Hermann Müller	discovery of the high efficiency of DDT as a contact poison against several arthropods
1949	Walter Rudolf Hess	discovery of the functional organization of the interbrain as a coordinator of the activities of the internal organs"
1949	Antonio Caetano de Abreu Freire Egas Moniz	discovery of the therapeutic value of leucotomy in certain psychoses
1950	Edward Calvin Kendall, Tadeus Reichstein and Philip Showalter Hench	discoveries relating to the hormones of the adrenal cortex, their structure and biological effects"
1951	Max Theiler	discoveries concerning yellow fever and how to combat it"
1952	Selman Abraham Waksman	discovery of streptomycin, the first antibiotic effective against tuberculosis"
1953	Hans Adolf Krebs	discovery of the citric acid cycle
1953	Fritz Albert Lipmann	discovery of co-enzyme A and its importance for intermediary metabolism"
1954	John Franklin Enders, Thomas Huckle Weller and Frederick Chapman Robbins	discovery of the ability of poliomyelitis viruses to grow in cultures of various types of tissue
1955	Axel Hugo Theodor Theorell	discoveries concerning the nature and mode of action of oxidation enzymes
1956	André Frédéric Cournand, Werner Forssmann and Dickinson W. Richards	discoveries concerning heart catheterization and pathological changes in the circulatory system
1957	Daniel Bovet	discoveries relating to synthetic compounds that inhibit the

Chapter 2 - Comments - Conventional Medicine - History of Medicine - What is Cancer?

Nobel Prize in Physiology or Medicine [8]		
Date	To	For the
		action of certain body substances, and especially their action on the vascular system and the skeletal muscles
1958	George Wells Beadle and Edward Lawrie Tatum, and	discovery that genes act by regulating definite chemical events
1958	Joshua Lederberg	discoveries concerning genetic recombination and the organization of the genetic material of bacteria
1959	Severo Ochoa and Arthur Kornberg	discovery of the mechanisms in the biological synthesis of ribonucleic acid and deoxyribonucleic acid
1960	Sir Frank Macfarlane Burnet and Peter Brian Medawar	discovery of acquired immunological tolerance
1961	Georg von Békésy	discoveries of the physical mechanism of stimulation within the cochlea
1962	Francis Harry Compton Crick, James Dewey Watson and Maurice Hugh Frederick Wilkins	discoveries concerning the molecular structure of nucleic acids and its significance for information transfer in living material
1963	Sir John Carew Eccles, Alan Lloyd Hodgkin and Andrew Fielding Huxley	discoveries concerning the ionic mechanisms involved in excitation and inhibition in the peripheral and central portions of the nerve cell membrane
1964	Konrad Bloch and Feodor Lynen	discoveries concerning the mechanism and regulation of the cholesterol and fatty acid metabolism
1965	François Jacob, André Lwoff and Jacques Monod	discoveries concerning genetic control of enzyme and virus synthesis
1966	Peyton Rous, and	discovery of tumour-inducing viruses
1966	Charles Brenton Huggins"	discoveries concerning hormonal treatment of prostatic cancer
1967	Ragnar Granit, Haldan Keffer Hartline and George Wald	discoveries concerning the primary physiological and chemical visual processes in the eye"
1968	Robert W. Holley, Har Gobind Khorana and Marshall W. Nirenberg	interpretation of the genetic code and its function in protein synthesis
1969	Max Delbrück, Alfred D. Hershey and Salvador E. Luria	discoveries concerning the replication mechanism and the genetic structure of viruses
1970	Sir Bernard Katz, Ulf	discoveries concerning the humoral transmittors in the nerve

Nobel Prize in Physiology or Medicine [8]		
Date	To	For the
	von Euler and Julius Axelrod	terminals and the mechanism for their storage, release and inactivation
1971	Earl W. Sutherland, Jr.	discoveries concerning the mechanisms of the action of hormones
1972	Gerald M. Edelman and Rodney R. Porter	discoveries concerning the chemical structure of antibodies
1973	Karl von Frisch, Konrad Lorenz and Nikolaas Tinbergen	discoveries concerning organization and elicitation of individual and social behaviour patterns
1974	Albert Claude, Christian de Duve and George E. Palade	discoveries concerning the structural and functional organization of the cell
1975	David Baltimore, Renato Dulbecco and Howard Martin Temin	discoveries concerning the interaction between tumour viruses and the genetic material of the cell
1976	Baruch S. Blumberg and D. Carleton Gajdusek	discoveries concerning new mechanisms for the origin and dissemination of infectious diseases
1977	Roger Guillemin and Andrew V. Schally, and	discoveries concerning the peptide hormone production of the brain
1977	Rosalyn Yalow	development of radioimmunoassays of peptide hormones
1978	Werner Arber, Daniel Nathans and Hamilton O. Smith	discovery of restriction enzymes and their application to problems of molecular genetics
1979	Allan M. Cormack and Godfrey N. Hounsfield	development of computer assisted tomography
1980	Baruj Benacerraf, Jean Dausset and George D. Snell	discoveries concerning genetically determined structures on the cell surface that regulate immunological reactions
1981	Roger W. Sperry. and	discoveries concerning the functional specialization of the cerebral hemispheres
1981	David H. Hubel and Torsten N. Wiesel	discoveries concerning information processing in the visual system
1982	Sune K. Bergström, Bengt I. Samuelsson and John R. Vane	discoveries concerning prostaglandins and related biologically active substances
1983	Barbara McClintock	discovery of mobile genetic elements
1984	Niels K. Jerne, Georges J.F. Köhler and César Milstein	theories concerning the specificity in development and control of the immune system and the discovery of the principle for production of monoclonal antibodies

45

Nobel Prize in Physiology or Medicine [8]		
Date	To	For the
1985	Michael S. Brown and Joseph L. Goldstein	discoveries concerning the regulation of cholesterol metabolism
1986	Stanley Cohen and Rita Levi-Montalcini	discoveries of growth factors
1987	Susumu Tonegawa	discovery of the genetic principle for generation of antibody diversity
1988	Sir James W. Black, Gertrude B. Elion and George H. Hitchings	discoveries of important principles for drug treatment
1989	J. Michael Bishop and Harold E. Varmus	discovery of the cellular origin of retroviral oncogenes
1990	Joseph E. Murray and E. Donnall Thomas	discoveries concerning organ and cell transplantation in the treatment of human disease
1991	Erwin Neher and Bert Sakmann	discoveries concerning the function of single ion channels in cells
1992	Edmond H. Fischer and Edwin G. Krebs	discoveries concerning reversible protein phosphorylation as a biological regulatory mechanism
1993	Richard J. Roberts and Phillip A. Sharp	discoveries of split genes
1994	Alfred G. Gilman and Martin Rodbell	discovery of G-proteins and the role of these proteins in signal transduction in cells
1995	Edward B. Lewis, Christiane Nüsslein-Volhard and Eric F. Wieschaus	discoveries concerning the genetic control of early embry-onic development
1996	Peter C. Doherty and Rolf M. Zinkernagel	discoveries concerning the specificity of the cell mediated immune defence
1997	Stanley B. Prusiner	discovery of Prions - a new biological principle of infection
1998	Robert F. Furchgott, Louis J. Ignarro and Ferid Murad	discoveries concerning nitric oxide as a signalling molecule in the cardiovascular system
1999	Günter Blobel	discovery that proteins have intrinsic signals that govern their transport and localization in the cell
2000	Arvid Carlsson, Paul Greengard and Eric R. Kandel	discoveries concerning signal transduction in the nervous system
2001	Leland H. Hartwell, Tim Hunt and Sir Paul M. Nurse	discoveries of key regulators of the cell cycle

Chapter 2 - Comments - Conventional Medicine - History of Medicine - What is Cancer?

Nobel Prize in Physiology or Medicine [8]		
Date	To	For the
2002	Sydney Brenner, H. Robert Horvitz and John E. Sulston	discoveries concerning genetic regulation of organ development and programmed cell death
2003	Paul C. Lauterbur and Sir Peter Mansfield	discoveries concerning magnetic resonance imaging"
2004	Richard Axel and Linda B. Buck	discoveries of odorant receptors and the organization of the olfactory system"
2005	Barry J. Marshall and J. Robin Warren	discovery of the bacterium Helicobacter pylori and its role in gastritis and peptic ulcer disease
2006	Andrew Z. Fire and Craig C. Mello	discovery of RNA interference - gene silencing by double-stranded RNA
2007	Mario R. Capecchi, Sir Martin J. Evans and Oliver Smithies	discoveries of principles for introducing specific gene modifications in mice by the use of embryonic stem cells
2008	Harald zur Hausen and	discovery of human papilloma viruses causing cervical cancer
2008	Françoise Barré-Sinoussi and Luc Montagnier	discovery of human immunodeficiency virus
2009	Elizabeth H. Blackburn, Carol W. Greider and Jack W. Szostak	discovery of how chromosomes are protected by telomeres and the enzyme telomerase
2010	Robert G. Edwards	development of in vitro fertilization
2011	Bruce A. Beutler and Jules A. Hoffmann, and	discoveries concerning the activation of innate immunity
2011	Ralph M. Steinman	discovery of the dendritic cell and its role in adaptive immunity
2012	Sir John B. Gurdon and Shinya Yamanaka	discovery that mature cells can be reprogrammed to become pluripotent
2013	James E. Rothman, Randy W. Schekman and Thomas C. Südhof	for their discoveries of machinery regulating vesicle traffic, a major transport system in our cells
2014	John O'Keefe, May-Britt Moser and Edvard I. Moser	discoveries of cells that constitute a positioning system in the brain.

Chapter 2 - Comments - Conventional Medicine - History of Medicine - What is Cancer?

For further information on the history of medicine see:

http://en.wikipedia.org/wiki/History_of_medicine

and

http://en.wikipedia.org/wiki/Timeline_of_medicine_and_medical_technology

Wikipedia.org is used as major reference in the writing of this book. It is a contributor-based Internet encyclopedia (the 5th most visited site on the Internet) and a most valuable source of information. It warrants your use and contribution.

Cancer - What Is It?

Cancer is an abnormal growth of one's own tissue. Although it behaves somewhat like an "infection", it is an infection by your own cells (not foreign entities like bacteria or viruses). Therefore, it escapes recognition and destruction by your immune system. It is a disease of uncontrolled cell division that is caused by a defect in cellular control and due to the damage of specific genes or segments of a cell's DNA and the ageing of the cellular micro-environment, as will be discussed in Chapter 11. Since 2000, there has been a general consensus about the cause of cancer at its molecular level:

"The hallmarks of cancer comprise six biological capabilities acquired during the multi-step development of human tumors. The hallmarks constitute an organizing principle for rationalizing the complexities of neoplastic disease. They include sustaining proliferative signaling, evading growth suppressors, resisting cell death, enabling replicative immortality, inducing angiogenesis, and activating invasion and metastasis. Underlying these hallmarks are genome instability, which generates the genetic diversity that expedites their acquisition, and inflammation, which fosters multiple hallmark functions. Conceptual progress in the last decade has added two emerging hallmarks of potential generality to this list— of energy metabolism and evading immune destruction. In addition to cancer cells, tumors exhibit another dimension of complexity: they contain a repertoire of recruited, ostensibly normal cells that contribute to the acquisition of hallmark traits by creating the "microenvironment." Recognition of the widespread applicability of these concepts will increasingly affect the development of new means to treat human cancer." [9]

---

[9] Hanahan D and Weinberg RA; Hallmarks of Cancer: The Next Generation; Cell, Vol. 144, pg. 646, March 4, 2011. And their original article: Hanahan D and Weinberg

48

Chapter 2 - Comments - Conventional Medicine - History of Medicine - What is Cancer?

Each one of these "biological capabilities" or defects must take place, and they are regulated by many different genes. Thus, cancer is a very rare event, even though, as part of normal metabolism, one routinely gets numerous cellular mutations; but those mutations almost always never lead to cancer - they self-destruct because of various control mechanisms within cells or because they are identified and destroyed by one's own immune system. It is now understood that all cancers begin with one, single cell which experiences damage to certain segments of its DNA which control cell division. That genetically damaged, single cell then goes through several stages of development, escaping "apoptosis" (self destruction) and immune surveillance; and a cluster of such cells develops in the tissue of its origin. Thus, it is said: cancer of the stomach, cancer of the bone, cancer of the pancreas, etc. - i.e., labeling the type of cancer by the organ in which it originates. The medical community and general public commonly used the term "cancer" - that being Latin for crab and coming from the ancient observation that many such tumors have a jagged blood vessel formation, resembling a crab. The scientific community uses the term "neoplasm" (new formation) for cancer, and according to that taxonomy, there are 177 different types of neoplasm or cancer as identified in the Medical Subject Heading dictionary of the National Library of Medicine. Another way of classifying cancer is by tissue type - e.g., **1) carcinoma** (a cancer that begins in the skin or in tissues that line or cover internal organs. There are a number of subtypes of carcinoma, including adenocarcinoma, basal cell carcinoma, squamous cell carcinoma, and transitional cell carcinoma), **2) sarcoma** (cancer that begins in bone, cartilage, fat, muscle, blood vessels, or other connective or supportive tissue), **3) leukemia** (cancer that starts in blood-forming tissue such as the bone marrow and causes large numbers of abnormal white blood cells to be produced and enter the blood), **4) lymphoma and myeloma** (cancers that begin in the cells of the immune system), and **5) central nervous system cancers** (cancers that begin in the tissues of the brain and spinal cord). However, in the near future, this nomenclature will probably be augmented by classification of neoplasms according the specific types of DNA damage that has caused the particular type of cancer in a particular person - personal genetic medicine. This should lead to the design of individual treatments for one's particular cancer.

Because a large number of mutated cells occur during normal metabolism, each of us is potentially getting cancer all of the time; and it is remarkable that full-blown cancer is not occurring in everyone on a daily basis, particularly during early development, when cell division is at its greatest. There are benign forms of cancer which do not invade surrounding tissue, remain encapsulated, and are usually easy to treat or do not need treatment. And there are malignant forms which do invade surrounding tissue, can migrate

RA; The Hallmarks of Cancer, Cell Vol. 100, pg. 57-70, January 7, 2000.

Chapter 2 - Comments - Conventional Medicine - History of Medicine - What is Cancer?

through-out the body, and will lead to death. Some cancers might develop rapidly and continue on that course or some might become dormant, while others might undergo "spontaneous remission". Cancer is highly idiosyncratic. If person "A's" cancer were to be transplanted to person "B", it would be immediately eliminated by person "B's" immune system. Thus, at its basic level, each person gets one's own unique type of cancer.

Although all cancers are caused by genetic damage, less that 10% have a hereditary basis, about 10% are caused by the chronic exposure to environmental agents (viruses and toxins), and about 80% are spontaneous or random mistakes in normal metabolism.

To understand cancer more fully, some basic concepts of developmental biology are essential. The human body is constructed from about 50 trillion cells, all of which come from one single cell that is created when the sperm cell from the father fuses with the ovum cell from the mother (oocyte) to create the complete single cell, "zygote" or embryonic stem cell. That single cell then divides into a cluster or "morula" of cells that are called "totipotent" - meaning that they are able to create the total fetus and all of the kinds of differentiated cells which construct the various types of tissues that make the different organs that are integrated into systems which make functional the complete body.

This process of development is graphically represented as follows: [10]

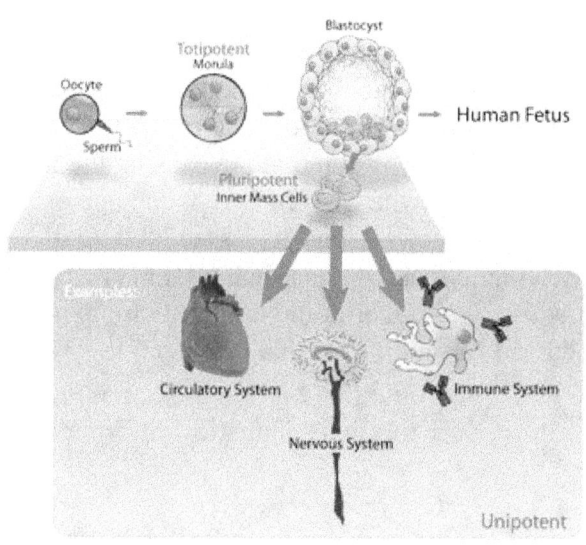

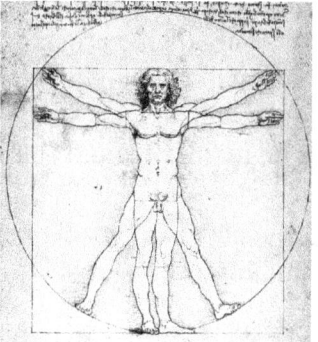

<hr />

[10]   Graphic from Wikipedia - "Stem Cell".

In the early stage of development, the "totipotent" embryonic stems cells transform into "pluripotent" stem cells, which means that they are capable of differentiating into nearly all cell types to form the three germ layers of tissue-types. Those pluripotent cells then transform into "multipotent" stem sells, a step which further commits that cell line to certain types of tissues. Those, in turn, differentiate into "oligopotent" stems cells, which finally differentiate into "unipotent" cells that produce only one cell type that are the functional cells of specific tissues.

This process of transforming from the very general to the increasingly more specific type of cells is represented below.

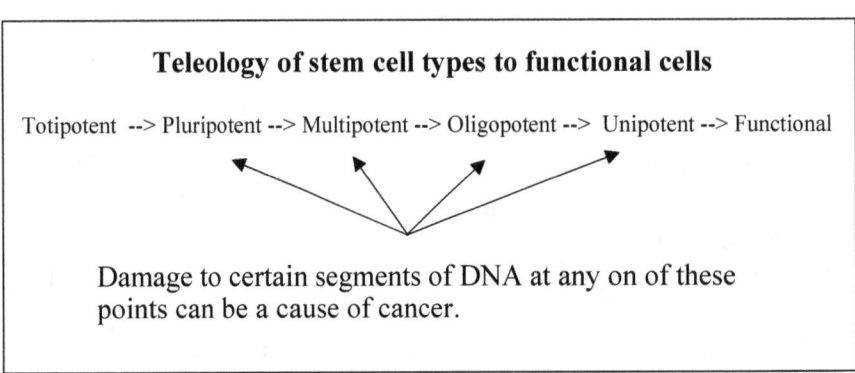

Teleology of stem cell types to functional cells

Totipotent --> Pluripotent --> Multipotent --> Oligopotent --> Unipotent --> Functional

Damage to certain segments of DNA at any on of these points can be a cause of cancer.

The conventional approach to cancer therapy is to kill the cells which have become cancerous. Usually, this is done by surgery, chemotherapy, and radiation, each of which has their limitations. Given the new understanding of the disease at the level of molecular biology, the challenge of research is held to be, ultimately, to identify the damaged segments of DNA of a particular tumor in a particular person that are causing the uncontrolled cell division and to design a targeted therapy which reverses that damage or destroys only those particular, pathological cells. For reasons discussed later, that approach will probably be even more problematic than conventional treatments; but nonetheless that seems to be the current, scientific Zeitgeist; and a lot of work is now going on in this regard. This will be discussed further in the final Chapter 11.

To put cancer in a broader perspective, consider the following statistical information from epidemiology.

Chapter 2 - Comments - Conventional Medicine - History of Medicine - What is Cancer?

The incidence of cancer in the U.S. over the last 30+ years has increased somewhat. This is surprising given the billions of dollars that have been spent on research and prevention. The U.S. statistics are probably comparable to the statistics for the European Union.

Cancer Incidence - all invasive types - 1975-2010. SEER Cancer Statistics - Table 2.5 [11]	
Year of Diagnosis	Incidence per 100,000 people
1975	400
1980	418
1985	449
1990	482
1995	477
2000	486
2005	472
2010	458

The above data are graphically represented below.

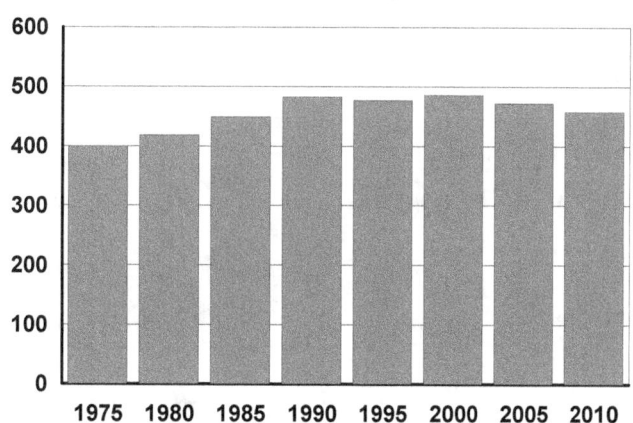

Cancer Incidence - all invasive types.
1975-2010

---

[11]   Howlader N, Noone AM, Krapcho M, Garshell J, Neyman N, Altekruse SF, Kosary CL, Yu M, Ruhl J, Tatalovich Z, Cho H, Mariotto A, Lewis DR, Chen HS, Feuer EJ, Cronin KA (eds). SEER Cancer Statistics Review, 1975-2010, National Cancer Institute. Bethesda, MD, http://seer.cancer.gov/csr/1975_2010/, based on November 2012 SEER data submission, posted to the SEER web site, April 2013.

Chapter 2 - Comments - Conventional Medicine - History of Medicine - What is Cancer?

Also, the mortality or death rate from cancer in the U.S. over the last 30+ years has remained fairly constant. Again, this is surprising given the billions of dollars that have been spent on therapy and research. And this is comparable to the statistics in the European Union.

Cancer Mortality - all invasive types - 1975-2010. SEER Cancer Statistics - Table 2.6 [12]	
Year of Diagnosis	Mortality per 100,000
1975	199
1980	207
1985	211
1990	215
1995	210
2000	199
2005	185
2010	172

These data are graphically represented below.

Cancer Mortality - all invasive types.
1975-2010

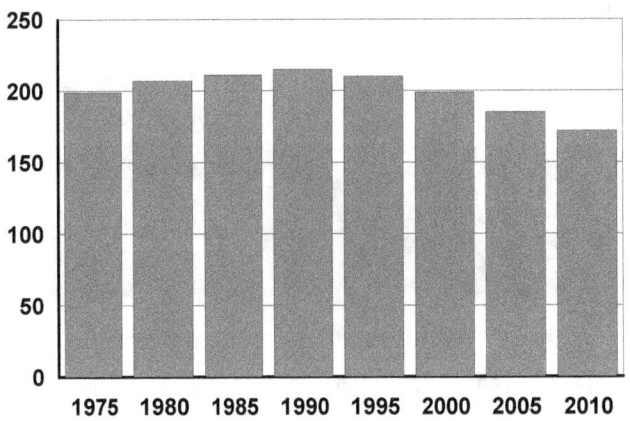

---

12   Ibidem.

Chapter 2 - Comments - Conventional Medicine - History of Medicine - What is Cancer?

Here you see the Incidence of and the mortality from cancer as correlated with age category. Cancer is associated with ageing; indeed, as will be discussed more fully in Chapter 11, we will be taking the position that biological ageing is one of the most important factors that actually cause cancer. Indeed, if biological ageing is not cured, then cancer can never be prevented or really cured. **B**iological ageing begins at about the age of 35 and from that point biological vitality (cell number, rate, and quality) decline exponentially while the incidence of cancer increases commensurately. This is graphically represented below in numbers per 100,000 population.

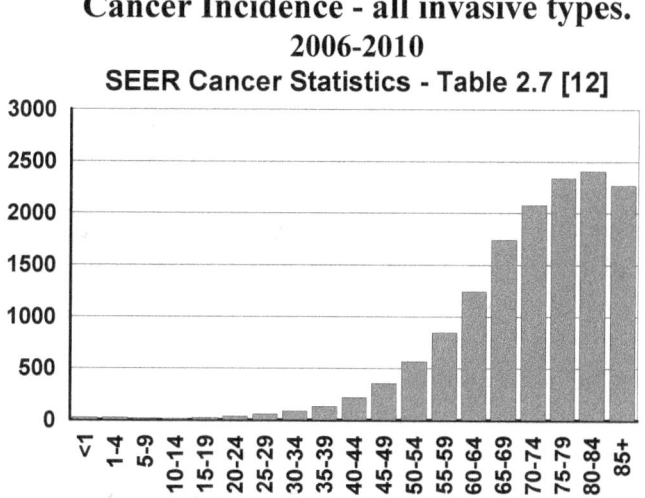

Cancer Incidence - all invasive types.
2006-2010
SEER Cancer Statistics - Table 2.7 [12]

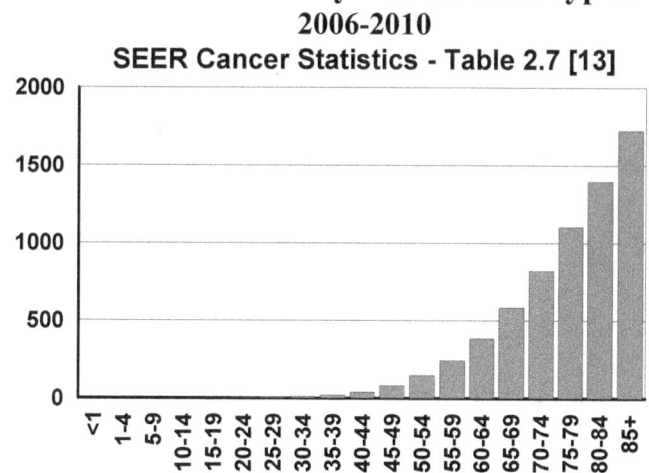

Cancer Mortality - all invasive types.
2006-2010
SEER Cancer Statistics - Table 2.7 [13]

Chapter 2 - Comments - Conventional Medicine - History of Medicine - What is Cancer?

A common notion is that cancer is caused by environmental toxins from industry. This needs to be dispelled. As already stated, cancer is a malfunction in cell division that is caused by damage to certain segments of the DNA in a particular cell and the ageing of the micro-environment. DNA damage happens all of the time; but >99% of damage is repaired by the DNA regulatory genes or the cells self-destructs. Usually, such cancer forming DNA damage occurs during normal metabolism when stem cells divide to replace their targeted func-tional cells; and it is believed that some 80% of cancer results from such natural, spontaneous processes. However, this spontaneous cause of DNA damage is amplified by any process that induces cell division such as irritation, exposure to toxins, or inflammation. Further, DNA damage, itself, can also occur from toxic chemicals which pass through the cell membrane and chemically interact directly with DNA, such as: "Benzo(a)pyrene", which is a potent mutagen and carcinogen and which is a public health concern because of its possible effects on industrial workers, as an environmental pollutant, and as a consequence of tobacco smoke. According to government classification, there are 57 substances which are labeled "Known To Be Human Carcino-gens" (some of which are drugs that are used in the treatment of cancer) and 189 substances which are labeled "Reasonably Anticipated To Be Human Carcinogens". [Ref. "Report on Carcinogens - Twelfth Edition 2011"; U.S. Department of Health and Human Services; Public Health Service; National Toxicology Program.] [13] That would seem low given the large number of artificial chemicals which are introduced into our environment but industrial processes. However, the toxicity of those artificial chemicals is minuscule when compared to the toxic chemicals in natural food sources which we routinely eat. The work of Bruce Ames (former Professor of Biochemistry at U.C. Berkeley and an expert on ageing and cancer) is insightful with respect to carcinogens. See his lecture which was given around 1990 on this subject. Although out of date in some respects, the basic information is foundational on this subject.

http://www.youtube.com/watch?v=F1EEscgMF14

At this point, let us return to the main theme of this book and proceed with dealing with one's treatment and where to find scientific information on specific types of cancer.

---

13   "Report on Carcinogens - Twelfth Edition 2011"; U.S. Department of Health and Human Services; Public Health Service; National Toxicology Program
  http://ntp.niehs.nih.gov/pubhealth/roc/index-4.html

55

Chapter 2 - Comments - Conventional Medicine - History of Medicine - What is Cancer?

Chapter 3
Medical Records

As previously said, you, yourself, should have a copy of all of your medical records; and in most governmental jurisdictions, those records are legally your property. Over-come any intimidation you might have about asking for such copies - your physician should not be offended by this. You need this information to understand better your situation, do research, and seek secondary opinions. The more you learn the medical terms, concepts, and procedures, the better a patient you will become and gain greater respect for and from the medical professionals with whom you are dealing. Managing your medical informa-tion is not as difficult as it might, at first, seem; but it does need some practice. It is very much like accounting - collecting the clinical documents, maintaining a journal of events, and posting information to ledgers, and, if you want, making graphic representations. In fact, medical record keeping is essentially the same as normal accounting - A General Journal in which all relevant transactions are recorded; and then the posting from that Journal to particular Ledgers on specific conditions. There is no need to have any elabo-rate, computerized medical records system, at least at first; and we will provide some basic forms, of which you may make as many copies as desired. If you are adroit at your word processor, you can make your own forms. For technical terms related to cancer see: http://www.cancer.gov/dictionary . It is a dictionary of some 7,500 terms that are related to cancer and with their pronunciation.

We recommend a three-ring binder with a set of blank tabs. You can use pre-punched, three-hole paper; or if you use regular paper, then you will need a three-punch device to make such holes. The suggested divisions are as follows.

Section 1 - General Journal. Other than the clinical data which you collect, this is the most important record; and it will be of considerable help to you and the physician(s). It is simply a running diary of all significant medical events, your thoughts and feelings, a synopsis of findings and progress, and anything you feel is worth noting. Other than recording the date of each entry, the narrative usually is free-form. People say that such journalizing is psychologically very beneficial; and your physician can add this to the clinical notes of your case. While your physician will be paying attention mostly to clini-cal parameters associated with the cancer, one might miss such things as depression and subtle signs and symptoms which you mention in your Journal and which, if over-looked, could result in significant problems if not medically addressed early. Thus, the General Journal is a major component of your clinical portfolio.

Section 2 - Ledgers of Specific Problems. You will keep a separate Ledger for each particular problem and post from your General Journal items that pertain to that condition. Obviously, there will be a Ledger for the primary medical problem or type of cancer which is diagnosed and being treated. There might also be a Ledger for a particular sign or symptom or any other conditions for which you wish to account.

Section 3 - Data. Here, include copies of all laboratory and other clinical testing data as well as clinical reports of the various physicians who are rendering opinions about your case. Organize these in a chronological manner - oldest to most recent. Physicians usually organize information in reverse chronology (i.e., most recent to oldest), however, normal chronology is the most logical and will enable anyone to go through your case in an orderly, sequential manner. You will make reference to and use these data in the comments in your General Journal and Ledger of Specific Problem.

Section 4 - Graphic Representations. You can graph any parameter that is significant including signs, symptoms, and laboratory information.

Again, the following forms may be used or you can keep your information in any type of recording system that works for you. The general idea is to record events as they occur in a chronological fashion and then to organize the information into problem-oriented segments so that you can see trends and evaluate progress.

Identification: _____

Date	General Journal: Events, Data, and Comments

Identification: _____

Ledger of Specific Problem: _____	
Date	**Description & Comments**

Chapter 3 - Medical Records

Longitudinal Tracking of Bio-Medical Parameters [1]

Parameter Name, units and range	Date	Date	Date	Date	Date	Date	Date
	Value	Value	Value	Value	Value	Value	Value

[1] First, record the particular **Date**. Next, recorder the **Parameter Name** which is being evaluated, the **Units** of measurement of the parameter, if applicable and the reference **Range**. This can be a laboratory test, or a condition such as: tumor size, or a symptom such as fatigue or pain. Finally, record the **Value** of the parameter such as: Tumor size in centimeters or PSA in ng/mL; Fatigue by "mild" "moderate" "severe". Record any parameter that you think is relevant.

Chapter 3 - Medical Records

Parameter Graph [2]

Parameter (a):

Units of Measure (b):

Scale (c)	Date	Date	Date	Date	Date	Date	Date	Date	Date	Date	Date
Normal Range											

---

[2] Make one graph for a desired "Parameter", which is the thing being measured and trended and identify it in section (a). "Units of Measure" is how the Parameter is measured and identify that in section (b). "Normal Range" will be the normal range of the Units of Measure of the particular Parameter. Put those values in section (c) and then "Scale" that up and down in some relative fashion from high to low, according to your best judgment. Finally, graph the data by connecting the values with a line.

61

Chapter 3 - Medical Records

Chapter 4 - MedlinePlus

Having studied the PDQ Summaries and worked on your medical records, it is appropriate to move out into the wider Internet resources. The best place to start is with MedlinePlus, which is a collection of Internet resources that is compiled by experts at the National Library of Medicine.

The National Library of Medicine is the world's largest and most authoritative source of information on health and medicine; and later, we will use their scientific research database called PubMed a.k.a. MEDLINE.

In the MedlinePlus site, the information from the National Institutes of Health and other sources, which are trusted by the Library, are organized in sections for over 800 diseases. It is advised to ground yourself in this information before jumping into the usual Internet search engines which can be quite chaotic and uncertain about their authenticity.

Expert Summary

- ❦ *Go to:*   http://www.nlm.nih.gov/medlineplus
- ❦ In the Search box, type in your subject of interest
- ❦ Or go to the category of interest button and search.

There are only a few instructions that are necessary to guide you through these procedures, and they are as follows.

MedlinePlus has three main sections: **Health Topics**, **Drugs & Supplements**, **Videos**. Select the one of interest to you and proceed from there.

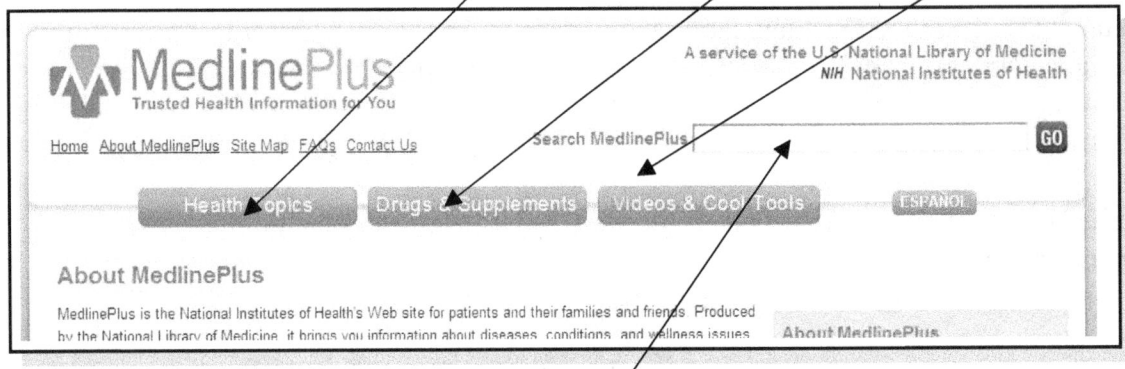

Or you can type in a specific topic in the **Search MedlinePlus** box.

Selecting the **Health Topics** section, you may search by using the alphabetical **Index** or **List of All Topics** or type in your subject in the **Search MedlinePlus** box.

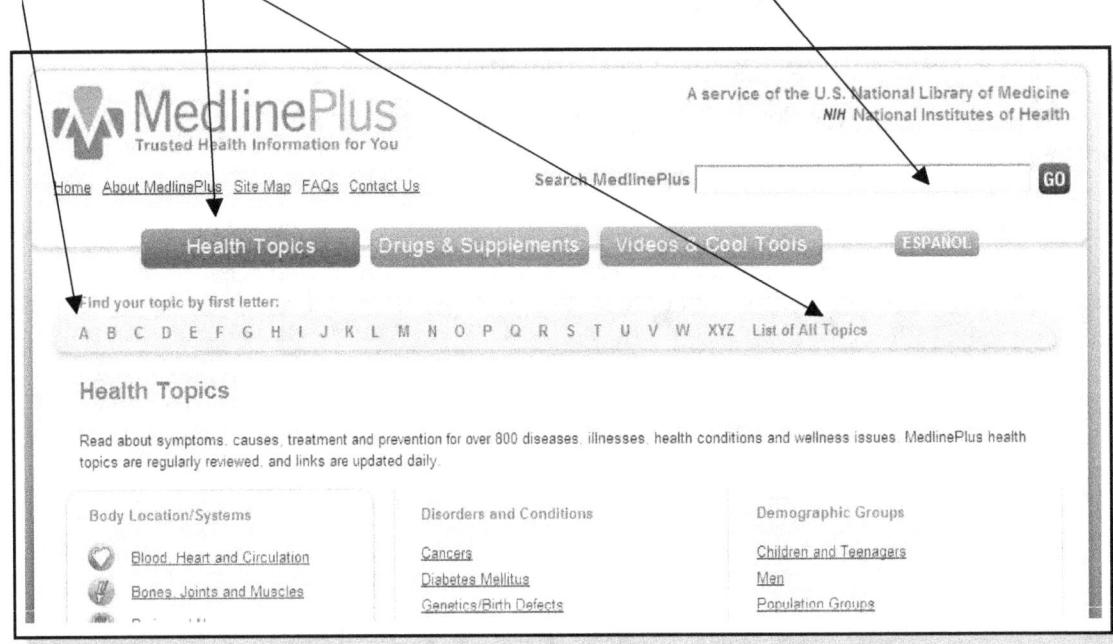

Again, this will not need much explanation; and each subject will have its unique set of links to resources on the Internet that relate to your subject.

63

Chapter 4 - MedlinePlus

One useful feature is to subscribe to e-mail up-dates on specific subjects.

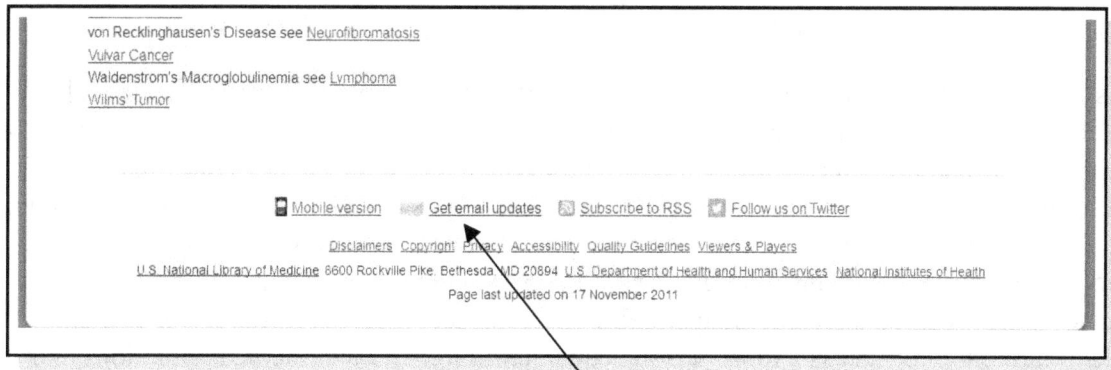

When you find a topic on which you would like to received automatic notices of new postings, at the bottom of a page, select the "**Get email updates**" and follow the instructions.

CHAPTER 5

SECONDARY OPINIONS AND PATHOLOGY CONFIRMATION

Usually, cancer is discovered when a person seeks a medical evaluation for some health related complaint, during a routine check-up, or self examination. This happens with one's primary medical provider, who will do the initial diagnosis after having done a battery of examinations - e.g., physical, radiological, and tissue sample. The diagnosis and treatment of cancer can be somewhat of an art. And if possible, before treatment is initiated, a secondary opinion and confirmation of pathology is a good idea because mistakes can be made or there can be different analyses and different, recommended courses of action. The treatment of cancer is a more serious consideration than most medical situations and should be well considered. Do not be concerned about hurting people's feelings by seeking confirmation even if you are initially satisfied with your first practitioner.

If a secondary opinion is desired, investigate different centers. The National Cancer Institute "designated cancer centers" or academic institutions are reasonable places to consider, a list of which is provided below.

http://www.cancer.gov/researchandfunding/extramural/cancercenters/find-a-cancer-center

After having interviewed and decided upon a prospective clinic for a second opinion, they will have a Medical Records Release Form, which you can use to have a copy of your prior records sent to them. Preferably, you, yourself, should already have a copy of all of your medical records, as discussed previously. This process of having a secondary opinion and correlating the findings between the first and second evaluations will constitute a period of "Watchful Waiting", which gives an idea about the rate of progression of the tumor, and this was previously discussed.

If a complete re-evaluation is not appropriate, then it still might be useful to have your initial pathology slides sent to a different laboratory to have the cell type confirmed. Critical to the proper diagnosis and treatment of any cancer is the "Cellular Classification". This is particularly true as we move into more advanced therapies and the design of individualized treatments because, as previously said, each person's cancer is genetically and molecularly unique, and specific treatments are emerging which target specific tumor markers. For some background on pathology reports, see:

http://www.cancer.gov/cancertopics/factsheet/detection/pathology-reports

The freezing and storage of biopsy tissue

One additional recommendation would be to have some of your biopsy tissue preserved cryogenically so that it can be analyzed later as new diagnostic methods and treatments arise in the future from the advancement of research. Getting your physician to do this may be problematic because this is not a customary procedure; but the tissue is available after the biopsy, and the cost of storage should not be great.

Chapter 6

CANCER STATISTICS

Some insight regarding one's personal cancer can be gained by understanding the broader, demographic statistics. Like the PDQ (Physicians Data Query), the National Cancer Institute sponsors such a cancer, statistical database, called: SEER (Surveillance, Epidemiology and End Results Program).

The SEER Program collects and publishes cancer data in order to assemble and report estimates of cancer incidence, survival, mortality, other measures of the cancer burden, and patterns of care in the US, including information that is specific to race/ethnic populations as well as other populations defined by age, gender, and geography.

Some 17 geographic zones in the United States are studied in detail; and this represents about 28 percent of the entire population. These statistics can be held to represent the United States, in general, as well as similar societies elsewhere. To obtain a perspective on your cancer of interest, this will give you a generalized, statistical picture.

SEER is a complex, professional level, database that is mostly intended for experts in public health with a background in statistics. However, with some patience and directions, as provided here, some of the information is accessible to most people.

Expert Summary

♆ *Go to:*   http://seer.cancer.gov
This takes you to the "Cancer Statistics page.

♆ *Go to:*   **"Cancer Stat Fact Sheets"** and *Select* "**All Sites**" and then the "**View**" button.

♆ *Select:*   From there, select the type of cancer of interest. The most common cancers are listed in the box on the left; but to see all types, select the "**More Cancer Types**". Select the appropriate type. This leads to a general overview "Statistics at a Glance" and by scrolling down the "**Survival Statistics**" link, that will be expanded. Note "How Many People Survive 5 Years ....".

Key Terms

"Cancer Incidence Rate". The cancer incidence rate is the number of <u>new</u> cancers of a specific site/type that occurs in a specified population during a year. This is expressed as the number of cancers per 100,000 population.

"Cancer Mortality Rate". The cancer mortality rate is the number of <u>deaths</u>, with cancer as the underlying cause of death, occurring in a specified population during a year. Cancer mortality is expressed as the number of deaths due to cancer per 100,000 population.

"Cancer Prevalence". Prevalence is defined as the number or percent of people alive on a certain date in a population who previously had a diagnosis of the disease. It includes new (incidence) and pre-existing cases and is a function of both past incidence and survival. Information on prevalence can be used for health planning, resource allocation, and an estimate of cancer survivorship.

"Cancer Survival Statistics". Cancer survival statistics are typically expressed as the proportion of patients alive at some point subsequent to the diagnosis of their cancer. Relative survival is an estimate of the percentage of patients who would be expected to survive the effects of their cancer. Observed survival is the actual percentage of patients still alive at some specified time after diagnosis of cancer. It considers deaths from all causes, cancer or otherwise.

"Lifetime risk". This is the probability of developing or dying from cancer in the course of one's life-span. Statistical models are used to compute the probability of developing or dying of cancer from birth or a certain age.

"Cancer Statistics by Race/Ethnicity". This helps to define the cancer burden by race and ethnicity and includes: White; Black; American Indian / Alaska Native; Asian / Pacific Islander; Hispanic (including any race); and Non-Hispanic White (Non-Hispanic White were calculated by subtracting the Hispanic White from total White).

SEER has many features, and instructions to only a few will be given here. Of interest to most people will be the 5 year survival rate after diagnosis for a particular type of cancer because 5 years is considered to be the threshold for being cured. And that will be the main focus here, although other sectors are informative and can be found by using instructions on the site. To find the 5 year survival rate do the following.

Go to the home page at: **http://seer.cancer.gov** .

First, use the section "**Cancer Stat Fact Sheets**".

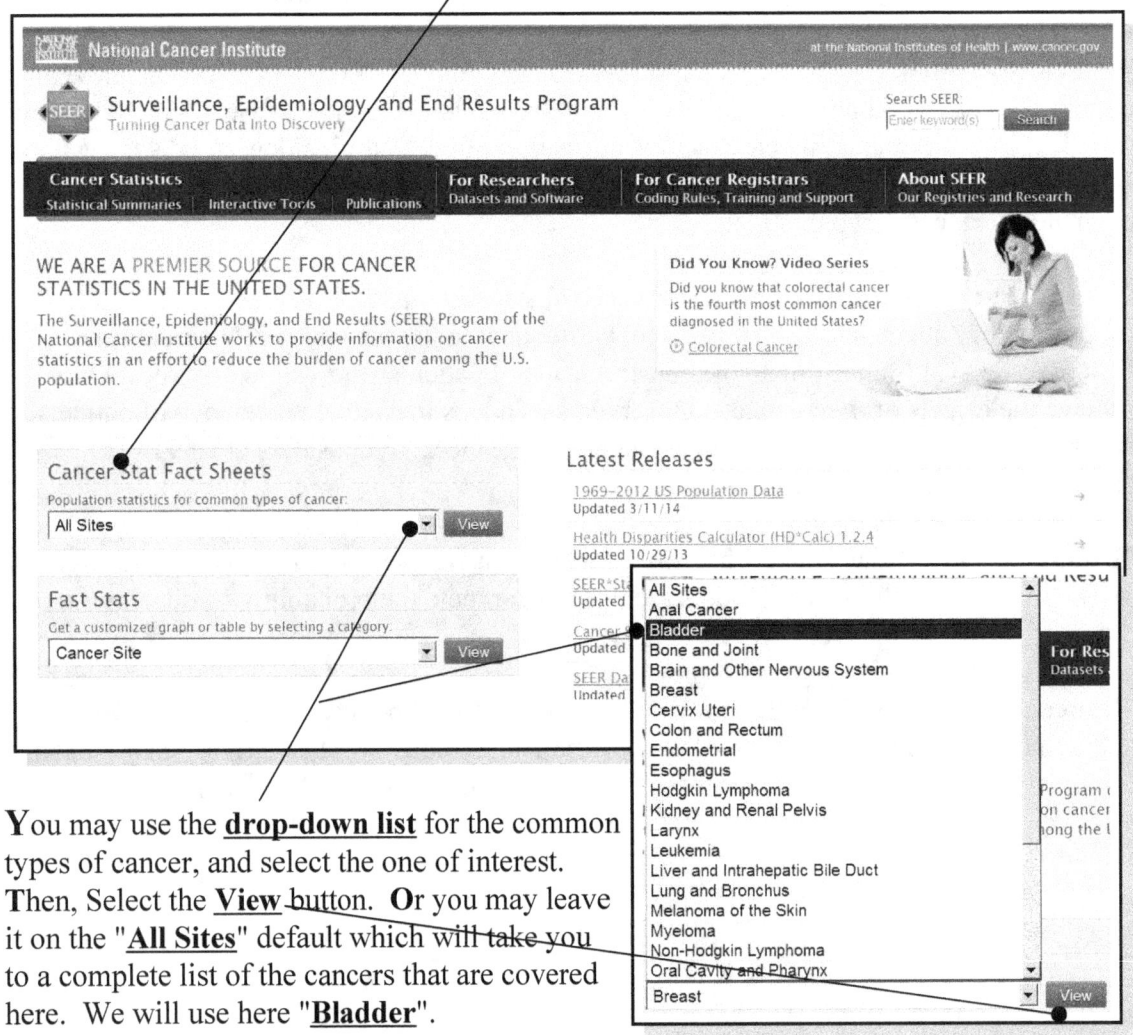

You may use the **drop-down list** for the common types of cancer, and select the one of interest. Then, Select the **View** button. Or you may leave it on the "**All Sites**" default which will take you to a complete list of the cancers that are covered here. We will use here "**Bladder**".

Chapter 6 - CANCER STATISTICS

You will be taken to the page on the type of cancer desired - here, "**Bladder Cancer**".

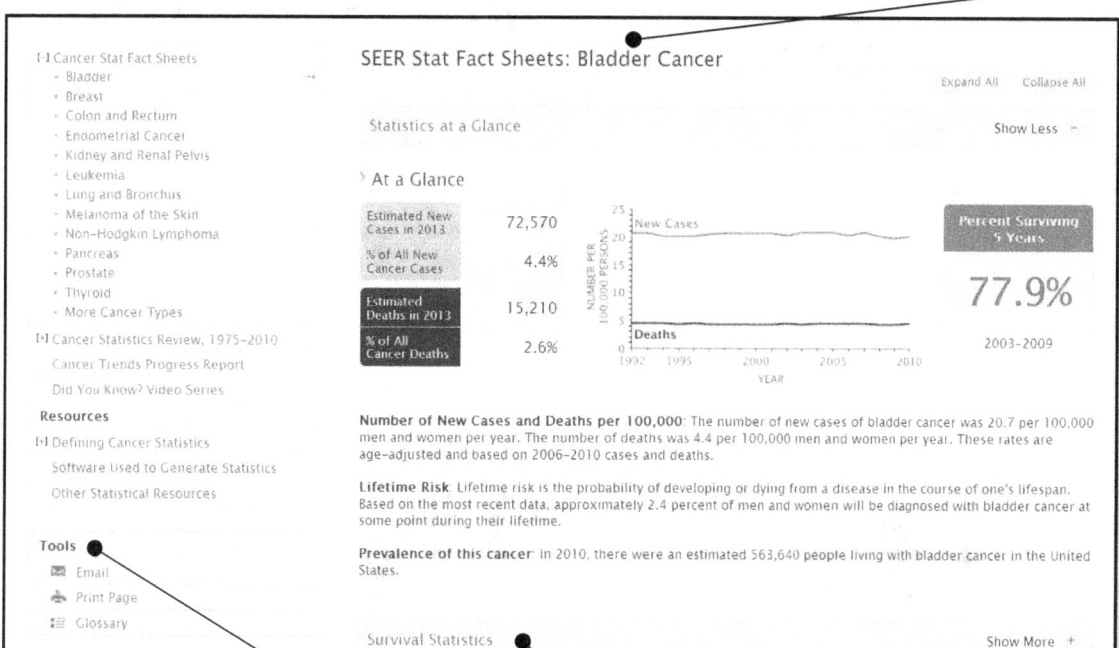

Two columns are presented - the one on the right is the subject information and in the left column there are links to other resources.

To retrieve more detailed information, Select the "**Survival Statistics**". The additional information will be appended to the page below. (This can happen so rapidly that it appears that nothing changed, in which case scroll down to see the information.)

You will notice in the left column, that there is a section entitled "**Tools**" in which there are procedures for Email, Print Page, and Glossary of terms.

In the Survival Statistics section and of particular interest, there is the "**5-year Relative Survival (%)**" and the "**Percent of Cases by Stage**". Again, five year survival is significant because it is taken as the threshold for being "cured".

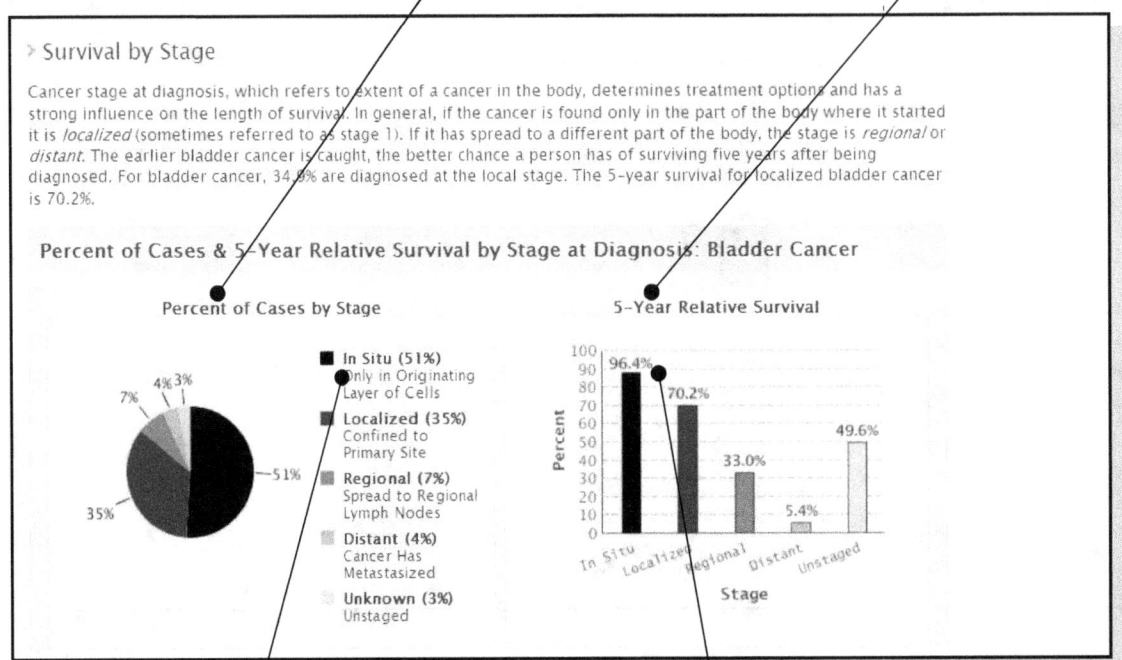

> Survival by Stage

Cancer stage at diagnosis, which refers to extent of a cancer in the body, determines treatment options and has a strong influence on the length of survival. In general, if the cancer is found only in the part of the body where it started it is *localized* (sometimes referred to as stage 1). If it has spread to a different part of the body, the stage is *regional* or *distant*. The earlier bladder cancer is caught, the better chance a person has of surviving five years after being diagnosed. For bladder cancer, 34.0% are diagnosed at the local stage. The 5-year survival for localized bladder cancer is 70.2%.

Percent of Cases & 5-Year Relative Survival by Stage at Diagnosis: Bladder Cancer

For cancer of the Bladder, the interplay between these two survival statistics is as follows:

Percent of Cases by Stage	5-Year Relative Survival
51% of the cases are diagnosed when the tumor was "**In Situ**" or in place,	in which "**96.4%**" survived for 5 years or longer;
35% of the cases are diagnosed when the tumor was "**Localized** (confined to primary site)",	of which **70.2%** survived for 5 years or longer;
7% of the cases are diagnosed at the stage of "**Regional** (spread to regional lymph nodes)",	of which **33%** survived for 5 years of longer;
4% of the cases are diagnosed at the stage "**Distant** (cancer has metastasized),	of which **5.4%** survived for 5 years or longer;
3% of the cases are diagnosed with the stage being "**Unknown** (unstaged)",	of which **49.6%** survived for 5 years or longer;

71

Below the previous section ("Survival by Stage"), there are three other sections of interest: "**Number of New Cases and Deaths**", "**Trends in Rates**", and "**More About This Cancer**". Select the title and browse the contents.

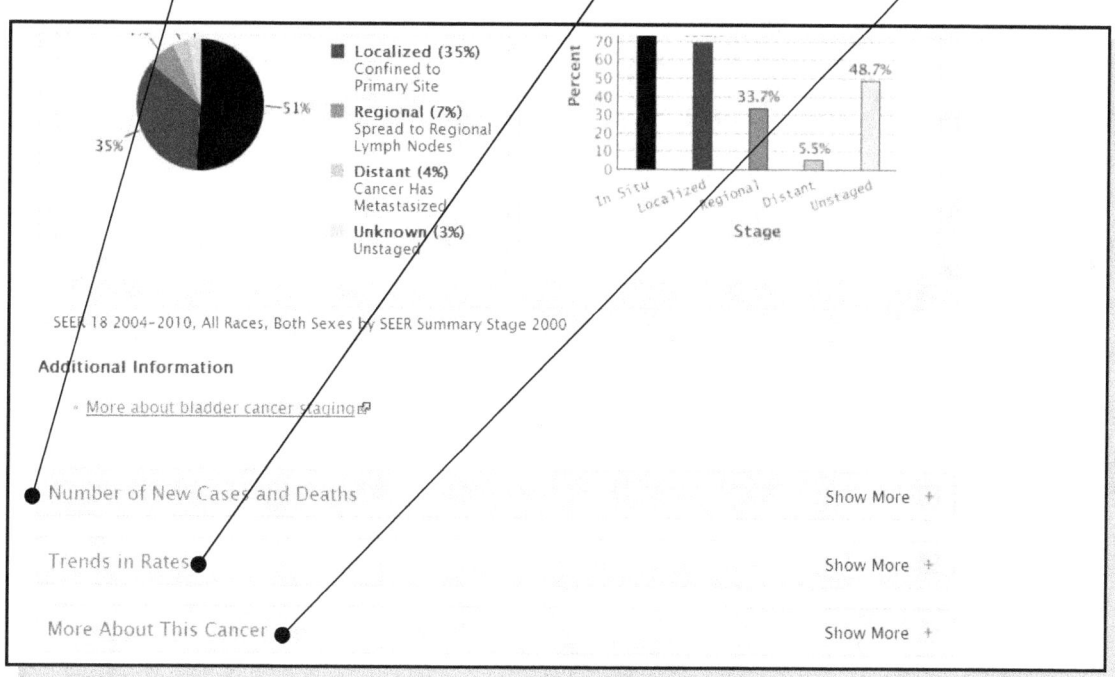

Just browse these sections for other pages in which there is valuable information.

Going back to the home page, the "**Fast Stats**" section will broaden the scope of the previous statistics. Go to the home page - http://www.seer.cancer.gov/ and in the "Fast Stats" section, Select the **Menu button**; identify the desired database, select "View", and proceed according to your interest.

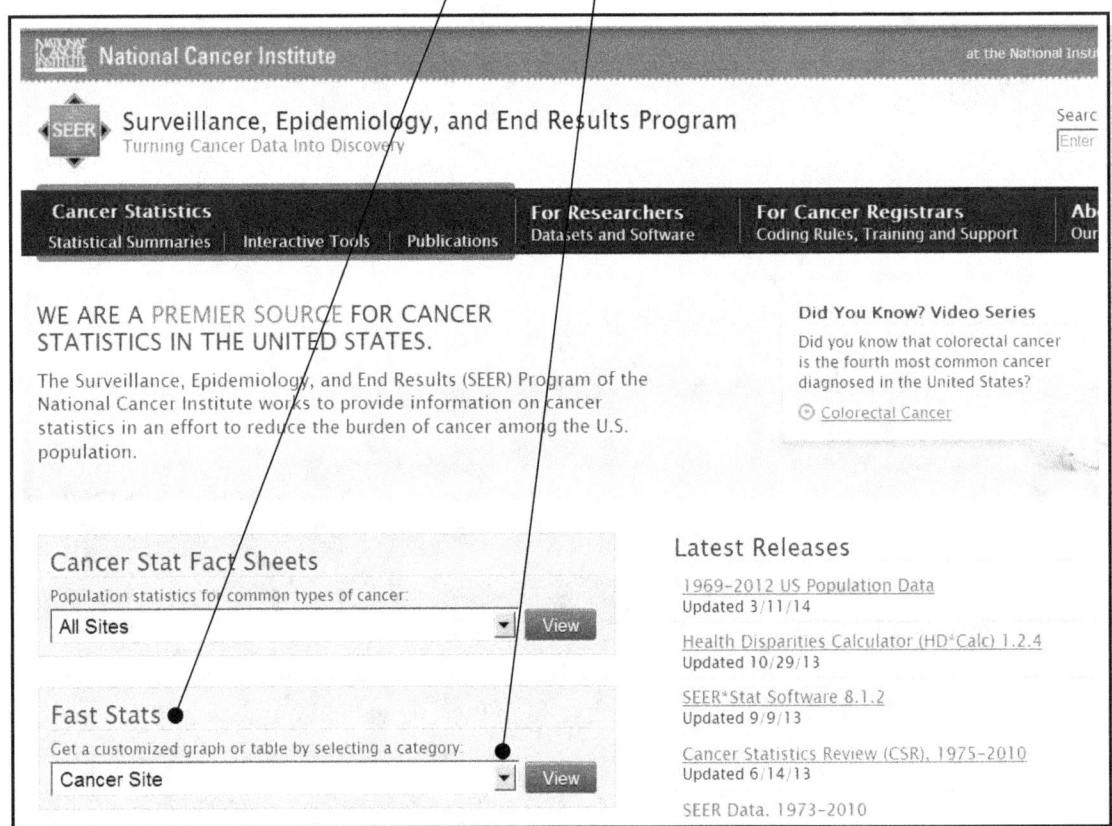

From there, select the data-set of interest to you and navigate accordingly from that point.

73

Chapter 6 - CANCER STATISTICS

Chapter 7
The National Library of Medicine and the
PubMed, Search Program

Thus far, we have covered the following: Chapter 1) how to obtain the state-of-the-art, conventional, medical treatment for any type of cancer using PDQ - Physician Data Query; Chapter 2) putting the PDQ protocols in a broader context with comments on "conventional medicine", the history of medicine, and what cancer is; Chapter 3) keeping one's medical records; Chapter 4) finding additional information from various sources on the Internet, using MedlinePlus; Chapter 5) comments on obtaining a secondary opinion; and Chapter 6) cancer statistics using the SEER database. Now, we will move into the bio-medical research information.

The National Library of Medicine is one of the many Institutes within the umbrella of the National Institutes of Health. The Library runs the National Center for Biotechnology Information which manages the MEDLINE database, which is accessible by the PubMed search program, and which is the one on which we will focus in this Chapter. This is the largest and most authoritative source of bio-medical information in the world. And it is impossible to grasp the quantitative immensity and the qualitative importance of the work which is done by the National Library of Medicine, the MEDLINE database, and the PubMed search program.

To approach an understanding of the importance of this data-base, consider how scientific information is generated and reported. Research projects are being conducted all over the world by scientist, most of who are affiliated with universities and other publicly funded organizations. (The basic research is usually too costly and uncertain to be funded by commercial enterprises.) As a scientific study is completed, the investigator(s) report the findings to professional societies and other scientific publishers who specialize in the relevant areas of interest. New reports are reviewed by peer groups in an attempt to make sure that the information is significant and authentic. Those reports, which are approved by the peer-review committees, are scheduled for publication in journals, which are published by these societies. The system is not nearly perfect. Some of the information is wrong, and most of it is made progressively obsolete by new findings. A lot of the research is political and economically driven rather than a pure pursuit of mission-oriented knowledge. And usually, there is a considerable lag-time between doing the research, presenting the information for publication, and its actual publication. Further, there is a lot of inertia within regulatory agencies and the medical profession against adopting new information; and it can take a decade or longer for new information to be incorporated into new therapies. Efforts in such areas as "Translational Medicine" and the electronic publishing of research via the Internet are now expediting this process. And in our own efforts, we hope to play a major role in accelerating the process from "bench to bedside", as it is called; and funds from the sale of this book are applied to that effort.

Irrespective of its short-comings, the scientific enterprise is a monumental achievement and will continue to expand exponentially. All of this scientific publishing represents a massive and overwhelming amount of disparate information, which would be essentially useless unless it was not made coherent and accessible by painstaking indexing and retrieval which is done by the National Library of Medicine and the PubMed search engine. The library has a vast collection of books, journals, photos, audio-visual materials, and electronic databases, but if that material were not indexed by highly trained specialists and cataloged by title, author, subjects, and summaries, it would be a mountain of fairly useless material. A person would never be able to find anything that was relevant to one's purpose. Thus, the indexing and cataloging functions, as mundane as they may seem, are the foundation of the entire library - of equal importance to or greater than the individual documents themselves.

The MEDLINE database contains records or articles from over 12,000 scientific journals (mostly bio-medical) of which 5,600 are currently being indexed. Presently, this consti-tutes from 2,000 to 4,000 new articles every day or 30,000 per month. In 2012, the program served 2.2 billion searches from all over the world, mostly from scientists but also from the scientifically adept public. The electronic database now goes back to 1946 and covers journals in over 39 different languages with a total of over 20 million citations that have taken millions of man-hours to build over decades. When you go on to the PubMed Internet site and search a medical topic, you are zipping through all of this information at the speed of light and getting results to your special inquiry within a couple of seconds. Some appreciation of the monumentality of this accomplishment is warranted. It takes some training to use the database; but for those who want to be in touch with the flow of scientific progress, it is best to spend a little time to learn how to use this resource.

Before going into the details of the search procedures, I want to give the reader a slight impression about the immensity of this resource. What follows is a brief review of the history of the National Library of Medicine using vignettes on a background of a listing of the journals which are currently indexed. The names of the journals have been abbreviated and the font reduced to the lowest size possible - otherwise the listing would take some 150 pages. So, the background is intended to be just a "wall-paper" to create an impres-sion of the immensity.

If you want to find specific journals, then go to the full index:

http://wwwcf.nlm.nih.gov/serials/journals/index.cfm

Flip through the following pages; get the idea; and do keep in mind that when you place a search command in PubMed you will be scanning through all of these journals (actually many more because the journals that are no longer indexed are also included in the database). The primary references for the historical information have been: 1) A History of The National Library of Medicine - The Nation's Treasury of Medical Knowledge" by Wyndham D. Miles, 1982. NIH Pub. # 85-1904, U.S. Dept. of Health and Human Services; 2) Images from the History of Medicine [http://wwwihm.nlm.nih.gov]; and 3) An Online Art and Architecture Tour of the U.S. National Library of Medicine, which you can take at [http://www.nlm.nih.gov/exhibition/tour/tour.html].

List Of Journals, Currently Indexed by NLM as Organized By Subject (November 2013)

A

ACQUIRED IMMUNODEFICIENCY SYNDROME (39)
J Int Assoc Provid AIDS Care
Top Antivir Med
J Watch AIDS Clin Care
Curr Opin HIV AIDS
Curr HIV/AIDS Rep
HIV AIDS Policy Law Rev
J Int AIDS Soc
SAHARA J
Curr HIV Res
HIV Clin Trials
IAPAC Mon
AIDS Rev
HIV Clin
HIV Med
J Acquir Immune Defic Syndr
HRSA Careaction
J HIV Ther
AIDS Behav
Proj Inf Perspect
AIDS Patient Care STDS
IAVI Rep
Res Initiat Treat Action
GMHC Treat Issues
HIV AIDS Surveill Rep
AIDS Read
BETA
Int J STD AIDS
Posit Aware
AIDS Care
AIDS Educ Prev
J Assoc Nurses AIDS Care
TreatmentUpdate
AIDS Res Hum Retroviruses
AIDS
AIDS Alert
AIDS Policy Law
AIDS Public Policy J
Focus
HIV Inside

AEROSPACE MEDICINE (4)
Air Med J
Aviakosm Ekolog Med
Adv Space Biol Med
Aviat Space Environ Med

ALLERGY AND IMMUNOLOGY (150) - includes Hypersensitivity, Lymphology, Serology, Serotherapy, And Interferons - see also Transplantation
Monoclon Antib Immunodiagn Immunother
Hum Vaccin Immunother
Int Forum Allergy Rhinol
Am J Rhinol Allergy
Arb Paul Ehrlich Inst Bundesinstitut Impfstoffe Biomed
Arzneim Langen Hess
Immunotherapy
J Innate Immun
MAbs
Innate Immun
Mucosal Immunol
Zhongguo Yi Miao He Mian Yi
Recent Pat Endocr Metab Immune Drug Discov
Recent Pat Inflamm Allergy Drug Discov
Ross Immunol Zhurnal
Semin Immunopathol
Antiinflamm Antiallergy Agents Med Chem
Clin Vaccine Immunol
Endocr Metab Immune Disord Drug Targets
Inflamm Allergy Drug Targets
J Neuroimmune Pharmacol
Expert Rev Clin Immunol
Int J Immunogenet
Cell Mol Immunol
Iran J Immunol
J Immunotoxicol
Postepy Hig Med Dosw (Online)
Chem Immunol Allergy
Clin Dev Immunol
Eur Ann Allergy Clin Immunol
Lymphat Res Biol
Autoimmun Rev
Expert Rev Vaccines
Cancer Immun
Curr Allergy Asthma Rep
Curr Opin Allergy Clin Immunol
Int Immunopharmacol
J Immunoassay Immunochem
Nat Rev Immunol
Trends Immunol
BMC Immunol
Dev Biol (Basel)
Iran J Allergy Asthma Immunol
Nat Immunol
Clin Immunol
Curr Dir Autoimmun
Microbes Infect
J Microbiol Immunol Infect
BioDrugs

Hum Antibodies
J Immunother
Allergol Int
Allergy Asthma Proc
Cytokine Growth Factor Rev
Sarcoidosis Vasc Diffuse Lung Dis
Xi Bao Yu Fen Zi Mian Yi Xue Za Zhi
Ann Allergy Asthma Immunol
Clin Rev Allergy Immunol
Exerc Immunol Rev
Inflamm Res
J Interferon Cytokine Res
Acta Microbiol Immunol Hung
Clin Allergy Immunol
Epidemiol Mikrobiol Imunol
Immunity
Neuroimmunomodulation
Infez Med
Ocul Immunol Inflamm
Rev Alerg Mex
Transpl Immunol
Curr Protoc Immunol

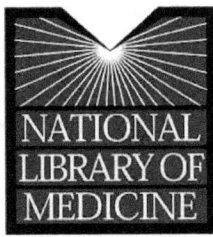

Int Arch Allergy Immunol
Fish Shellfish Immunol
J Investig Allergol Clin Immunol
Pneumonol Alergol Pol
Roum Arch Microbiol Immunol
Biologicals
Egypt J Immunol
Eur Cytokine Netw
Genes Immun
J Leukoc Biol Suppl
Pediatr Allergy Immunol
Photodermatol Photoimmunol Photomed
Am J Reprod Immunol
Clin Exp Allergy
Cytokine
Int Immunol
Semin Immunol
APMIS
APMIS Suppl
Autoimmunity
Curr Opin Immunol
Immunol Suppl
Int J Immunopathol Pharmacol
J Autoimmun
Brain Behav Immun
Immunol Allergy Clin North Am
Immunol Cell Biol
Immunopharmacol Immunotoxicol
Viral Immunol
Immunol Res
Int Rev Immunol
Immunol Invest
Immunohematology
J Leukoc Biol
Annu Rev Immunol
Asian Pac J Allergy Immunol
Vaccine
Cancer Immunol Immunother
J Asthma
J Clin Immunol
J Neuroimmunol
Crit Rev Immunol
Hum Immunol
Immunobiology
Immunol Lett
J Reprod Immunol
Mol Immunol
Parasite Immunol
Vet Immunol Immunopathol
Allergy
Comp Immunol Microbiol Infect Dis
J Clin Lab Immunol
Nihon Rinsho Meneki Gakkai Kaishi
Dev Comp Immunol
Immunol Rev
Microbiol Immunol
Inflammation
Immunogenetics
Allergol Immunopathol (Madr)
Infection
Scand J Immunol
Eur J Immunol
J Allergy Clin Immunol
J Immunol Methods
Med Microbiol Immunol
Tissue Antigens
Cell Immunol
Infect Immun

Lymphology
Curr Top Microbiol Immunol
Clin Exp Immunol
Arch Immunol Ther Exp (Warsz)
Adv Immunol
Immunology
Arerugi
J Immunol
Zh Mikrobiol Epidemiol Immunobiol
Antonie Van Leeuwenhoek
J Exp Med
ALTERNATIVE MEDICINE see Complementary Therapies

ANATOMY (21) - includes Morphology
Anat Rec (Hoboken)
Anat Sci Educ
Anat Sci Int
Cells Tissues Organs
Morphologie
Adv Anat Pathol
Ann Anat
Dev Dyn

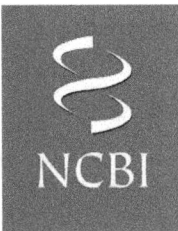

Ital J Anat Embryol
Morfologiia
Rom J Morphol Embryol
Clin Anat
J Chem Neuroanat
Surg Radiol Anat
Adv Anat Embryol Cell Biol
Anat Histol Embryol
Okajimas Folia Anat Jpn
Folia Morphol (Warsz)
Kaibogaku Zasshi
J Anat
J Morphol

ANESTHESIOLOGY (40) - includes Resuscitation
Anesthesiol Clin
Acta Anaesthesiol Taiwan
Anaesthesiol Intensive Ther
Best Pract Res Clin Anaesthesiol
Vet Anaesth Analg
Ann Card Anaesth
Reg Anesth Pain Med
Semin Cardiothorac Vasc Anesth
J Perianesth Nurs
Bull Anesth Hist
Anaesthesiol Intensivmed Notfallmed Schmerzther
Int J Obstet Anesth
J Cardiothorac Vasc Anesth
Paediatr Anaesth
J Neurosurg Anesthesiol
Curr Opin Anaesthesiol
J Clin Anesth
Can J Anaesth
Eur J Anaesthesiol Suppl
J Anesth
Eur J Anaesthesiol
Middle East J Anesthesiol
Ann Fr Anesth Reanim
Anesteziol Reanimatol
AANA J
Anaesth Intensive Care
Rev Esp Anestesiol Reanim
Anesth Prog
Int Anesthesiol Clin
Acta Anaesthesiol Scand Suppl
Acta Anaesthesiol Scand
Anesth Analg
Minerva Anestesiol
Anaesthesist
Masui
Rev Bras Anestesiol
Acta Anaesthesiol Belg
Anaesthesia
Anesthesiology
Br J Anaesth

ANTHROPOLOGY (12)
J Physiol Anthropol
J Anthropol Sci
Anthropol Med
Evol Anthropol
Med Anthropol Q
Coll Antropol
Med Anthropol
Paleopathol Newsl
J Hum Evol
Curr Anthropol
Anthropol Anz
Am J Phys Anthropol
ANTI-BACTERIAL AGENTS (10)
Expert Rev Anti Infect Ther
Drug Resist Updat

Microb Drug Resist
Int J Antimicrob Agents
Antibiot Khimioter
J Antimicrob Chemother
Antimicrob Agents Chemother
Jpn J Antibiot
Hindustan Antibiot Bull
J Antibiot (Tokyo)
ANTINEOPLASTIC AGENTS (10)
Anticancer Agents Med Chem
Curr Cancer Drug Targets
Mol Cancer Ther
Drug Resist Updat
Anticancer Drugs
J Chemother
Invest New Drugs
Cancer Chemother Pharmacol
Cancer Treat Rev
Gan To Kagaku Ryoho
AUDIOLOGY (19)
J Soc Bras Fonoaudiol
Int J Audiol
Cochlear Implants Int
Noise Health
J Speech Lang Hear Res
Audiol Neurootol
J Deaf Stud Deaf Educ
Trends Amplif
Int Tinnitus J
Am J Audiol
Kulak Burun Bogaz Ihtis Derg
J Am Acad Audiol
Ear Hear
Hear Res
S Afr J Commun Disord
Lang Speech Hear Serv Sch
J Commun Disord
J Acoust Soc Am
Am Ann Deaf

B

BACTERIOLOGY (6)
Innate Immun
Surg Infect (Larchmt)
Helicobacter
Bacteriol Virusol Parazitol Epidemiol
Nihon Saikingaku Zasshi
J Bacteriol
BEHAVIORAL SCIENCES (82) Includes Child Behavior, Sex Behavior, And Suicide - See Also Psychiatry; Psychology
Cyberpsychol Behav Soc Netw
Appl Psychol Health Well Being
Curr Top Behav Neurosci
Brain Imaging Behav
Integr Psychol Behav Sci
Sex Dev
Behav Res Methods
Behav Brain Funct
Int J Behav Nutr Phys Act
Behav Sleep Med
Evol Psychol
Learn Behav
Cogn Behav Ther
Genes Brain Behav
J Nutr Educ Behav
Cogn Affect Behav Neurosci
J Comp Physiol A Neuroethol Sens Neural Behav Physiol
Adv Life Course Res
Eat Behav
Epilepsy Behav
Attach Hum Dev
Cult Health Sex
J Behav Health Serv Res
AIDS Behav
Appl Psychophysiol Biofeedback
Health Educ Behav
J Lesbian Stud
Am J Health Behav
Arch Suicide Res
Neurobiol Learn Mem
Neurocase
Int J Behav Med
Behav Cogn Psychother
Anxiety Stress Coping
J Child Sex Abus
Crim Behav Ment Health
Behav Pharmacol
Behav Med
Behav Neurol
Violence Vict
Ann Behav Med
Behav Neurosci
Behav Sci Law
Int J Eat Disord
Appetite
Behav Brain Res
Crisis
J Dev Behav Pediatr
Behav Brain Sci
Infant Behav Dev
J Behav Med
Neurosci Biobehav Rev
Behav Modif
Law Hum Behav
Behav Processes
Suicide Life Threat Behav
Addict Behav
J Exp Psychol Anim Behav Process
Aggress Behav
J Homosex

A Perspective On The National Library of Medicine

J Sex Marital Ther
Pharmacol Biochem Behav
Int J Offender Ther Comp Criminol
J Youth Adolesc
Arch Sex Behav
Behav Genet
Behav Ther
J Behav Ther Exp Psychiatry
Horm Behav
Brain Behav Evol
J Appl Behav Anal
J Health Soc Behav
Physiol Behav
J Sex Res
J Hist Behav Sci
Cortex
Adv Child Dev Behav
Behav Res Ther
J Exp Anal Behav
J Genet Psychol
Nebr Symp Motiv
Psychometrika
BIOCHEMISTRY (194) - Includes Biochemical
Techniques, Enzymes, Lipids, Nucleic Acids, And Proteins -
See Also Molecular Biology
Adv Biol Regul
Nucleic Acid Ther
Annu Rev Chem Biomol Eng
Artif DNA PNA XNA
Food Funct
Protein Cell
Small GTPases
Curr Protoc Chem Biol
Metallomics
Adv Protein Chem Struct Biol
BMB Rep
J Proteomics
Mitochondrial DNA
Biomark Med
Channels (Austin)
J Clin Lipidol
Prion
Proteomics Clin Appl
ACS Chem Biol
Chem Biol Drug Des
Comp Biochem Physiol Part D Genomics Proteomics
Met Ions Life Sci
Cancer Biomark
FEBS J
Mol Biosyst
Acta Biochim Biophys Sin (Shanghai)
Cancer Genomics Proteomics
Chem Biodivers
Expert Rev Proteomics
Nucleic Acids Symp Ser (Oxf)
Protein Eng Des Sel
Protein J
Purinergic Signal
Biomed Khim
Cell Commun Signal
Chem Immunol Allergy
Genomics Proteomics Bioinformatics
Nucl Recept Signal
Org Biomol Chem
DNA Repair (Amst)
J Enzyme Inhib Med Chem
J Proteome Res
Lipids Health Dis
Mol Cell Proteomics
BMC Struct Biol
Curr Protoc Protein Sci
Dokl Biochem Biophys
J Oleo Sci
Macromol Biosci
Proteomics
Biochem Mol Biol Educ
Bioelectrochemistry
Biomacromolecules
BMC Biochem
Chembiochem
Curr Protein Pept Sci
Curr Protoc Nucleic Acid Chem
Int J Mol Sci
Nucleosides Nucleotides Nucleic Acids
IUBMB Life
Luminescence
Org Lett
Physiol Biochem Zool
J Biochem Mol Toxicol
J Physiol Biochem
Mol Genet Metab
Curr Opin Chem Biol
Nitric Oxide
Biol Chem
Biomarkers
Cell Biochem Biophys
Cytokine Growth Factor Rev
Exp Mol Med
J Biol Inorg Chem
Prep Biochem Biotechnol
Arch Physiol Biochem
Int J Biochem Cell Biol
J Pept Sci
J Recept Signal Transduct Res
Amyloid
Chem Biol
Comp Biochem Physiol B Biochem Mol Biol
Free Radic Res
Macromol Rapid Commun
Matrix Biol

Mol Membr Biol
Protein Pept Lett
Redox Rep
Biochem Med (Zagreb)
Biol Pharm Bull
Bioorg Med Chem
Structure
Biometals
Biosci Biotechnol Biochem
Insect Biochem Mol Biol
Mediators Inflamm
Protein Sci
Amino Acids
Bioorg Med Chem Lett

Cancer Epidemiol Biomarkers Prev
Cell Physiol Biochem
Curr Opin Struct Biol
Curr Top Membr
Bioconjug Chem
Biodegradation
Curr Opin Lipidol
Glycobiology
J Nutr Biochem
J Steroid Biochem Mol Biol
Methods
Crit Rev Biochem Mol Biol
Biofactors
J Liposome Res

Free Radic Biol Med
J Biol Regul Homeost Agents
Plant Physiol Biochem
Biochem Cell Biol
Biotechnol Appl Biochem
Fish Physiol Biochem
Int J Biol Markers
Proteins
Z Naturforsch C
Glycoconj J
J Comp Physiol B
Adv Biochem Eng Biotechnol
Arch Insect Biochem Physiol
Cell Biochem Funct
Dis Markers
J Biomol Struct Dyn
J Pharm Biomed Anal
Physiol Chem Phys Med NMR
J Cell Biochem
Appl Biochem Biotechnol
Carbohydr Polym
Chem Senses
Mol Biochem Parasitol
Neuropeptides
Peptides
Regul Pept
Enzyme Microb Technol
Int J Biol Macromol
J Biosci
J Inorg Biochem
Prog Lipid Res
Ukr Biokhim Zh
J Bioenerg Biomembr
Trends Biochem Sci
Bioorg Khim
Nucleic Acids Res
Rev Physiol Biochem Pharmacol
Biochem Soc Trans
Biophys Chem
Life Sci
Mol Cell Biochem
Pharmacol Biochem Behav
Biochimie
Bioorg Chem
Indian J Biochem Biophys
Subcell Biochem
Adv Carbohydr Chem Biochem
Ann Clin Biochem
Chem Biol Interact
Prog Mol Subcell Biol
FEBS Lett
Adv Enzymol Relat Areas Mol Biol
Clin Biochem
Chem Phys Lipids
Lipids
Carbohydr Res
Essays Biochem
Prikl Biokhim Mikrobiol
Zh Evol Biokhim Fiziol
Biopolymers
Steroids
Biochemistry
Photochem Photobiol
Anal Biochem
Biochem Biophys Res Commun
J Lipid Res
Biochem Pharmacol
Perspect Biol Med
Biochemistry (Mosc)
Methods Enzymol
Postepy Biochem
Acta Biochim Pol
Methods Biochem Anal
Arch Biochem Biophys
Biochem Soc Symp
Seikagaku
Biochim Biophys Acta
Annu Rev Biochem
J Biochem
Biochem J
J Biol Chem
BIOLOGY (156) - Includes Evolution And Marine Biology -
See Also Botany; Microbiology; Zoology
Wiley Interdiscip Rev Dev Biol
Theor Biol Forum
Biol Aujourdhui
Nat Commun
Sci China Life Sci
Ann Rev Mar Sci
Cold Spring Harb Perspect Biol
Front Biosci (Elite Ed)
Front Biosci (Landmark Ed)
Front Biosci (Schol Ed)
Genome Biol Evol
Integr Biol (Camb)
Adv Protein Chem Struct Biol
Biodemography Soc Biol
BMC Res Notes
Mar Genomics
Biosci Trends
Dev Neurobiol
J Biol Dyn
ACS Chem Biol
Bioinspir Biomim
Biol Direct
J Vis Exp
Biol Lett
J Zhejiang Univ Sci B
Nat Chem Biol
SEB Exp Biol Ser

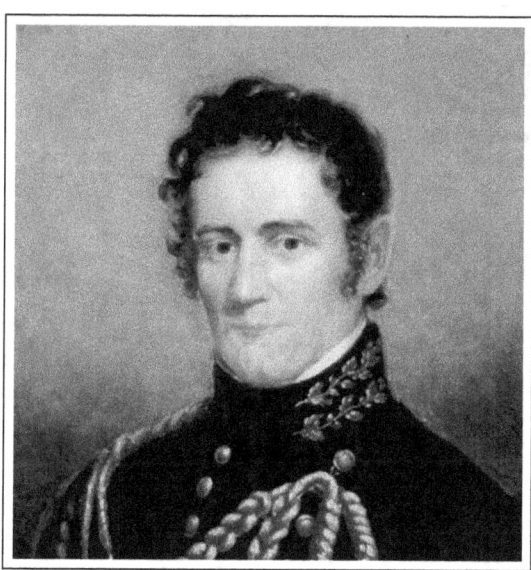

Joseph Lovell, M.D. - Surgeon General, U.S. Army from 1818 to 1836. Aristotle pondered on the phenomenon that, from a small acorn, a giant oak tree evolved. He called this "teleology". The gigantic National Library of Medicine of today grew from a small collection of medical books, mostly from the personal collection of General Lovell. His library comprised a few dozen books, journals, and pamphlets. In 1836 both Lovell and his wife died, leaving orphaned 11 children. His successors maintained and expanded the collection.

Chapter 7 - The National Library of Medicine

A Perspective On The National Library of Medicine

Int J Biol Sci
J R Soc Interface
Math Biosci Eng
Organogenesis
Phys Biol
Theor Biol Med Model
BMC Biol
Commun Agric Appl Biol Sci
Econ Hum Biol
Evol Psychol
Geobiology
Mar Drugs
Math Med Biol
Nat Prod Res
PLoS Biol
C R Biol
Electromagn Biol Med
Integr Comp Biol
Photochem Photobiol Sci
Astrobiology
BMC Evol Biol
Exp Biol Med (Maywood)
Expert Opin Biol Ther
Infect Genet Evol
Braz J Biol
High Alt Med Biol
Biol Res Nurs
Evol Dev
Mar Biotechnol (NY)
Alkaloids Chem Biol
Pak J Biol Sci
Protist
Extremophiles
Iran Biomed J
Nonlinear Dynamics Psychol Life Sci
Theory Biosci
Dev Genes Evol
Molecules
Annu Rev Cell Dev Biol
Glob Chang Biol
Neurobiol Learn Mem
Artif Life
Chem Biol
Br J Biomed Sci
Evol Comput
Nucl Med Biol
Biol Res
Izv Akad Nauk Ser Biol
Mol Phylogenet Evol
Syst Biol
Adv Space Biol Med
Curr Biol
Curr Opin Neurobiol
Proc Biol Sci
Am J Hum Biol
Genet Sel Evol
Int J Dev Biol
Biofouling
Growth Factors
Development
Eur J Protistol
FASEB J
J Biol Regul Homeost Agents
J Evol Biol
J Photochem Photobiol B
Phys Med
Dev Biol (N Y 1985)
Dis Aquat Organ
Bioessays
Orig Life Evol Biosph
Acta Biol Hung
Biomed Pharmacother
Aquat Toxicol
Braz J Med Biol Res
Prilozi
Cryo Letters
Hist Philos Life Sci
J Biosci
Mar Environ Res
Proc Jpn Acad Ser B Phys Biol Sci
Neuropathol Appl Neurobiol
Ann Hum Biol
Biosystems
J Math Biol
Bull Math Biol
Life Sci
Prog Neurobiol
Chemosphere
J Hum Evol
Acta Neurobiol Exp (Wars)
Comput Biol Med
Mar Pollut Bull
Biologist (London)
Dev Growth Differ
Pathol Biol (Paris)
Brain Behav Evol
J Hist Biol
Adv Exp Med Biol
Zh Evol Biokhim Fiziol
Cryobiology
Dokl Biol Sci
Adv Mar Biol
Indian J Exp Biol
Photochem Photobiol
J Theor Biol
Dev Biol
Int Rev Neurobiol
Perspect Biol Med
Bull Exp Biol Med
Phys Med Biol

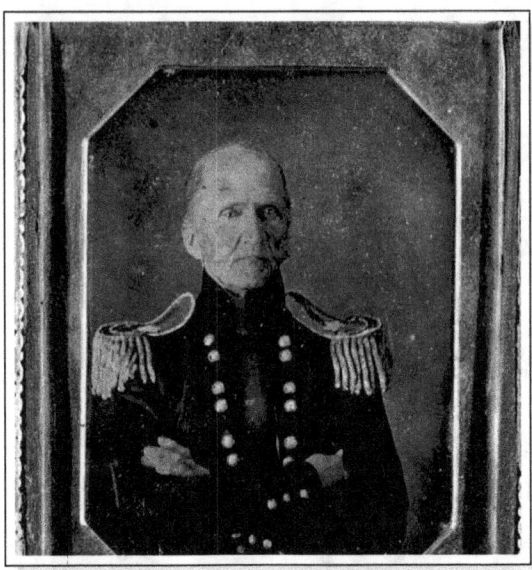

Thomas Lawson, M.D. - Surgeon General, U.S. Army from 1836 to 1861. In his notes, he recorded a budget of $150 for "medical books for office". In 1840, a brief listing of the library's contents included: 134 titles of which 8 were journals. The entire collection was in 1 four-shelf book case, measuring 6 ft. x 7 ft. The budget for the Library for 2013 is $372 million.

Folia Biol (Praha)
Folia Biol (Krakow)
Rev Biol Trop
Homo
Evolution
Ann Biol Clin (Paris)
Zh Obshch Biol
Acta Biotheor
Biol Rev Camb Philos Soc
Philos Trans R Soc Lond B Biol Sci
Cold Spring Harb Symp Quant Biol
J Exp Biol
Hum Biol
Yale J Biol Med
Protoplasma
Q Rev Biol
Biol Bull
Arch Ital Biol
Am Nat
BIOMEDICAL ENGINEERING (76) Includes Biocompatible Materials, Biomechanics, And Prostheses - See Also Technology
IEEE J Biomed Health Inform
IEEE Trans Cybern
Adv Healthc Mater
Bioengineered
J Appl Biomater Funct Mater
Biomatter

IEEE Pulse
Int j numer method biomed eng
J Healthc Eng
ACS Appl Mater Interfaces
IEEE Rev Biomed Eng
IEEE Trans Haptics
J Mech Behav Biomed Mater
Mater Sci Eng C Mater Biol Appl
N Biotechnol
IEEE Trans Biomed Circuits Syst
Bioinspir Biomim
Biointerphases
Biomed Mater
Acta Biomater
Mol Cell Biomech
Small
Conf Proc IEEE Eng Med Biol Soc
J Neural Eng
J Neuroeng Rehabil
J R Soc Interface
Math Biosci Eng
J Biomed Mater Res A
J Biomed Mater Res B Appl Biomater
Biomech Model Mechanobiol
Biomed Eng Online
J Chromatogr B Analyt Technol Biomed Life Sci
Bioprocess Biosyst Eng
Cardiovasc Eng

IEEE Trans Neural Syst Rehabil Eng
Acta Bioeng Biomech
Annu Rev Biomed Eng
J Biosci Bioeng
Metab Eng
Biomed Microdevices
J Artif Organs
Comput Methods Biomech Biomed Engin
J Biomed Opt
Philos Trans A Math Phys Eng Sci
Med Eng Phys
J Appl Biomech
Physiol Meas
Technol Health Care
Biomed Mater Eng
Bioresour Technol
J Mater Sci Mater Med
Biomed Instrum Technol
Int J Neural Syst
J Biomater Sci Polym Ed
Proc Inst Mech Eng H
J Comput Aided Mol Des
Clin Biomech (Bristol, Avon)
J Biomater Appl
Biotechnol Genet Eng Rev
J Rehabil Res Dev
Sheng Wu Yi Xue Gong Cheng Xue Za Zhi
Crit Rev Biomed Eng
Australas Phys Eng Sci Med
Biomaterials
J Biomech Eng
J Med Eng Technol
Med Biol Eng Comput
Prosthet Orthot Int
Ann Biomed Eng
Biomed Tech (Berl)
Polim Med
IEEE Trans Biomed Eng
Biomed Sci Instrum
Biotechnol Bioeng
ISA Trans
Rev Sci Instrum
BIOPHYSICS (47) Includes Acoustics And Rheology
Annu Rev Biophys
J Biophotonics
Radiol Phys Technol
Acta Biochim Biophys Sin (Shanghai)
J R Soc Interface
Phys Life Rev
Dokl Biochem Biophys
Phys Rev E Stat Nonlin Soft Matter Phys
Chemphyschem
Eur Phys J E Soft Matter
Igaku Butsuri
J Appl Clin Med Phys
Luminescence
Phys Chem Chem Phys
Opt Express
Cell Biochem Biophys
Philos Trans A Math Phys Eng Sci
Med Eng Phys
Physiol Meas
J Fluoresc
Adv Mater
J Phys Condens Matter
Phys Med
J Microw Power Electromagn Energy
Eur Biophys J
Physiol Chem Phys Med NMR
Gen Physiol Biophys
Australas Phys Eng Sci Med
Bioelectromagnetics
Med Phys
Radiat Environ Biophys
Biophys Chem
J Biol Phys
Indian J Biochem Biophys
Q Rev Biophys
Prog Biophys Mol Biol
Biorheology
Int J Biometeorol
Biophys J
Biochem Biophys Res Commun
Biofizika
Phys Med Biol
Arch Biochem Biophys
Biochim Biophys Acta
Rep Prog Phys
J Chem Phys
Rev Sci Instrum
BIOTECHNOLOGY (69) See Also Nanotechnology; Technology
Artif Cells Nanomed Biotechnol
ACS Synth Biol
Bioengineered
Biomed Res Int
GM Crops Food
Biomatter
ACS Appl Mater Interfaces
Biofabrication
Microb Biotechnol
Tissue Eng Part A
Tissue Eng Part B Rev
Tissue Eng Part C Methods
Wiley Interdiscip Rev Nanomed Nanobiotechnol
IEEE Trans Biomed Circuits Syst
IET Nanobiotechnol
J Tissue Eng Regen Med
Recent Pat Biotechnol
Biointerphases

Chapter 7 - The National Library of Medicine

A Perspective On The National Library of Medicine

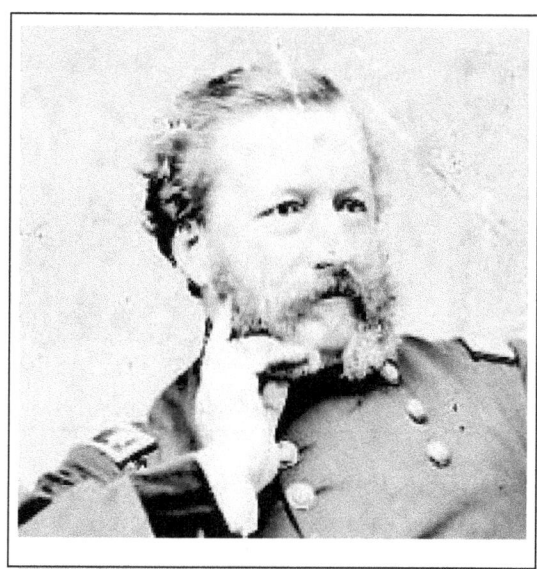

Joseph K. Barnes, M.D. - Surgeon General, U.S. Army (1864-1882). The Surgeon General's collection of books starts to become a true library when Gen. Barnes appoints a young assistant surgeon by the name of John Shaw Billings to organize and catalog the collection Although Billings is credited with creating the library, it was Barnes who supported the project and sustained the effort.

C

A Perspective On The National Library of Medicine

Zhonghua Xin Xue Guan Bing Za Zhi
Heart Lung
Turk Kardiyol Dern Ars
Adv Cardiol
Cardiology
J Mol Cell Cardiol
Ann Cardiol Angeiol (Paris)
J Electrocardiol
Cardiovasc Res
Kardiologia
J Cardiovasc Surg (Torino)
J Thorac Cardiovasc Surg
Am J Cardiol
Prog Cardiovasc Dis
Kardiol Pol
Circ Res
Minerva Cardioangiol
Circulation
Indian Heart J
Arq Bras Cardiol
Rev Esp Cardiol (Engl Ed)
Acta Cardiol
Am Heart J
CELL BIOLOGY (136)
Monoclon Antib Immunodiagn Immunother
Cell Rep
Cell Oncol (Dordr)
Front Cell Infect Microbiol
Open Biol
Stem Cells Transl Med
Anal Cell Pathol (Amst)
Bioarchitecture
Cell Death Dis
Cell Reprogram
Cytoskeleton (Hoboken)
Nucleus
Protein Cell
Small GTPases
Stem Cell Res Ther
Int Rev Cell Mol Biol
Oxid Med Cell Longev
Pigment Cell Melanoma Res
Sci Signal
Cell Adh Migr
Cell Stem Cell
Curr Protoc Stem Cell Biol
Stem Cell Res
CBE Life Sci Educ
Curr Stem Cell Res Ther
J Stem Cells
Autophagy
Cell Metab
Med Mol Morphol
Mol Cell Biomech
Stem Cell Rev
Stem Cells Dev
Cell Commun Signal
Cytometry A
Cytometry B Clin Cytom
Aging Cell
Cell Cycle
Mol Cancer Res
Mol Cell Proteomics
Neurosignals
Cell Commun Adhes
Curr Protoc Cell Biol
Dev Cell
Eur Cell Mater
Mitochondrion
BMC Cell Biol
Cell Tissue Bank
J Cell Mol Med
Cells Tissues Organs
Cell Microbiol
Cytotherapy
Nat Cell Biol
Curr Protoc Cytom
Cell Mol Life Sci
Mol Cell
Apoptosis
Cell Biochem Biophys
Cell Stress Chaperones
Cell Mol Biol Lett
Genes Cells
Semin Cell Dev Biol
Annu Rev Cell Dev Biol
Histochem Cell Biol
Int J Biochem Cell Biol
J Recept Signal Transduct Res
Biocell
Cell Death Differ
Virchows Arch
Cell Biol Int
In Vitro Cell Dev Biol Anim
Stem Cells
Cell Transplant
Cell Mol Biol (Noisy-le-grand)
Mol Biol Cell
Cell Prolif
Cell Physiol Biochem
Curr Top Membr
Plant J
Trends Cell Biol
Cell Res
Cytopathology
DNA Cell Biol
J Struct Biol
Mech Dev
Mol Cell Neurosci
Mol Cells

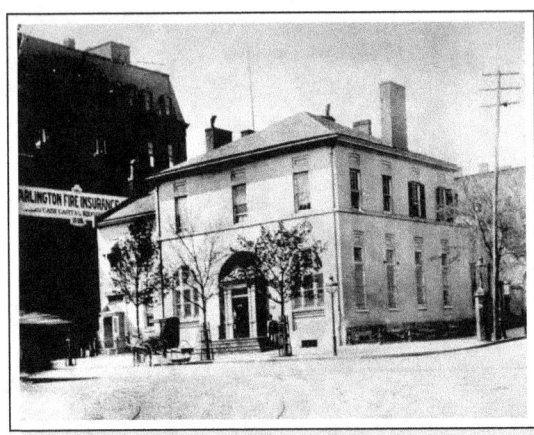

The Riggs Bank. For 26 years (1862 to 1888), the Library of the Surgeon General's Office was housed in the parlor of the small building on the left side of the Riggs Bank building. An inventory of 1887 showed that the library had 5 chairs, 10 desks, 9 tables, 9 stools, 8 spittoons, 7 book and file cases, 5 ladders, 2 library tables, 2 manuscript cases, 1 negative case, 1 map chest, an umbrella stand, wash bowl and pitcher, and a clock.

CBE Life Sci Educ
Curr Stem Cell Res Ther
J Stem Cells
Autophagy
Cell Metab
Med Mol Morphol
Mol Cell Biomech
Stem Cell Rev
Stem Cells Dev
Cell Commun Signal
Cytometry A
Cytometry B Clin Cytom
Aging Cell
Cell Cycle
Mol Cancer Res
Mol Cell Proteomics
Neurosignals
Cell Commun Adhes
Curr Protoc Cell Biol
Dev Cell
Eur Cell Mater
Mitochondrion
BMC Cell Biol
Cell Tissue Bank
J Cell Mol Med
Cells Tissues Organs
Cell Microbiol
Cytotherapy
Nat Cell Biol
Curr Protoc Cytom
Cell Mol Life Sci
Mol Cell
Apoptosis
Cell Biochem Biophys
Cell Stress Chaperones
Cell Mol Biol Lett
Genes Cells
Semin Cell Dev Biol
Annu Rev Cell Dev Biol
Histochem Cell Biol
Int J Biochem Cell Biol
J Recept Signal Transduct Res
Biocell
Cell Death Differ
Virchows Arch
Cell Biol Int
In Vitro Cell Dev Biol Anim
Stem Cells
Cell Transplant
Cell Mol Biol (Noisy-le-grand)
Mol Biol Cell
Cell Prolif
Cell Physiol Biochem
Curr Top Membr
Plant J
Trends Cell Biol
Cell Res
Cytopathology
DNA Cell Biol
J Struct Biol
Mech Dev
Mol Cell Neurosci
Mol Cells
Am J Physiol Lung Cell Mol Physiol
Am J Respir Cell Mol Biol
Cell Signal
Curr Opin Cell Biol
Plant Cell
Arch Histol Cytol
Hum Cell
J Submicrosc Cytol Pathol
Immunol Cell Biol
Mol Cell Probes
Biochem Cell Biol
Anal Quant Cytol Histol
Diagn Cytopathol
Bioessays
Cell Biol Toxicol
Folia Histochem Cytobiol
Cell Biochem Funct
Eur J Cell Biol Suppl
J Cell Biochem
Biol Cell
Biosci Rep
Cell Mol Neurobiol
Mol Cell Biol
Cell Calcium
J Muscle Res Cell Motil
Eur J Cell Biol
Plant Cell Environ
Scanning
Am J Physiol Cell Physiol
Cell Struct Funct
Cell Tissue Res
Cell
Mol Cell Endocrinol
Adv Anat Embryol Cell Biol
Differentiation
Methods Cell Biol
Mol Cell Biochem
Subcell Biochem
Cell Immunol
J Mol Cell Cardiol
Monogr Clin Cytol
Tissue Cell
Results Probl Cell Differ
J Cell Sci
J Cell Physiol
J Cell Biol
Plant Cell Physiol

Am J Physiol Lung Cell Mol Physiol
Am J Respir Cell Mol Biol
Cell Signal
Curr Opin Cell Biol
Plant Cell
Arch Histol Cytol
Hum Cell
J Submicrosc Cytol Pathol
Immunol Cell Biol
Mol Cell Probes
Biochem Cell Biol
Anal Quant Cytol Histol
Diagn Cytopathol
Bioessays
Cell Biol Toxicol
Folia Histochem Cytobiol
Cell Biochem Funct
Eur J Cell Biol Suppl
J Cell Biochem
Biol Cell
Biosci Rep
Cell Mol Neurobiol
Mol Cell Biol
Cell Calcium
J Muscle Res Cell Motil
Eur J Cell Biol
Plant Cell Environ
Scanning
Am J Physiol Cell Physiol
Cell Struct Funct
Cell Tissue Res
Cell
Mol Cell Endocrinol
Adv Anat Embryol Cell Biol
Differentiation
Methods Cell Biol
Mol Cell Biochem

Subcell Biochem
Cell Immunol
J Mol Cell Cardiol
Monogr Clin Cytol
Tissue Cell
Results Probl Cell Differ
J Cell Sci
J Cell Physiol
J Cell Biol
Plant Cell Physiol
Tsitologiia
Acta Cytol
Exp Cell Res
CHEMISTRY (136) See Also Biochemistry; Histocytochemistry; Pharmacy Monoclon Antib Immunodiagn Immunother
Cell Rep
Cell Oncol (Dordr)
Front Cell Infect Microbiol
Open Biol
Stem Cells Transl Med
Anal Cell Pathol (Amst)
Bioarchitecture
Cell Death Dis
Cell Reprogram
Cytoskeleton (Hoboken)
Nucleus
Protein Cell
Small GTPases
Stem Cell Res Ther
Int Rev Cell Mol Biol
Oxid Med Cell Longev
Pigment Cell Melanoma Res
Sci Signal
Cell Adh Migr
Cell Stem Cell
Curr Protoc Stem Cell Biol
Stem Cell Res

81

Chapter 7 - The National Library of Medicine

A Perspective On The National Library of Medicine

Tsitologiia
Acta Cytol
Exp Cell Res
CHEMISTRY TECHNIQUES, ANALYTICAL (38)
Acta Crystallogr B Struct Sci Cryst Eng Mater
Bioanalysis
Curr Protoc Chem Biol
Drug Test Anal
Annu Rev Anal Chem (Palo Alto Calif)
Expert Opin Drug Discov
Acta Crystallogr Sect F Struct Biol Cryst Commun
Profiles Drug Subst Excip Relat Methodol
Anal Bioanal Chem
Assay Drug Dev Technol
J Chromatogr B Analyt Technol Biomed Life Sci
J Sep Sci
Curr Protoc Nucleic Acid Chem
Eur J Mass Spectrom (Chichester, Eng)
J Capill Electrophor Microchip Technol
Microsc Microanal
J Mass Spectrom
Acta Crystallogr D Biol Crystallogr
J Chromatogr A
J AOAC Int
J Fluoresc
J Am Soc Mass Spectrom
Rapid Commun Mass Spectrom
Biomed Chromatogr
Anal Sci
Se Pu
Acta Crystallogr A
Acta Crystallogr C
Mass Spectrom Rev
Guang Pu Xue Yu Guang Pu Fen Xi
Electrophoresis
J Chromatogr Sci
Adv Chromatogr
Talanta
Appl Spectrosc
Anal Chim Acta
Anal Chem
Analyst
CHEMISTRY, CLINICAL (4)
Clin Chem Lab Med
Adv Clin Chem
Clin Chim Acta
Clin Chem
CHIROPRACTIC (1)
J Manipulative Physiol Ther
CLINICAL LABORATORY TECHNIQUES (27) See Also
Histocytochemistry Monoclon Antib Immunodiagn
Immunother
Ann Lab Med
J Lab Autom
Cold Spring Harb Protoc
Expert Opin Med Diagn
Clin Vaccine Immunol
Mol Diagn Ther
Nat Protoc
Transl Res
Nat Methods
Clin Chem Lab Med
J Clin Densitom
Clin Lab
Lab Hematol
Br J Biomed Sci
Klin Lab Diagn
Clin Lab Sci
J Clin Lab Anal
Clin Lab Med
Crit Rev Clin Lab Sci
Ann Clin Lab Sci
J Immunol Methods
MLO Med Lab Obs
Lab Invest
Appl Spectrosc
Scand J Clin Lab Invest Suppl
Scand J Clin Lab Invest
COMMUNICABLE DISEASES (53) - see also Acquired
Immunodeficiency Syndrome; Allergy And Immunology;
Epidemiology; Sexually Transmitted Diseases; Tropical
Medicine
Pathog Dis
Pathog Glob Health
Front Cell Infect Microbiol
Ticks Tick Borne Dis
Can Commun Dis Rep Wkly
Emerg Health Threats J
J Infect Public Health
J Infect Dev Ctries
Infect Disord Drug Targets
Expert Rev Anti Infect Ther
Travel Med Infect Dis
BMC Infect Dis
Commun Dis Intell Q Rep
Infect Genet Evol
Lancet Infect Dis
Vector Borne Zoonotic Dis
Jpn J Infect Dis
Braz J Infect Dis
Int J Infect Dis
Clin Microbiol Infect
Emerg Infect Dis
Euro Surveill
Klin Mikrobiol Infekc Lek
J Travel Med
Infect Dis Obstet Gynecol
Can Commun Dis Rep
Clin Infect Dis
Curr Opin Infect Dis

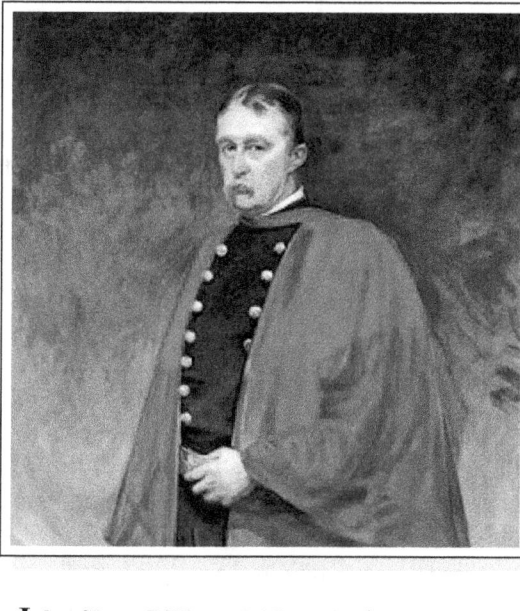

Eur J Clin Microbiol Infect Dis
Infect Control Hosp Epidemiol
Epidemiol Infect
Infect Dis Clin North Am
Pediatr Infect Dis J
Microb Pathog
Enferm Infecc Microbiol Clin
Rev Chilena Infectol
Diagn Microbiol Infect Dis
Rev Sci Tech
Zhonghua Liu Xing Bing Xue Za Zhi
Am J Infect Control
J Hosp Infect
J Infect
Comp Immunol Microbiol Infect Dis
Infection
Med Mal Infect
Infect Immun
Kansenshogaku Zasshi
Scand J Infect Dis Suppl
J Commun Dis
Scand J Infect Dis
Zhonghua Yu Fang Yi Xue Za Zhi
Indian J Tuberc
J Infect Dis
COMPLEMENTARY THERAPIES (35) Includes
Acupuncture; Medicine, Traditional; Phytotherapy, And
Spiritual Therapy
J Integr Med
J Acupunct Meridian Stud
Forsch Komplementmed
J Nat Med
Complement Ther Clin Pract
Explore (NY)
Afr J Tradit Complement Altern Med
J Complement Integr MedChin J Integr Med
Chin J Nat Med
Homeopathy
BMC Complement Altern Med
Int J Med Mushrooms
Int J Yoga Therap
Adv Mind Body Med
Altern Med Rev
Altern Ther Health Med
J Altern Complement Med
Phytomedicine
Complement Ther Med
Zhongguo Zhong Xi Yi Jie He Za Zhi
Chin Med Sci J
Zhongguo Zhong Yao Za Zhi
Phytother Res
Acupunct Med
J Tradit Chin Med
Zhongguo Zhen Jiu
Zhen Ci Yan Jiu
Am J Chin Med
Zhong Yao Cai
Acupunct Electrother Res
Chin Med J (Engl)
J Music Ther
Zhonghua Yi Xue Za Zhi
Fitoterapia
COMPUTATIONAL BIOLOGY (30) includes Bioinfor-
matics and Systems Biology
Database (Oxford)
Interdiscip Sci
Wiley Interdiscip Rev Syst Biol Med
Int J Comput Biol Drug Des
Syst Biol Reprod Med
BMC Syst Biol
IET Syst Biol
Comput Intell Neurosci
Comput Syst Bioinformatics Conf
Int J Data Min Bioinform
Int J Bioinform Res Appl
Mol Syst Biol
PLoS Comput Biol
IEEE/ACM Trans Comput Biol Bioinform
J Integr Bioinform
Comput Biol Chem
Genomics Proteomics Bioinformatics
J Bioinform Comput Biol
Curr Protoc Bioinformatics
OMICS
Genome Inform
BMC Bioinformatics
Brief Bioinform
Bioinformatics
In Silico Biol
Pac Symp Biocomput
J Comput Biol
J Comput Neurosci
J Comput Chem
Biosystems
CRITICAL CARE (32)
Zhonghua Wei Zhong Bing Ji Jiu Yi Xue
AACN Adv Crit Care
Neurocrit Care
Anaesthesiol Intensive Ther
J Vet Emerg Crit Care (San Antonio)
Pediatr Crit Care Med
Crit Care Resusc
Crit Care
Nurs Crit Care
Curr Opin Crit Care
Am J Respir Crit Care Med
Semin Respir Crit Care Med
Am J Crit Care
Aust Crit Care
Intensive Crit Care Nurs

John Shaw Billings, M.D. - Assistant Surgeon and eventual Director of the library (1864-1895). Billings is the person, who is most credited with establishing The Library. Billings studied medicine at the Medical College of Ohio and in 1861 entered the Army where he spent four years of service as a surgeon, becoming Lieutenant Colonel and Medical Inspector of the Army of the Potomac. In the battles of Chancellorsville and Gettysburg, he performed many operations in the field. After the war, Barnes appointed him to catalog the Surgeon General's Library, launching his thirty years of leadership, during which the collection grew from 602 titles into the largest collection of medical literature in the world. In 1879 he published the first volume of the index to current literature, Index Medicus, the precursor to MEDLINE, and, in 1880, the first volume of the Index-Catalog of the full collection. Among Billings' other accomplishments were the planning of the Johns Hopkins Hospital in Baltimore and the New York Public Library.

Chapter 7 - The National Library of Medicine

A Perspective On The National Library of Medicine

Anasthesiol Intensivmed Notfallmed Schmerzther
Crit Care Nurs Clin North Am
Rev Bras Ter Intensiva
Enferm Intensiva
Crit Care Nurs Q
J Crit Care
J Intensive Care Med
Crit Care Clin
Ann Fr Anesth Reanim
Dimens Crit Care Nurs
Crit Care Nurse
Intensive Care Med
Crit Care Med
Anaesth Intensive Care
Heart Lung
Med Intensiva
J Safety Res

D

DENTISTRY (176) includes Pedodontics, Periodontics, Stomatology, Tooth Diseases, And Mouth Diseases - see also Orthodontics
Rev Stomatol Chir Maxillofac Chir Orale
Oral Surg Oral Med Oral Pathol Oral Radiol
Prim Dent J
Oral Health Dent Manag
Orthodontics (Chic.)
HDA Now
J Investig Clin Dent
Mol Oral Microbiol
Int J Oral Sci
J Prosthodont Res
Eur J Oral Implantol
Jpn Dent Sci Rev
Oral Maxillofac Surg
Eur Arch Paediatr Dent
Eur J Esthet Dent
Head Face Med
Annals N Y Acad Dent
Braz Oral Res
J Oral Biosci
Med Oral Patol Oral Cir Bucal
Int J Dent Hyg
J Appl Oral Sci
J Dent Child (Chic)
Oral Health Prev Dent
Int J Orthod Milwaukee
Orthod Craniofac Res
BMC Oral Health
Dent Traumatol
J Esthet Restor Dent
J Evid Based Dent Pract
Odontology
Eur J Paediatr Dent
J Orthod
Prog Orthod
Clin Implant Dent Relat Res
J Adhes Dent
J Contemp Dent Pract
J Int Acad Periodontol
Stomatologija
Aust Endod J
Chin J Dent Res
Evid Based Dent
Front Oral Biol
Int J Comput Dent
J Oral Sci
SADJ
Clin Oral Investig
Eur J Dent Educ
J Med Dent Sci
J Orofac Orthop
J Hist Dent
Compend Contin Educ Dent
Eur J Oral Sci
Oral Dis
Dent Assist
Atlas Oral Maxillofac Surg Clin North Am
J Orofac Pain
Periodontol 2000
Refuat Hapeh Vehashinayim
Eur J Prosthodont Restor Dent
Implant Dent
J Prosthodont
Shanghai Kou Qiang Yi Xue
Cleft Palate Craniofac J
Harv Dent Bull
Int J Paediatr Dent
Braz Dent J
Clin Oral Implants Res
Dent Implantol Update
J Clin Pediatr Dent
J Craniofac Surg
Indian J Dent Res
J Oral Pathol Med
Oral Maxillofac Surg Clin North Am
Todays FDA
Am J Dent
Int J Prosthodont
J Clin Dent
J Dent Hyg
J Calif Dent Assoc
J Vet Dent
Adv Dent Res
J Craniomaxillofac Surg
Schweiz Monatsschr Zahnmed
Zhonghua Kou Qiang Yi Xue Za Zhi

Am J Orthod Dentofacial Orthop
Int J Oral Maxillofac Surg
Int J Oral Maxillofac Implants
Cranio
Dent Hist
Dent Mater
Quintessence Int
Acta Odontol Latinoam
Br J Oral Maxillofac Surg
Community Dent Health
Facial Plast Surg
Hua Xi Kou Qiang Yi Xue Za Zhi
J Forensic Odontostomatol
J Indian Soc Pedod Prev Dent
Rev Belge Med Dent (1984)
Dent Mater J
Gerodontology
J Oral Maxillofac Surg
Int J Periodontics Restorative Dent
Spec Care Dentist
Dent Today
Int Endod J
Int J Orofacial Myology
Eur J Orthod
J Can Dent Assoc
Pediatr Dent
J Okla Dent Assoc
Odontostomatol Trop
Ann R Australas Coll Dent Surg
J Oral Implantol
J N Z Soc Periodontol
Oper Dent Suppl
Swed Dent J Suppl
Swed Dent J

Bull Group Int Rech Sci Stomatol Odontol
Gen Dent
J West Soc Periodontol Periodontal Abstr
Oper Dent
J Endod
Dent Update
J Clin Periodontol
J Oral Rehabil
J Indiana Dent Assoc
Singapore Dent J
CDS Rev
Community Dent Oral Epidemiol
LDA J
Dentomaxillofac Radiol
J Dent
Monogr Oral Sci
J Clin Orthod
J Periodontol
J N J Dent Assoc
J Tenn Dent Assoc
SAAD Dig
J Mich Dent Assoc
Aust Orthod J
Caries Res
Anesth Prog
J Periodontal Res
J Public Health Dent
J Ir Dent Assoc
Ned Tijdschr Tandheelkd
Bull Tokyo Dent Coll
Arch Oral Biol
Dent Clin North Am
Aust Dent J
J Mass Dent Soc

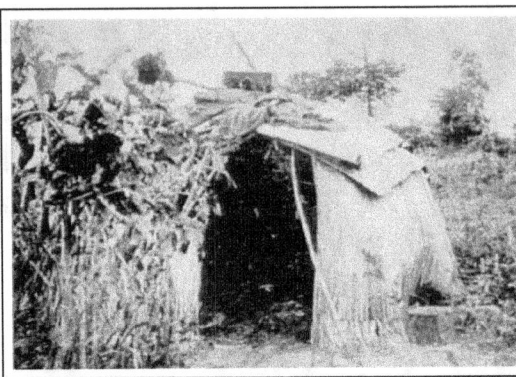

Bibliographic indexing in the wild. In the early days of the Library, Billings faced a chronic shortage of qualified personnel to index scientific journals. Undaunted, he used the Surgeon General's medical officers in the field. The following is correspondence from one of those officers, Wm. Steinmetz, M.D., who took with him 13 volumes of a German medical journal to index while he was stationed in Indian Territory and living in a tent similar to the one above. (See the next page for an excerpt from one of his letters.)

Minerva Stomatol
J Prosthet Dent
Int Dent J
Pa Dent J (Harrisb)
N Y State Dent J
Acta Odontol Scand
J Am Dent Assoc
Stomatologiia (Mosk)
J Dent Educ
J Am Coll Dent
Northwest Dent
Angle Orthod
Kokubyo Gakkai Zasshi
Orthod Fr
J Dent Res
Alpha Omegan
Fogorv Sz
N Z Dent J
Br Dent J
Penn Dent J (Phila)
Tex Dent J
DERMATOLOGY (55) see also Sexually Transmitted Diseases
JAMA Dermatol
Cutan Ocul Toxicol
Dermatitis
Skin Pharmacol Physiol
J Dtsch Dermatol Ges
J Cosmet Dermatol
J Drugs Dermatol
Skinmed
BMC Dermatol
J Cosmet Laser Ther
Am J Clin Dermatol
Dermatol Ther
J Cutan Med Surg
J Investig Dermatol Symp Proc
Semin Cutan Med Surg
Dermatol Surg
Dermatol Online J
Skin Res Technol
Skin Therapy Lett
Acta Dermatovenerol Croat
Wound Repair Regen
Acta Dermatovenerol Alp Panonica Adriat
Dermatology
Exp Dermatol
J Eur Acad Dermatol Venereol
Eur J Dermatol
J Dermatol Sci
Photodermatol Photoimmunol Photomed
J Dermatolog Treat
Vet Dermatol
Clin Dermatol
Dermatol Clin
Pediatr Dermatol
G Ital Dermatol Venereol
Am J Dermatopathol
Int J Cosmet Sci
J Am Acad Dermatol
Arch Dermatol Res
Ann Dermatol Venereol
Clin Exp Dermatol
Indian J Dermatol Venereol Leprol
Contact Dermatitis
J Cutan Pathol
J Dermatol
Int J Dermatol
Curr Probl Dermatol
Australas J Dermatol
Cutis
An Bras Dermatol
Br J Dermatol
Hautarzt
J Invest Dermatol
Acta Derm Venereol Suppl (Stockh)
Acta Derm Venereol
Actas Dermosifiliogr
DIAGNOSTIC IMAGING (71) includes Endoscopy, Magnetic Resonance Imaging, Microscopy, Nuclear Magnetic Resonance, And Ultrasonics - see also Radiology
Microscopy (Oxf)
Diagn Interv Imaging
Eur Heart J Cardiovasc Imaging
Theranostics
Jpn J Radiol
Asian J Endosc Surg
Circ Cardiovasc Imaging
JACC Cardiovasc Imaging
J Med Imaging Radiat Oncol
Med Ultrason
Brain Imaging Behav
Expert Opin Med Diagn
Contrast Media Mol Imaging
Diagn Interv Radiol
Expert Rev Med Devices
Photodiagnosis Photodyn Ther
Cardiovasc Ultrasound
Magn Reson Med Sci
Mol Imaging Biol
Mol Imaging
BMC Med Imaging
Int J Cardiovasc Imaging
Cancer Imaging
Surg Laparosc Endosc Percutan Tech
J Cardiovasc Magn Reson
Med Image Comput Comput Assist Interv
J Magn Reson
Med Image Anal
Biocell

Chapter 7 - The National Library of Medicine

A Perspective On The National Library of Medicine

Ultrason Sonochem
Abdom Imaging
MAGMA
Magn Reson Imaging Clin N Am
Micron
Microsc Res Tech
Neuroimage
Vet Radiol Ultrasound
Gastrointest Endosc Clin N Am
J Magn Reson Imaging
J Neuroimaging
Neuroimaging Clin N Am
Ultrasound Obstet Gynecol
Fetal Diagn Ther
Clin Imaging
Dig Endosc
Comput Med Imaging Graph
J Digit Imaging
J Am Soc Echocardiogr
NMR Biomed
Top Magn Reson Imaging
Ultrasound Q
Surg Endosc
J Thorac Imaging
Echocardiography
Magn Reson Med
Semin Ultrasound CT MR
IEEE Trans Med Imaging
J Ultrasound Med
Magn Reson Imaging
Inf Process Med Imaging
Ultraschall Med
Ultrason Imaging
Rofo
Ultramicroscopy
J Clin Ultrasound
Ultrasound Med Biol
Endoscopy
J Microsc
Gastrointest Endosc
Rontgenpraxis
Ultrasonics
DISASTER MEDICINE (5)
Disaster Med Public Health Prep
Am J Disaster Med
Biosecur Bioterror
Prehosp Disaster Med
Disasters
DRUG THERAPY (84) see also Anti-bacterial Agents;
Antineoplastic Agents
Drug Res (Stuttg)
Nucleic Acid Ther
J Popul Ther Clin Pharmacol
Ther Deliv
J Aerosol Med Pulm Drug Deliv
Drug Des Devel Ther
Drug Discov Ther
Recent Pat Endocr Metab Immune Drug Discov
Antiinflamm Antiallergy Agents Med Chem
Cardiovasc Hematol Disord Drug Targets
CNS Neurol Disord Drug Targets
Curr Drug Saf
Endocr Metab Immune Disord Drug Targets
Infect Disord Drug Targets
Inflamm Allergy Drug Targets
Recent Pat Anticancer Drug Discov
Recent Pat Antiinfect Drug Discov
Recent Pat Cardiovasc Drug Discov
Recent Pat CNS Drug Discov
J Opioid Manag
AAPS J
Curr Drug Deliv
Drug Discov Today Technol
Expert Opin Drug Deliv
Harm Reduct J
Am J Geriatr Pharmacother
Expert Opin Drug Saf
J Pain Palliat Care Pharmacother
Nat Rev Drug Discov
Treat Guidel Med Lett
Am J Cardiovasc Drugs
Expert Opin Emerg Drugs
Curr Drug Targets
Drugs R D
Paediatr Drugs
Drugs Today (Barc)
BioDrugs
Antivir Ther
Drug Discov Today
J Exp Ther Oncol
Clin Drug Investig
J Infect Chemother
J Ocul Pharmacol Ther
Microb Drug Resist
CNS Drugs
Expert Opin Investig Drugs
Int J Clin Pharmacol Ther
Drug Deliv
Ann Pharmacother
Pharmacoeconomics
Pharmacoepidemiol Drug Saf
Prescrire Int
Drugs Aging
Inflammopharmacology
Antivir Chem Chemother
Drug Saf
J Chemother
Antibiot Khimioter
Magnes Res
Rev Esp Quimioter

Adv Drug Deliv Rev
Aliment Pharmacol Ther
Cardiovasc Drugs Ther
Crit Rev Ther Drug Carrier Syst
Biomed Pharmacother
Int J Clin Pharmacol Res
Pharmacotherapy
Pharmacol Ther
Ther Drug Monit
Med Monatsschr Pharm
Clin Ther
J Antimicrob Chemother
Antimicrob Agents Chemother
Drugs
Eur J Clin Pharmacol
Chemotherapy
Drug Ther Bull
Prog Med Chem
Clin Pharmacol Ther
Med Lett Drugs Ther
Clin Ter

J Pharm Belg
J Pharmacol Exp Ther
Ann Clin Microbiol Antimicrob

E

EDUCATION (45) includes Dental, Medical and Nursing education
Glob Health Promot
Anat Sci Educ
CBE Life Sci Educ
J Physician Assist Educ
GMS Z Med Ausbild
Clin Teach
Int J Nurs Educ Scholarsh
J Nutr Educ Behav
J R Coll Physicians Edinb
Nurs Educ Perspect
BMC Med Educ

Educ Prim Care
Nurse Educ Pract
Biochem Mol Biol Educ
Eur J Dent Educ
Health Educ Behav
Adv Health Sci Educ Theory Pract
Educ Health (Abingdon)
J Deaf Stud Deaf Educ
Med Educ Online
Compend Contin Educ Dent
Nurs N Z
Sch Psychol Q
Acad Med
Adv Physiol Educ
AIDS Educ Prev
J Contin Educ Health Prof
Med Princ Pract
Health Educ Res
J Cancer Educ
J Health Adm Educ
Nurse Educ Today
Gerontol Geriatr Educ
Med Teach
Med Educ
Nurse Educ
J Vet Med Educ
J Allied Health
J Drug Educ
J Contin Educ Nurs
J Sch Psychol
J Nurs Educ
Am J Pharm Educ
J Dent Educ
Br J Educ Psychol
EMBRYOLOGY (24) includes Prenatal Developmental
Biology - see also Teratology
Birth Defects Res C Embryo Today
BMC Dev Biol
Dev Cell
Dev Genes Evol
Semin Cell Dev Biol
Hum Reprod Update
Stem Cells
Zygote
Ital J Anat Embryol
Mech Dev
Rom J Morphol Embryol
Int J Dev Biol
Development
Reprod Toxicol
Dev Biol (N Y 1985)
Placenta
Early Hum Dev
Adv Anat Embryol Cell Biol
Anat Histol Embryol
Differentiation
Ontogenez
Dev Growth Differ
Curr Top Dev Biol
Dev Biol
EMERGENCY MEDICINE (34)
Zhonghua Wei Zhong Bing Ji Jiu Yi Xue
EMS World
Int Emerg Nurs
Scand J Trauma Resusc Emerg Med
Adv Emerg Nurs J
Intern Emerg Med
J Bus Contin Emer Plan
Australas Emerg Nurs J
Emerg Med Australas
Pediatr Emerg Med Pract
J Emerg Manag
BMC Emerg Med
Emerg Med J
J Vet Emerg Crit Care (San Antonio)
CJEM
Emerg Med Pract
Int J Emerg Ment Health
Prehosp Emerg Care
Acad Emerg Med
Eur J Emerg Med
Air Med J
Emerg Nurse
Anasthesiol Intensivmed Notfallmed Schmerzther
ED Manag
Prehosp Disaster Med
Pediatr Emerg Care
Am J Emerg Med
Emerg Med Clin North Am
J Emerg Med
Ann Emerg Med
JEMS
J Emerg Nurs
Resuscitation
ENDOCRINOLOGY (90) includes Hormones And Diabetes
Mellitus - see also Reproductive Medicine
J Diabetes Res
Horm Res Paediatr
Horm Cancer
Islets
J Diabetes
Nat Rev Endocrinol
J Clin Res Pediatr Endocrinol
Curr Opin Endocrinol Diabetes Obes
Diabetes Metab Syndr
J Diabetes Sci Technol
Pediatr Endocrinol Diabetes Metab
Recent Pat Endocr Metab Immune Drug Discov
Endocr Metab Immune Disord Drug Targets

On July 5, 1875, Steinmetz writes to Billings: "We are right amongst the Cheyennes & Arapahoes. The first tribe was very troublesome ... this spring, giving our troops a skirmish about a mile from our camp .... Our command consists of three Cos. of Calvary and two of Infantry; all in tents on the south bank of the north fork of the Canadian river." Completing the indexing, he returns the journals to Billings with the following letter of August 14, 1875: "I return to you today per express the thirteen books, you sent me sometime ago, and hope that the indexing is done to your satisfaction .... During the last six weeks, our mail ... frequently arrived here in a fearful condition, & thoroughly soaked owing to the high water and heavy rains, and I was under apprehension, that the books might share the same fate. One of the severest thunder showers & storms, I ever witnessed, passed over this section of the country last Monday night .... The wind was so strong, that within a few minutes, all the hospital tents ... were blown down and torn to pieces .... During last winter, in order to keep from freezing to death, this Command dug holes in the bank of the river, and ... we will have to do the same thing unless something is done before the cold season sets in."

A Perspective On The National Library of Medicine

Curr Diabetes Rev
Diab Vasc Dis Res
Rev Diabet Stud
Pediatr Endocrinol Rev
Reprod Biol Endocrinol
Can J Diabetes
Cardiovasc Diabetol
Hormones (Athens)
Best Pract Res Clin Endocrinol Metab
Curr Diab Rep
Pancreatology
JOP
Pediatr Diabetes
Prim Care Diabetes
Rev Endocr Metab Disord
Diabetes Metab Res Rev
Diabetes Obes Metab
Diabetes Technol Ther
Endocr Dev
Endocrinol Nutr
Growth Horm IGF Res
Pituitary
Prostaglandins Other Lipid Mediat
Diabetes Metab
Endocr Pract
Exp Clin Endocrinol Diabetes
J Pediatr Endocrinol Metab
Endocr Relat Cancer
Endocrine
Eur J Endocrinol
Endocr J
Breast
J Diabetes Complications
Acta Diabetol
Endocr Regul
Endocr Pathol
Thyroid
J Neuroendocrinol
Trends Endocrinol Metab
J Mol Endocrinol
Prostaglandins Leukot Essent Fatty Acids
Endocrinol Metab Clin North Am
Gynecol Endocrinol
Mol Endocrinol
Diabetes Res Clin Pract
Diabet Med
Domest Anim Endocrinol
Endocr Res
J Pineal Res
Diabetes Self Manag
Am J Physiol Endocrinol Metab
Endocr Rev
Neuro Endocrinol Lett
Diabetes Care
J Endocrinol Invest
Minerva Endocrinol
Diabetes Educ
Psychoneuroendocrinology
Diabetes Forecast
Mol Cell Endocrinol
Clin Endocrinol (Oxf)
Front Horm Res
Front Neuroendocrinol
Horm Metab Res
Horm Behav
Diabetologia
Neuroendocrinology
Gen Comp Endocrinol
Journ Annu Diabetol Hotel Dieu
Arq Bras Endocrinol Metabol
Diabetes
J Clin Endocrinol Metab
Endokrynol Pol
Vitam Horm
Ann Endocrinol (Paris)
J Endocrinol
Endocrinology
ENVIRONMENTAL HEALTH (117) includes Ecology,
Pollution, Radiation, And Radioactivity
Environ Sci Process Impacts
Int J Occup Environ Med
Environ Microbiol Rep
Food Environ Virol
J Environ Public Health
Mol Ecol Resour
ISME J
Geospat Health
J Expo Sci Environ Epidemiol
Arch Environ Occup Health
Integr Environ Assess Manag
Ecohealth
Int J Environ Res Public Health
J Environ Sci Eng
J Occup Environ Hyg
Commun Agric Appl Biol Sci
Geobiology
J Water Health
Environ Health
BMC Ecol
Healthc Hazard Manage Monit
Int J Hyg Environ Health
Environ Microbiol
Environ Toxicol
Int J Phytoremediation
Ecol Lett
J Toxicol Environ Health A
J Toxicol Environ Health B Crit Rev
Environ Health Prev Med
Environ Toxicol Pharmacol
Glob Chang Biol

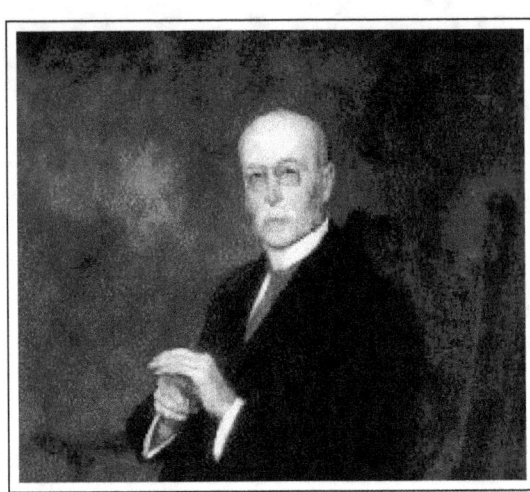

Robert Fletcher, M.D. - Principal Assistant Librarian (1876-1912). Fletcher assisted Billings in compiling the Library's Index- Catalogue of the whole collection, the first volume of which appeared in 1880. From 1879-1899 he served as co-editor and later (1903-1911) as editor-in-chief of the Index Medicus (the index to current periodicals and the precursor to MEDLINE). He devoted thirty-five years of work to The Library and can rightfully be called one of the founders.

Int J Occup Environ Health
Isotopes Environ Health Stud
J Occup Environ Med
J Air Waste Manag Assoc
J Trace Elem Med Biol
J Vector Ecol
Wilderness Environ Med
Ann Agric Environ Med
Environ Sci Pollut Res Int
Int J Occup Med Environ Health
Microbiol Res
Occup Environ Med
Appl Radiat Isot
SAR QSAR Environ Res
Aviakosm Ekolog Med
Ecotoxicology
Mol Ecol
Water Environ Res
Ecol Appl
Indoor Air
Int J Environ Health Res
J Environ Sci Health C Environ Carcinog Ecotoxicol Rev
Biodegradation
Environ Technol
New Solut
Ying Yong Sheng Tai Xue Bao
J Environ Sci (China)
Waste Manag

Biomed Environ Sci
Conserv Biol
Environ Mol Mutagen
Environ Pollut
Rev Environ Contam Toxicol
Mutagenesis
Trends Ecol Evol
Environ Geochem Health
FEMS Microbiol Ecol
Res Rep Health Eff Inst
J Environ Pathol Toxicol Oncol
J Environ Radioact
Waste Manag Res
Environ Toxicol Chem
Environ Monit Assess
Water Sci Technol
J Environ Biol
Biol Trace Elem Res
J UOEH
Neurotoxicology
Environ Int
Huan Jing Ke Xue
Mar Environ Res
Ann ICRP
Ecotoxicol Environ Saf
J Food Prot
Environ Manage
J Environ Sci Health B

WHO Reg Publ Eur Ser
Aviat Space Environ Med
Int Arch Occup Environ Health
J Chem Ecol
J Hazard Mater
Scand J Work Environ Health
Radiat Environ Biophys
Arch Environ Contam Toxicol
J Environ Manage
Ambio
Chemosphere
Environ Health Perspect
J Environ Qual
Rev Environ Health
Sci Total Environ
Mar Pollut Bull
Oecologia
Environ Res
Environ Sci Technol
Water Res
Zhonghua Yu Fang Yi Xue Za Zhi
Bull Environ Contam Toxicol
Ground Water
Ind Health
J Environ Health
J Radiat Res
Health Phys
Schriftenr Ver Wasser Boden Lufthyg
J Anim Ecol
Ecology
EPIDEMIOLOGY (54)
Chronic Dis Inj Can
Epidemiol Psychiatr Sci
J Epidemiol Glob Health
Western Pac Surveill Response J
Cancer Epidemiol
Epidemics
Spat Spatiotemporal Epidemiol
Biodemography Soc Biol
Can Commun Dis Rep Wkly
J Expo Sci Environ Epidemiol
World Health Popul
Vector Borne Zoonotic Dis
J Urban Health
Rev Bras Epidemiol
Health Place
MSMR
Epidemiol Mikrobiol Imunol
J Med Screen
Ophthalmic Epidemiol
Cent Eur J Public Health
Can Commun Dis Rep
Pharmacoepidemiol Drug Saf
Cancer Epidemiol Biomarkers Prev
Eur J Public Health
J Epidemiol
Ann Epidemiol
Bacteriol Virusol Parazitol Epidemiol
Cancer Causes Control
Epidemiology
N S W Public Health Bull
Infect Control Hosp Epidemiol
J Clin Epidemiol
Soc Psychiatry Psychiatr Epidemiol
Epidemiol Infect
Paediatr Perinat Epidemiol
Eur J Epidemiol
Genet Epidemiol
Neuroepidemiology
Zhonghua Liu Xing Bing Xue Za Zhi
Epidemiol Bull
Epidemiol Rev
J Epidemiol Community Health
Epidemiol Prev
Rev Epidemiol Sante Publique
Community Dent Oral Epidemiol
Int J Epidemiol
Local Popul Stud
Am J Epidemiol
Popul Stud (Camb)
Przegl Epidemiol
Zh Mikrobiol Epidemiol Immunobiol
Wkly Epidemiol Rec
Int J Health Geogr
J Registry Manag
ETHICS (42) includes Medical Philosophy
Narrat Inq Bioeth
J Empir Res Hum Res Ethics
Philos Ethics Humanit Med
Indian J Med Ethics
J Bioeth Inq
Organ Ethic
Am J Bioeth
Dev World Bioeth
J Philos Sci Law
Yale J Health Policy Law Ethics
BMC Med Ethics
Med Humanit
Nurs Philos
JONAS Healthc Law Ethics Regul
Virtual Mentor
Hum Reprod Genet Ethics
Med Health Care Philos
Stud Hist Philos Biol Biomed Sci
Theor Med Bioeth
Sci Eng Ethics
Health Hum Rights
Monash Bioeth Rev
Nurs Ethics
J Law Med Ethics

A Perspective On The National Library of Medicine

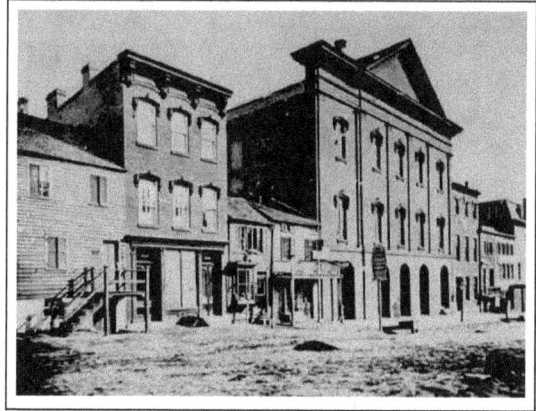

The Library Moves to Ford's Theatre.

After the assassination of President Lincoln at Ford's Theatre, there was such an onus on the building that it became impossible for the owner to use. The federal government bought it for $100,000; and for 20 years (1866 to 1886), it served as the first permanent home of the Army Surgeon General's Library. Concerned about fire hazard and structural integrity, Billings lobbied for appropriations to build a new facility for the rapidly expanded collection. Fortunately, he was successful because several years after that move, the interior of the theatre collapsed, killing 22 persons. Such a catastrophe, during its formative years, might have permanently thwarted the evolution of The Library.

A Perspective On The National Library of Medicine

Eur J Cardiothorac Surg
J Craniomaxillofac Surg
Surg Endosc
Acta Cir Bras
Ann Vasc Surg
Arq Bras Cir Dig
Clin Pediatr Med Surg
Int J Oral Maxillofac Surg
Int J Oral Maxillofac Implants
J Card Surg
Pediatr Surg Int
Rev Bras Cir Cardiovasc
Surg Radiol Anat
Eur J Surg Oncol
Ophthal Plast Reconstr Surg
Br J Oral Maxillofac Surg
Dig Surg
J Reconstr Microsurg
J Vasc Surg
Ann Chir Plast Esthet
Facial Plast Surg
Microsurgery
Plast Surg Nurs
Presse Med
Handchir Mikrochir Plast Chir
J Oral Maxillofac Surg
Orbit
Otolaryngol Head Neck Surg
G Chir
Lasers Surg Med
Pediatr Med Chir
Thorac Cardiovasc Surg
Ann Plast Surg
Vet Surg
Am J Surg Pathol
Ann R Australas Coll Dent Surg
J Oral Implantol
Oper Dent Suppl
World J Surg
Aesthetic Plast Surg
J Hand Surg Am
Oper Dent
Clin Plast Surg
Rev Col Bras Cir
Cir Esp
Eur Surg Res
J Surg Oncol
J Extra Corpor Technol
Int Surg
J Pediatr Surg
Adv Surg
Ann Thorac Surg
Curr Probl Surg
Plast Reconstr Surg
S Afr J Surg
J Surg Res
J Cardiovasc Surg (Torino)
Acta Chir Plast
J Thorac Cardiovasc Surg
Can J Surg
Rev Med Chir Soc Med Nat Iasi
Acta Chir Iugosl
Zhonghua Wai Ke Za Zhi
Am Surg
Khirurgiia (Sofiia)
Magy Seb
J Bone Joint Surg Am
Kyobu Geka
Ann R Coll Surg Engl
Acta Chir Belg
Minerva Chir
Rozhl Chir
Khirurgiia (Mosk)
Surgery
Vestn Khir Im I I Grek
Cir Cir
Chirurg
Ann Ital Chir
Pol Przegl Chir
Surg Clin North Am
Bull Am Coll Surg
Br J Surg
Nihon Geka Gakkai Zasshi
Am J Surg
Zentralbl Chir
Ann Surg
GENETICS (70) includes Cytogenetics, Genetic Psychology, And Heredity
G3 (Bethesda)
Brief Funct Genomics
Epigenomics
Genet Test Mol Biomarkers
Genet Res (Camb)
J Nutrigenet Nutrigenomics
Mar Genomics
Forensic Sci Int Genet
J Exp Zool A Ecol Genet Physiol
J Genet Genomics
Recent Pat DNA Gene Seq
Comp Biochem Physiol Part D Genomics Proteomics
Epigenetics
Genome Dyn
Int J Immunogenet
PLoS Genet
Genomics Proteomics Bioinformatics
Hum Genomics
Cytogenet Genome Res
Genes Brain Behav
Genet Mol Res
Stat Appl Genet Mol Biol

Curr Protoc Hum Genet
Genome Inform
Infect Genet Evol
Mol Genet Genomics
Annu Rev Genomics Hum Genet
BMC Genomics
Funct Integr Genomics
Genome Biol
J Struct Funct Genomics
Nat Rev Genet
Hum Reprod Genet Ethics
Neurogenetics
Fungal Genet Biol
Genome Res
J Appl Genet
DNA Res
Rev Derecho Genoma Hum
Radiats Biol Radioecol
J Assist Reprod Genet
Curr Opin Genet Dev
Mamm Genome
Psychiatr Genet
Genet Sel Evol
Genome
Genomics
Anim Genet
J Anim Breed Genet
Trends Genet
Curr Genet
Genet Eng (N Y)
Yi Chuan
Plasmid
Immunogenetics
Behav Genet
Mendel Newsl
Theor Appl Genet
Annu Rev Genet
Tsitol Genet
Genetika
Mutat Res
J Genet Psychol
Radiat Res
Hereditas (Edinb)
Hereditas
Genetica
Genetics
J Hered
J Genet
GENETICS, BIOCHEMICAL - see Molecular Biology
GENETICS, MEDICAL (45) includes Eugenics And Twins
Hum Gene Ther Clin Dev
Hum Gene Ther Methods
Cancer Genet
BMC Med Genomics
Circ Cardiovasc Genet
Public Health Genomics
Eur J Med Genet
Pharmacogenet Genomics

Twin Res Hum Genet
Cancer Genomics Proteomics
Am J Med Genet A
Am J Med Genet B Neuropsychiatr Genet
Am J Med Genet C Semin Med Genet
Curr Gene Ther
Annu Rev Genomics Hum Genet
BMC Med Genet
Pharmacogenomics
J Gene Med
Genet Med
Int J Mol Med
J Hum Genet
BioDrugs
J Mol Med (Berl)
Cancer Gene Ther
Gene Ther
Ophthalmic Genet
Eur J Hum Genet
Hum Mol Genet
Hum Mutat
J Genet Couns
Nat Genet
Zhonghua Yi Xue Yi Chuan Xue Za Zhi
Genet Couns
Hum Gene Ther
Mutagenesis
Genet Epidemiol
J Neurogenet
Hum Genet
Clin Genet
Theor Popul Biol
Hum Hered
J Med Genet
Ann Hum Genet
Am J Hum Genet
Adv Genet
GERIATRICS (70) includes Aging And The Aged
Geriatr Psychol Neuropsychiatr Vieil
J Nutr Gerontol Geriatr
J Geriatr Oncol
Aging (Albany NY)
Curr Aging Sci
Res Gerontol Nurs
Clin Interv Aging
Int J Older People Nurs
Age (Dordr)
Rejuvenation Res
Am J Geriatr Pharmacother
Ageing Res Rev
Aging Clin Exp Res
Natl Bur Econ Res Bull Aging Health
BMC Geriatr
Geriatr Gerontol Int
J Geriatr Phys Ther
Psychogeriatrics
Biogerontology
Nurs Older People

Aging Male
Australas J Ageing
J Alzheimers Dis
Aging Ment Health
Dement Geriatr Cogn Disord
J Nutr Health Aging
Neuropsychol Dev Cogn B Aging Neuropsychol Cogn
Soins Gerontol
J Gerontol A Biol Sci Med Sci
J Gerontol B Psychol Sci Soc Sci
Z Gerontol Geriatr
Am J Geriatr Psychiatry
J Aging Phys Act
Drugs Aging
Int Psychogeriatr
Johns Hopkins Med Lett Health After 50
J Aging Health
J Aging Soc Policy
J Elder Abuse Negl
J Geriatr Psychiatry Neurol
J Women Aging
J Aging Stud
Int J Geriatr Psychiatry
J Cross Cult Gerontol
Psychol Aging
Clin Geriatr Med
Arch Gerontol Geriatr
Can J Aging
Gerodontology
J Appl Gerontol
Tijdschr Gerontol Geriatr
Geriatr Nurs
Gerontol Geriatr Educ
Neurobiol Aging
Rev Esp Geriatr Gerontol
J Gerontol Soc Work
Maturitas
Perspectives
Gerontology
Exp Aging Res
J Gerontol Nurs
Int J Aging Hum Dev
Age Ageing
Mech Ageing Dev
Interdiscip Top Gerontol
Exp Gerontol
Nihon Ronen Igakkai Zasshi
Gerontologist
J Am Geriatr Soc
Adv Gerontol
GYNECOLOGY (54) see also Obstetrics; Reproductive Medicine; Women's Health
Female Pelvic Med Reconstr Surg
Int Urogynecol J
Menopause Int
J Minim Invasive Gynecol
J Sex Med
J Womens Health (Larchmt)
Best Pract Res Clin Obstet Gynaecol
J Obstet Gynaecol Can
BJOG
Gynecol Obstet Fertil
Climacteric
Int J Fertil Womens Med
J Low Genit Tract Dis
J Obstet Gynecol Res
J Pediatr Adolesc Gynecol
Ceska Gynekol
J Am Coll Surg
Menopause
Infect Dis Obstet Gynecol
Womens Health Data Book
Int J Gynecol Cancer
Ultrasound Obstet Gynecol
Womens Health Issues
Curr Opin Obstet Gynecol
Arch Gynecol Obstet
Breast Dis
Gynecol Endocrinol
Obstet Gynecol Clin North Am
J Obstet Gynecol Neonatal Nurs
Taiwan J Obstet Gynecol
Int J Gynecol Pathol
J Psychosom Obstet Gynaecol
Eur J Gynaecol Oncol
J Obstet Gynaecol
Rev Bras Ginecol Obstet
Gynecol Obstet Invest
Women Health
Clin Exp Obstet Gynecol
Eur J Obstet Gynecol Reprod Biol
Gynecol Oncol
J Gynecol Obstet Biol Reprod (Paris)
Int J Gynaecol Obstet
Akush Ginekol (Sofiia)
Aust N Z J Obstet Gynaecol
Clin Obstet Gynecol
Obstet Gynecol
Zhonghua Fu Chan Ke Za Zhi
Minerva Ginecol
Ginecol Obstet Mex
Obstet Gynecol Surv
Rozhl Chir
Acta Obstet Gynecol Scand
Ginekol Pol
Am J Obstet Gynecol

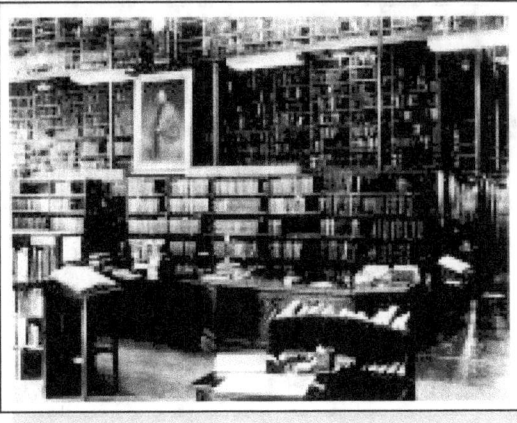

The reading room of the Library.
Note the painting of Billings in the background, which is the one presented previously and which is still on display.

H

Chapter 7 - The National Library of Medicine

A Perspective On The National Library of Medicine

HEALTH SERVICES (170)
Healthc Philanthr
Medicare Medicaid Res Rev
EMS World
J Healthc Eng
Disabil Health J
J (Inst Health Rec Inf Manag)
Patient
Popul Health Manag
Am J Mens Health
HERD
Prof Case Manag
Behav Healthc
Health Econ Policy Law
Profiles Healthc Commun
World Health Popul
Health Syst Transit
Healthc Policy
Int J Evid Based Healthc
Jt Comm J Qual Patient Saf
J Patient Saf
Commun Med
Healthc Q
Int J Electron Healthc
Perspect Health Inf Manag
Psychol Serv
Access Manag J
Hum Resour Health
J Health Organ Manag
Appl Health Econ Health Policy
Int J Equity Health
Issue Brief (Inst Health Care Costs Solut)
Afr Health Sci
BMC Int Health Hum Rights
Curr Probl Pediatr Adolesc Health Care
Eur J Health Econ
Health Info Libr J
Int J Health Care Finance Econ
J Hosp Mark Public Relations
MGMA Connex
Rural Remote Health
Adv Health Care Manag
Clin Leadersh Manag Rev
Healthc Hazard Manage Monit
Hisp Health Care Int
Telemed J E Health
Care Manag J
Health Care Manag (Frederick)
Healthc Pap
Health Care Law Mon
Health Care Manag Sci
Health Estate
J Behav Health Serv Res
J Healthc Inf Manag
J Healthc Manag
J Med Econ
J Ment Health Policy Econ
Rev Esp Sanid Penit
Health (London)
Manag Care Interface
Mark Health Serv
Medicare Brief
Perm J
Rural Policy Brief
Educ Health (Abingdon)
J Health Commun
J Prev Interv Community
Psychol Health Med
Am J Manag Care
Health Care Financ Rev Stat Suppl
J Public Health Manag Pract
J Telemed Telecare
Health Data Manag
Health Manag Technol
Int J Qual Health Care
J Correct Health Care
J Health Hum Serv Adm
J Health Care Finance
World Hosp Health Serv
Health Care Anal
Health Soc Care Community
Hosp Health Netw
Technol Health Care
Am J Med Qual
Dev Health Econ Public Policy
Health Econ
J Healthc Risk Manag
J Interprof Care
Manag Care
Mater Manag Health Care
Qual Manag Health Care
Q Rev Econ Finance
Future Child
Health Matrix Clevel
J AHIMA
J Sch Nurs
Qual Connect
Healthc Inform
J Health Care Poor Underserved
Rev Calid Asist
ED Manag
Health Commun
Adm Policy Ment Health
Health Facil Manage
Health Serv Manage Res
Healthc Manage Forum
J Contin Educ Health Prof
Jt Comm Perspect
J Econ Perspect

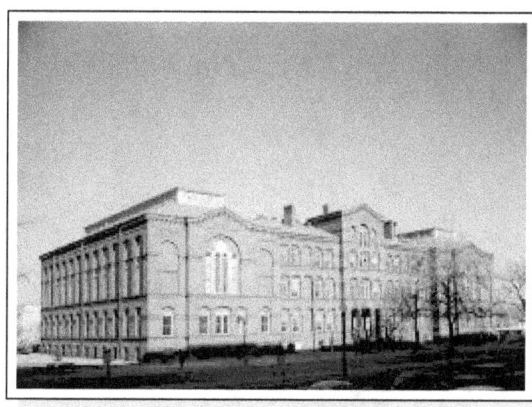

The New Library and Medical Museum.
Constructed on the Mall at Seventh and Independence Avenue, S.W., Washington, D.C., the facility was designed by John Shaw Billings and is where the collection was housed for 75 years (1886 to 1961). Below is a reading room and stacks.

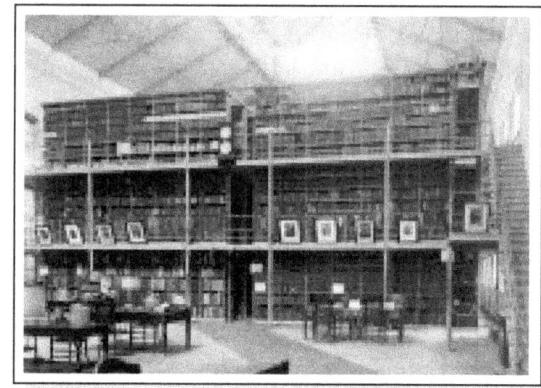

J Pediatr Health Care
Health Serv J
Milbank Q
Physician Exec
Provider
Benefits Q
Death Stud
Healthc Exec
Int J Health Plann Manage
J Med Pract Manage
Front Health Serv Manage
Health Care Women Int
Health Prog
J Healthc Prot Manage
Rand J Econ
Health Care Strateg Manage
Health Mark Q
Home Healthc Nurse

J Health Adm Educ
Can J Commun Ment Health
Caring
Healthc Financ Manage
Jpn Hosp
J Am Coll Health
J Health Econ
Med Ref Serv Q
Soc Sci Med
Int Q Community Health Educ
Health Law Can
JEMS
Home Health Care Serv Q
J Epidemiol Community Health
J Insur Med
Radiol Manage
Aust Health Rev
Fam Community Health

J Ambul Care Manage
Mod Healthc
Health Care Manage Rev
Hosp Peer Rev
Sante Ment Que
Soc Work Health Care
J Allied Health
Int J Health Serv
Lang Speech Hear Serv Sch
Rev Law Soc Change
Fund Raising Manage
Acad Manage J
Inquiry
Med Care
Child Welfare
J Sch Health
Fortune
Med Econ
Harv Bus Rev
Bull Am Coll Surg
Am Econ Rev
Capitation Manag Rep
EBRI Issue Brief
NIH Guide Grants Contracts
School Nurse News
Archit Rec
HEALTH SERVICES RESEARCH (93) includes Health
Services Planning, Evaluation, And Assessment
Patient
Tanzan J Health Res
Leadersh Health Serv (Bradf Engl)
Implement Sci
Int J Qual Stud Health Well-being
Simul Healthc
Global Health
Issue Brief George Wash Univ Natl Health Policy Forum
Organ Ethic
Health Res Policy Syst
Hum Resour Health
J Nepal Health Res Counc
Natl Bur Econ Res Bull Aging Health
NIH Consens State Sci Statements
Synth Proj Res Synth Rep
Track Rep
BMC Health Serv Res
Ont Health Technol Assess Ser
Policy Brief George Wash Univ Cent Health Serv Res Policy
Technol Eval Cent Assess Program Exec Summ
Policy Brief (Cent Home Care Policy Res)
Prim Health Care Res Dev
State Coverage Initiat Issue Brief
Evid Rep Technol Assess (Full Rep)
Issue Brief (Grantmakers Health)
Medi-Cal Policy Inst Issue Brief
Policy Anal Brief H Ser
Evid Based Nurs
Health Expect
Issue Brief George Wash Univ Cent Health Serv Res Policy
J Behav Health Serv Res
Policy Anal Brief W Ser
Sentinel Event Alert
Data Bull (Cent Stud Health Syst Change)
Health Technol Assess
Issues Emerg Health Technol
Find Brief
Issue Brief Cent Stud Health Syst Change
J Health Serv Res Policy
J Eval Clin Pract
Med Care Res Rev
Int J Qual Health Care
LDI Issue Brief
Policy Brief UCLA Cent Health Policy Res
Nurse Res
Annu Stat Suppl Soc Secur Bull
J Healthc Qual
Qual Manag Health Care
SMU Law Rev
Qual Health Res
Qual Connect
Stud Health Technol Inform
Cochrane Database Syst Rev
Health Commun
Vital Health Stat 21
Health Serv Manage Res
Int J Health Care Qual Assur
Health Policy Plan
Int J Health Plann Manage
Int J Technol Assess Health Care
Stand News
Health Policy
Vital Health Stat 5
Vital Health Stat Health Aff (Millwood)
Med Decis Making
Eval Rev
Eval Program Plann
Eval Health Prof
Res Nurs Health
J Med Eng Technol
Vital Health Stat 23
J Health Polit Policy Law
Hastings Cent Rep
Health Devices
Int J Health Serv
J Extra Corpor Technol
Cornell Law Rev
Health Serv Res
Vital Health Stat 13
Vital Health Stat Vital Health Stat 20
Vital Health Stat 11
Vital Health Stat 1

Chapter 7 - The National Library of Medicine

A Perspective On The National Library of Medicine

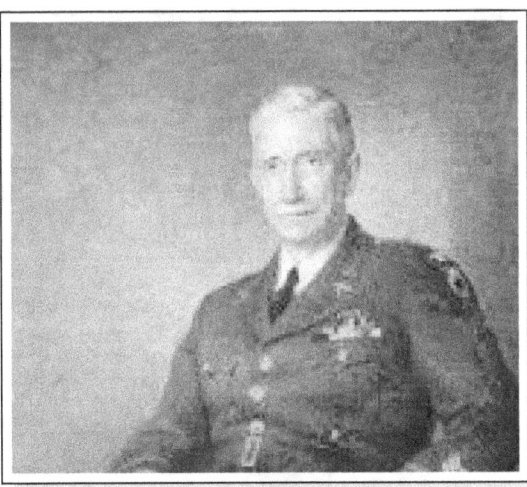

Harold W. Jones, **M.D.** - Director of the Library (1936-1944). Jones exemplifies the diverse background of the librarians. An Associate Professor of Orthopedic Surgery at St. Louis University Medical School, he become a Colonel in the Army Medical Corps assigned to the Army Medical School which was housed in the Army Medical Library and Museum Building. He also served as ship's surgeon, as commander of one of the largest hospital centers in World War I (the Beau Desert in France), as Secretary-General of the American delegation of an international congress of military medicine, and as chief of the surgical services of several military hospitals. In 1936 he returned to Washington and the Army Medical Library to serve for nine years as its Librarian and Director.

A Perspective On The National Library of Medicine

J Health Econ
J Hosp Infect
Gen Hosp Psychiatry
Aust Health Rev
Health Care Manage Rev
Hosp Peer Rev
Hist Hosp
Hosp Top
Trustee
Nig Q J Hosp Med
Archit Rec

I

IMMUNOLOGY see Allergy and Immunology
INTERNAL MEDICINE (21)
Clin Evid (Online)
Intern Emerg Med
Intern Med J
Intern Med
Rom J Intern Med
Eur J Intern Med
J Intern Med Suppl
J Intern Med
J Vet Intern Med
J Gen Intern Med
Korean J Intern Med
Rev Med Interne
Neth J Med
Internist (Berl)
Vnitr Lek
Zhonghua Nei Ke Za Zhi
Ann Intern Med
Pol Arch Med Wewn
Nihon Naika Gakkai Zasshi

J

JURISPRUDENCE (66)
J Forensic Leg Med
J Philos Sci Law
Yale J Health Policy Law Ethics
JONAS Healthc Law Ethics Regul
Leg Med (Tokyo)
Health Care Law Mon
Sci Justice
Rev Derecho Genoma Hum
J Law Med Ethics
Med Law Rev
Ann Health Law
Food Drug Law J
SMU Law Rev
Int J Risk Saf Med
HEC Forum
AIDS Policy Law
J Law Health
Fa Yi Xue Za Zhi
Issues Law Med
J Contemp Health Law Policy
Behav Sci Law
J Forensic Odontostomatol
Med Law
Am J Forensic Med Pathol
Health Law Can
J Leg Med
Forensic Sci Int
Law Hum Behav
State Legis
Rev Law Soc Change
Med Sci Law
Sud Med Ekspert
Am Univ Law Rev
Duke Law J
J Forensic Sci
Soud Lek
Albany Law Rev
Nihon Hoigaku Zasshi
Fed Regist
Arch Kriminol
Fordham Law Rev
Harv Law Rev

K
None

L

LABORATORY ANIMAL SCIENCE (8) includes Alterna-
tives To Laboratory Animals - see also Veterinary Medicine
J Am Assoc Lab Anim Sci
Comp Med
Exp Anim
ILAR J
ALTEX
Altern Lab Anim
Lab Anim (NY)
Lab Anim
LIBRARY SCIENCE (2)
J Med Libr Assoc
Natl Netw

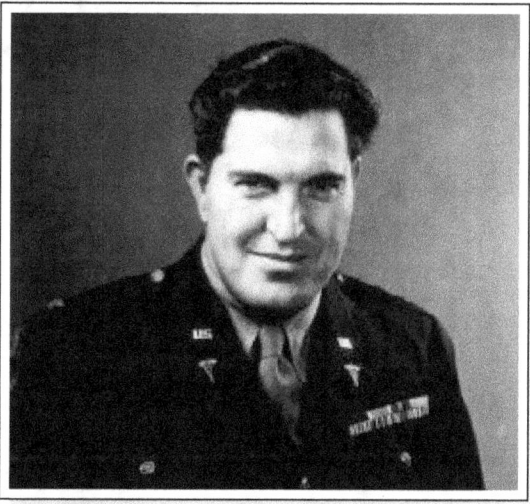

Joseph H. McNinch, M.D. - Director of the Library (1946-1949). McNinch taught in the Army Medical School, was Assistant Chief of the Medical Statistics Division of the Surgeon General's Office, and served in the European Theater during the World War II. In 1945, the Surgeon General appointed him to be the editor-in-chief of the Medical History of World War II. Among the important actions in which Dr. McNinch participated were those concerning the location of the proposed new building and the future of the Index-Catalogue.

M

MEDICAL INFORMATICS (51)
IEEE J Biomed Health Inform
IEEE Trans Neural Netw Learn Syst
Appl Clin Inform
Wiley Interdiscip Rev Syst Biol Med
Inform Health Soc Care
J (Inst Health Rec Inf Manag)
Comput Math Methods Med
Curr Comput Aided Drug Des
J Chem Inf Model
Perspect Health Inf Manag
AMIA Annu Symp Proc
Comput Biol Chem
Comput Inform Nurs
Inform Prim Care
Neuroinformatics
BMC Med Inform Decis Mak

Health Info Libr J
HIM J
J Biomed Inform
Telemed J E Health
J Med Internet Res
J Clin Monit Comput
J Healthc Inf Manag
Med Image Comput Comput Assist Interv
Health Informatics J
Int J Med Inform
IEEE Trans Vis Comput Graph
J Telemed Telecare
Health Manag Technol
J Am Med Inform Assoc
IEEE Trans Image Process
Yearb Med Inform
J AHIMA
Stud Health Technol Inform
Healthc Inform
Artif Intell Med
Int J Neural Syst

Neural Comput
Teach Learn Med
J Digit Imaging
Comput Methods Programs Biomed
IEEE Comput Graph Appl
Med Decis Making
Inf Process Med Imaging
IEEE Trans Pattern Anal Mach Intell
J Med Syst
Med Biol Eng Comput
J Biocommun
Medinfo
Comput Biol Med
Methods Inf Med
MEDICINE (339)
J Integr Med
Med Sci Monit Basic Res
R I Med J (2013)
Biomed Res Int
Biomed J
Dan J Med
Hawaii J Med Public Health
Syst Rev
Cold Spring Harb Perspect Med
Front Med
Med Klin Intensivmed Notfmed
Arb Paul Ehrlich Inst Bundesinstitut Impfstoffe Biomed
Arzneim Langen Hess Wiesbaden : Chmielorz
Glob J Health Sci
Sci Transl Med
Ann Adv Automot Med
BMC Res Notes
BMJ Case Rep
Clin Transl Sci
Dis Model Mech
J Evid Based Med
J Med Life
MD Advis
Pan Afr Med J
Z Evid Forthild Qual Gesundhwes
Biomark Med
Open Med
Acta Med Acad
Adv Med Sci
Dtsch Arztebl Int
Duke Med Health News
Ernst Schering Found Symp Proc
J Vis Exp
Libyan J Med
Orphanet J Rare Dis
PLoS One
Rev Recent Clin Trials
S D Med
Transl Res
Trials
Acute Med
Br J Hosp Med (Lond)
Chronic Illn
Clinics (Sao Paulo)
Contemp Clin Trials
Forensic Sci Med Pathol
Head Face Med
J Ethnobiol Ethnomed
J Zhejiang Univ Sci B
Nan Fang Yi Ke Da Xue Xue Bao
Rev Med Suisse
Clin Trials
Commun Med
Gend Med
Int J Med Sci
Med Glas (Zenica)
PLoS Med
Postepy Hig Med Dosw (Online)
Prague Med Rep
Theor Biol Med Model
Zhong Nan Da Xue Xue Bao Yi Xue Ban
BMC Med
Clin Med Res
Einstein (Sao Paulo)
Ger Med Sci
J Chin Med Assoc
J Transl Med
Kathmandu Univ Med J (KUMJ)
Math Med Biol
Sichuan Da Xue Xue Bao Yi Xue Ban
Acta Biomed
J Huazhong Univ Sci Technolog Med Sci
J Negat Results Biomed
J R Coll Physicians Edinb
NIH Consens State Sci Statements
Afr Health Sci
Beijing Da Xue Xue Bao
BMC Med Res Methodol
Clin Exp Med
Clin Med
Discov Med
Exp Biol Med (Maywood)
Swiss Med Wkly
Ann Afr Med
Comp Med
High Alt Med Biol
J Nippon Med Sch
J Am Med Dir Assoc
Md Med
ScientificWorldJournal
Isr Med Assoc J
MMW Fortschr Med
Zhejiang Da Xue Xue Bao Yi Xue Ban
Adv Clin Exp Med
Arch Iran Med

Chapter 7 - The National Library of Medicine

A Perspective On The National Library of Medicine

Bosn J Basic Med Sci
Ethiop J Health Sci
J Clin Monit Comput
Nepal Med Coll J
Niger J Clin Pract
Anthropol Med
Int J Circumpolar Health
Int J Clin Pract Suppl
Int J Clin Pract
Iran Biomed J
J Med Dent Sci
J Med Invest
Kokuritsu Iyakuhin Shokuhin Eisei Kenkyusho Hokoku
Perm J
WMJ
Acta Medica (Hradec Kralove)
Can J Rural Med
Harv Mens Health Watch
Kaohsiung J Med Sci
Pol Merkur Lekarski
Psychol Health Med
Tenn Med
East Mediterr Health J
Eur J Med Res
Evid Based Med
Hong Kong Med J
Med Sci Monit
Nat Med
Georgian Med News
JAAPA
J Biomed Sci
J Investig Med
Niger Postgrad Med J
Praxis (Bern 1994)
QJM
Sao Paulo Med J
J Law Med Ethics
Arch Med Res
Croat Med J
Lik Sprava
Mymensingh Med J
Rev Assoc Med Bras
Vestn Ross Akad Med Nauk
Acta Clin Croat
Acta Med Croatica
Enfermi Clin
J Coll Physicians Surg Pak
J Formos Med Assoc
Cochrane Database Syst Rev
Fortschr Med Orig
Harv Health Lett
Int J Risk Saf Med
Malawi Med J
Niger J Med
Ann Med
Johns Hopkins Med Lett Health After 50
J Assoc Acad Minor Phys
Teach Learn Med
BMJ
Jahresber Schweiz Akad Med Wiss
J Ayub Med Coll Abbottabad
Versicherungsmedizin
Cleve Clin J Med
Free Radic Biol Med
Phys Med
J Korean Med Sci
Ann Saudi Med
Biomed Pap Med Fac Univ Palacky Olomouc Czech Repub
CMAJ
Med Sci (Paris)
Iowa Med
Mayo Clin Health Lett
Presse Med
Rev Med Inst Mex Seguro Soc
Biomed Pharmacother
Lit Med
P R Health Sci J
Biomedica
Braz J Med Biol Res
West Afr J Med
Biomed Res
Prilozi
Acta Med Port
Clin Sci (Lond)
Dakar Med
J Insur Med
Saudi Med J
Zhongguo Yi Xue Ke Xue Yuan Xue Bao
Clin Invest Med
J R Soc Med
Med Monatsschr Pharm
Coll Antropol
Rev Fac Cien Med Univ Nac Cordoba
Afr J Med Med Sci
Rev Med Panama
Tokai J Exp Clin Med
Am J Law Med
Bangladesh Med Res Counc Bull
Bull Mem Acad R Med Belg
Med Hypotheses
Ir Med J
J S C Med Assoc
J Pak Med Assoc
Acta Med Okayama
Verh K Acad Geneeskd Belg
Ann Acad Med Singapore
Curr Med Res Opin
J Int Med Res
Med J Malaysia
Ups J Med Sci Suppl

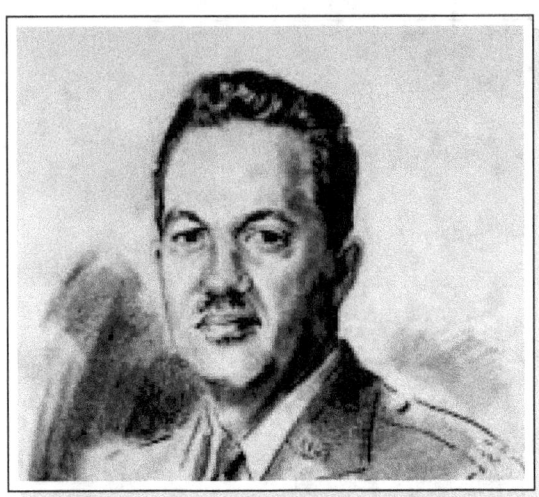

Frank Bradway Rogers, M.D. - Director of the Library (1949 to 1963). Through his leadership, the Library was given statutory authority and transferred to civilian control as the National Library of Medicine (1956). As the volume of information began to over-load the older methods of typesetting, he converted to a computerized system, from which, it was discovered, the information could be retrieved for research. This led to the Medical Literature Analysis and Retrieval System (MEDLARS), which was the precursor to MEDLINE (**MED**lars on-**LINE**) and the Internet system which you are using herein. In 1962, he moved the library into its current location in Bethesda.

Ups J Med Sci
Ir J Med Sci
Med Mal Infect
Wien Med Wochenschr Suppl
Comput Biol Med
Eur J Clin Invest
Acta Med Indones
Adv Exp Med Biol
J Med Assoc Thai
Tex Med
Acta Clin Belg Suppl

Lakartidningen
Mayo Clin Proc
Mich Med
JNMA J Nepal Med Assoc
Mali Med
Rev Med Univ Navarra
Ethiop Med J
Ghana Med J
J Relig Health
Acta Univ Carol Med Monogr
Del Med J

Glas Srp Akad Nauka Med
Invest Clin
JAMA
J Miss State Med Assoc
Singapore Med J
Wiad Lek
Yonsei Med J
Alaska Med
Folia Med Cracov
Folia Med (Plovdiv)
Panminerva Med
Conn Med
Phys Rev Lett
Ned Tijdschr Geneeskd
Perspect Biol Med
Acta Med Iran
Bull Exp Biol Med
Rev Med Chir Soc Med Nat Iasi
Scott Med J
Cent Afr J Med
J Postgrad Med
P N G Med J
Dis Mon
Fukushima J Med Sci
Kurume Med J
Osaka City Med J
J Assoc Physicians India
J La State Med Soc
Mo Med
Ceylon Med J
Keio J Med
Hiroshima J Med Sci
Kobe J Med Sci
Rev Prat
West Indian Med J
Annu Rev Med
J Med Liban
Med Dosw Mikrobiol
Med Pregl
Med Pr
Rev Invest Clin
Bull Acad Natl Med
Indian J Med Sci
Med Arh
Postgrad Med
Acta Clin Belg
Am J Med
Ann Univ Mariae Curie Sklodowska Med
Dtsch Med Wochenschr
Recenti Prog Med
Rev Med Liege
Wien Med Wochenschr
Przegl Lek
Rev Med Brux
Br Med Bull
Med Clin (Barc)
Nihon Rinsho
Fukuoka Igaku Zasshi
Medicina (B Aires)
N C Med J
Rev Clin Esp
East Afr Med J
S Afr Med J
Ulster Med J
J Indian Med Assoc
Tunis Med
N Engl J Med
Yale J Biol Med
Ann Intern Med
Nagoya J Med Sci
Postgrad Med J
Harefuah
J Clin Invest
Hokkaido Igaku Zasshi
Klin Med (Mosk)
Time
Medicine (Baltimore)
Bratisl Lek Listy
Medicina (Kaunas)
Tohoku J Exp Med
Minn Med
Med Clin North Am
Laeknabladid
Med J Aust
Indian J Med Res
J Med Assoc Ga
J Natl Med Assoc
Minerva Med
J Okla State Med Assoc
South Med J
J Ark Med Soc
W V Med J
Harvey Lect
Bol Asoc Med P R
Pharos Alpha Omega Alpha Honor Med Soc
Srp Arh Celok Lek
J Exp Med
Tidsskr Nor Laegeforen
Wien Klin Wochenschr
N Z Med J
Duodecim
An R Acad Nac Med (Madr)
Lijec Vjesn
Rev Med Chil
Bull Soc Sci Med Grand Duche Luxemb
Gac Med Mex
Cas Lek Cesk
Orv Hetil
Ugeskr Laeger
Am J Med Sci

Chapter 7 - The National Library of Medicine

A Perspective On The National Library of Medicine

Lancet
Trans Med Soc Lond
METABOLISM (66)
Pediatr Obes
Child Obes
J Obes
Obes Facts
Oxid Med Cell Longev
Curr Opin Endocrinol Diabetes Obes
Diabetes Metab Syndr
Drug Metab Lett
J Clin Lipidol
Obes Res Clin Pract
Pediatr Endocrinol Diabetes Metab
Recent Pat Endocr Metab Immune Drug Discov
Appl Physiol Nutr Metab
Arch Osteoporos
Endocr Metab Immune Disord Drug Targets
Obesity (Silver Spring)
Cell Metab
Expert Opin Drug Metab Toxicol
Int J Obes (Lond)
Surg Obes Relat Dis
Curr Osteoporos Rep
Metab Syndr Relat Disord
Drug Metab Pharmacokinet
Lipids Health Dis
Best Pract Res Clin Endocrinol Metab
Curr Drug Metab
Int J Sport Nutr Exerc Metab
Obes Rev
Rev Endocr Metab Disord
Antioxid Redox Signal
Diabetes Metab Res Rev
Diabetes Obes Metab
Metab Eng
Curr Opin Clin Nutr Metab Care
J Clin Densitom
Mol Genet Metab
Diabetes Metab
Eat Weight Disord
J Trace Elem Med Biol
Redox Rep
Clin Calcium
Nutr Metab Cardiovasc Dis
Obes Surg
Osteoporos Int
Trends Endocrinol Metab
J Bone Miner Metab
Magnes Res
Endocrinol Metab Clin North Am
J Bone Miner Res
Metab Brain Dis
Bone
Glycoconj J
J Comp Physiol B
Ann Nutr Metab
J Cereb Blood Flow Metab
Am J Physiol Endocrinol Metab
Cell Calcium
Photosynth Res
J Inherit Metab Dis
J Bioenerg Biomembr
Adv Carbohydr Chem Biochem
Horm Metab Res
Carbohydr Res
Arq Bras Endocrinol Metabol
J Clin Endocrinol Metab
Metabolism
MICROBIOLOGY (124) includes Mycology - see also
Bacteriology, Parasitology, Virology
Pathog Dis
Bioengineered
Pathog Glob Health
Benef Microbes
Fungal Biol
Gut Microbes
PLoS Pathog
Pol J Microbiol
BMC Microbiol
FEMS Yeast Res
J Biosci Bioeng
J Mol Microbiol Biotechnol
Contrib Microbiol
Curr Opin Microbiol
Int Microbiol
J Microbiol Immunol Infect
Med Mycol
J Appl Microbiol
Microbiol Mol Biol Rev
Biocontrol Sci
Fungal Genet Biol
J Ind Microbiol Biotechnol
Microbes Environ
J Infect Chemother
J Microbiol
Klin Mikrobiol Infekc Lek
Acta Microbiol Immunol Hung
Microbiol Res
Microbiology
J Eukaryot Microbiol
Mikrobiol Z
New Microbiol
Trends Microbiol
J Mycol Med
J Microbiol Biotechnol
Roum Arch Microbiol Immunol
Braz J Microbiol
Rev Iberoam Micol
World J Microbiol Biotechnol

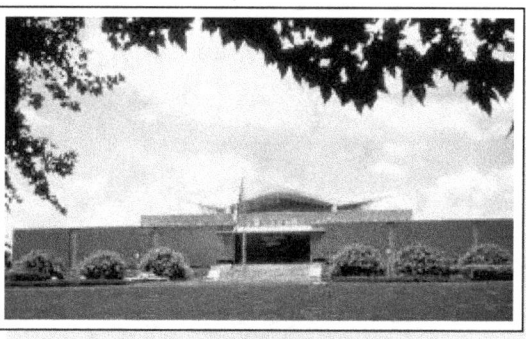

The National Library of Medicine, Bethesda, Maryland, completed in 1962, the current home of the Library. The unusual roof, portrayed as "art" is probably a shock wave deflector to protect from a nuclear blast, and the collection is protected by thick, Indiana limestone walls with most of it in underground floors with emergency supplies of water and food. The adjacent multi-story complex, below, was constructed about 1980 and is the Lister Hill Research Center of the Library.

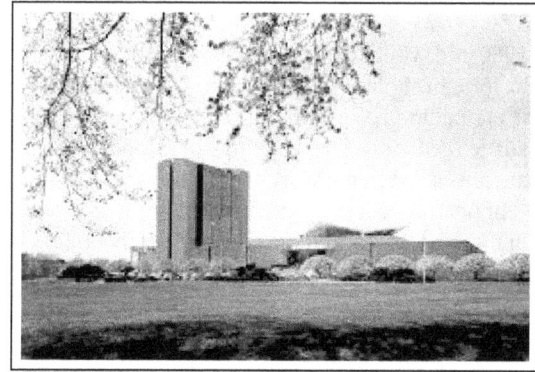

Ann Ig
Res Microbiol
APMIS
Eur J Clin Microbiol Infect Dis
Mol Plant Microbe Interact
Mycoses

Rinsho Biseibutshu Jinsoku Shindan Kenkyukai Shi
Mol Microbiol
Microb Pathog
FEMS Microbiol Ecol
FEMS Microbiol Rev
J Basic Microbiol

Lett Appl Microbiol
Mycotoxin Res
Yeast
Enferm Infecc Microbiol Clin
Food Microbiol
Int J Food Microbiol
Diagn Microbiol Infect Dis
Indian J Med Microbiol
J Microbiol Methods
Mol Gen Mikrobiol Virusol
Syst Appl Microbiol
Crit Rev Microbiol
Enzyme Microb Technol
Rev Argent Microbiol
Comp Immunol Microbiol Infect Dis
FEMS Microbiol Lett
Appl Environ Microbiol
J Clin Microbiol
Mycopathologia
Arch Microbiol
Microb Ecol
Med Microbiol Immunol
J Med Microbiol
Adv Microb Physiol
Curr Top Microbiol Immunol
Mikrobiyol Bul
Prikl Biokhim Mikrobiol
Adv Appl Microbiol
Folia Microbiol (Praha)
J Gen Appl Microbiol
Can J Microbiol
Wei Sheng Wu Xue Bao
Med Dosw Mikrobiol
Annu Rev Microbiol
Zh Mikrobiol Epidemiol Immunobiol
Antonie Van Leeuwenhoek
Mikrobiologiia
Mycologia
Ann Clin Microbiol Antimicrob
MILITARY MEDICINE (14) - includes Naval Medicine
Diving Hyperb Med
Biosecur Bioterror
J Spec Oper Med
Int Marit Health
Med Confl Surviv
MSMR
US Army Med Dep J
Undersea Hyperb Med
Ann Acad Med Stetin
Mil Med
Voen Med Zh
Vojnosanit Pregl
J R Nav Med Serv
J R Army Med Corps
MOLECULAR BIOLOGY (189) Includes Membrane
Dynamics - See Also Biotechnology
ACS Synth Biol
Adv Biol Regul
Cell Rep
GM Crops Food
G3 (Bethesda)
Nucleic Acid Ther
Open Biol
Genet Test Mol Biomarkers
Genome Biol Evol
J Mol Cell Biol
BMB Rep
Mol Brain
Mol Plant
Prog Mol Biol Transl Sci
Biomol NMR Assign
Mol Neurodegener
Med Mol Morphol
Mol Biosyst
Gene Expr Patterns
Genet Mol Res
OMICS
BMC Struct Biol
Biochem Mol Biol Educ
Biomacromolecules
BMC Genet
BMC Mol Biol
Genesis
Int J Mol Sci
Mol Plant Pathol
J Gene Med
Physiol Genomics
Comb Chem High Throughput Screen
Comp Biochem Physiol A Mol Integr Physiol
Int J Mol Med
J Biochem Mol Toxicol
Mol Genet Metab
J Mol Graph Model
Mol Cell
Exp Mol Med
Genes Genet Syst
Genes Cells
J Biomol Screen
Mol Psychiatry
J Mol Med (Berl)
Mol Model
Mol Hum Reprod
Mol Vis
Nat Med
RNA
Spectrochim Acta A Mol Biomol Spectrosc
Biocell
DNA Res
Macromol Rapid Commun
Matrix Biol

Chapter 7 - The National Library of Medicine

A Perspective On The National Library of Medicine

Mol Biotechnol
Mol Med
Res Commun Mol Pathol Pharmacol
Virchows Arch
Chromosome Res
Diagn Mol Pathol
Hum Mol Genet
Insect Biochem Mol Biol
Insect Mol Biol
Mol Biol Cell
Mol Ecol
Mol Phylogenet Evol
Curr Opin Struct Biol
Gene Expr
J Biomol NMR
Plant J
Transgenic Res
DNA Cell Biol
Genes Immun
J Steroid Biochem Mol Biol
J Struct Biol
Mol Cell Neurosci
Mol Cells
Protein Expr Purif
Am J Physiol Lung Cell Mol Physiol
Crit Rev Biochem Mol Biol
Genes Chromosomes Cancer
J Mol Neurosci
Curr Protoc Mol Biol
J Mol Endocrinol
J Mol Recognit
Mol Carcinog
Mol Plant Microbe Interact
Mol Reprod Dev
Environ Mol Mutagen
Genes Dev
J Comput Aided Mol Des
Mol Cell Probes
Mol Endocrinol
Mol Microbiol
Mol Neurobiol
Oncogene
Virus Genes
Z Naturforsch C
Bioessays
Biotechnol Genet Eng Rev
Methods Mol Biol
Orig Life Evol Biosph
J Biomol Struct Dyn
Mol Biol Evol
Mol Gen Mikrobiol Virusol
EMBO J
Biosci Rep
Mol Cell Biol
Plant Mol Biol
Mol Biochem Parasitol
Int J Biol Macromol
Mol Immunol
Gene
Bioorg Khim
Mol Aspects Med
Mol Cell Endocrinol
Mol Cell Biochem
Mol Biol Rep
J Mol Evol
J Mol Cell Cardiol
J Membr Biol
Prog Mol Subcell Biol
Adv Enzymol Relat Areas Mol Biol
Biochem Genet
Mol Biol (Mosk)
Mol Pharmacol
Prog Biophys Mol Biol
Exp Mol Pathol
J Mol Biol
Chromosoma

N

NANOTECHNOLOGY (21) Includes Nanomedicine - See
Also Biotechnology; Technology
Artif Cells Nanomed Biotechnol
J Appl Biomater Funct Mater
Theranostics
Nanoscale
Wiley Interdiscip Rev Nanomed Nanobiotechnol
ACS Nano
IET Nanobiotechnol
Nanotoxicology
Recent Pat Nanotechnol
Int J Nanomedicine
Nanomedicine (Lond)
Nat Nanotechnol
J Biomed Nanotechnol
Nanomedicine
Small
J Nanobiotechnology
IEEE Trans Nanobioscience
J Nanosci Nanotechnol
Nano Lett
Nanotechnology
J Phys Condens Matter
NEOPLASMS (206) Includes Medical And Experimental
Oncology Cancer Med
Cancer Discov
Cancer Genet
Cell Oncol (Dordr)
Anal Cell Pathol (Amst)

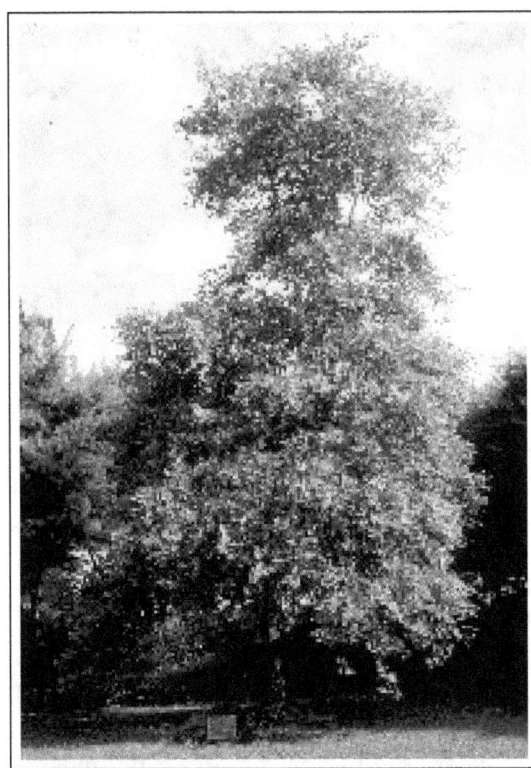

Commemorating Hippocrates. This tree (on the grounds of the Library) was grown from a cutting of the very tree under which Hippocrates is said to have conducted his classes some 2,500 years ago. It was planted at the library in 1960 and was a gift from the island of Cos, the historic birthplace of Hippocrates. Hippocrates is the father of Western, rational / non- spiritualistic medicine. The teachings of Hippocrates are preserved in the works known as the "Hippocratic Corpus," manuscripts of which are in the library. One of his ancient therapeutic maxims ("above all, cause no harm") is at the crux of intense controversy regarding the appropriateness of many current, conventional therapies.

Cancer Cytopathol
Clin Lymphoma Myeloma Leuk
Horm Cancer
Int J Surg Oncol
J Geriatr Oncol

Cancer Epidemiol
Head Neck Oncol
Nat Rev Clin Oncol
Oncotarget
Cancer Prev Res (Phila)

Chin J Cancer
Hematol Oncol Stem Cell Ther
J Hematol Oncol
J Med Imaging Radiat Oncol
Pigment Cell Melanoma Res
Rep Carcinog Backgr Doc
Gulf J Oncolog
Head Neck Pathol
J Cancer Surviv
J Gastrointest Cancer
Mol Oncol
ONS Connect
Curr Hematol Malig Rep
J Thorac Oncol
Radiat Oncol
Recent Pat Anticancer Drug Discov
Target Oncol
Asia Pac J Clin Oncol
Cancer Biomark
Clin Genitourin Cancer
Clin Lymphoma Myeloma
Clin Transl Oncol
Future Oncol
J Cancer Res Ther
J Oncol Pract
J Soc Integr Oncol
Exp Oncol
Pediatr Blood Cancer
Cancer Sci
Clin Adv Hematol Oncol
J Support Oncol
J Natl Compr Canc Netw
Vet Comp Oncol
World J Surg Oncol
Cancer Biol Ther
Cancer Cell
Integr Cancer Ther
Mol Cancer Res
Mol Cancer
Suppl Tumori
Technol Cancer Res Treat
BMC Cancer
Cancer Immun
Clin Colorectal Cancer
Curr Cancer Drug Targets
Expert Rev Anticancer Ther
Int J Gastrointest Cancer
Nat Rev Cancer
Asian Pac J Cancer Prev
Cancer Imaging
Cancer J
Clin Breast Cancer
Curr Treat Options Oncol
Fam Cancer
Lancet Oncol
Rep Carcinog
Breast Cancer Res
Clin Lung Cancer
Curr Oncol Rep
Neoplasia
Neuro Oncol
Eur J Oncol Nurs
Gastric Cancer
Zhongguo Fei Ai Za Zhi
Brain Tumor Pathol
Cancer Radiother
Clin J Oncol Nurs
J Immunother
Oral Oncol
Prostate Cancer Prostatic Dis
Cancer Biother Radiopharm
Int J Clin Oncol
J Exp Ther Oncol
J Mammary Gland Biol Neoplasia
Oncologist
Breast J
Clin Cancer Res
J Oncol Pharm Pract
Pathol Oncol Res
Urol Oncol
Ann Surg Oncol
Breast Cancer
Cancer Control
Cancer Gene Ther
Endocr Relat Cancer
Med Oncol
Oncol Rep
Support Care Cancer
Breast
Int J Oncol
Oncol Res
Psychooncology
Surg Oncol Clin N Am
Surg Oncol
Can Oncol Nurs J
Cancer Epidemiol Biomarkers Prev
Eur J Cancer Care (Engl)
Eur J Cancer Prev
Int J Gynecol Cancer
Melanoma Res
Semin Radiat Oncol
Ann Oncol
Cancer Causes Control
Eur J Cancer
J BUON
J Natl Cancer Inst Monogr
Semin Cancer Biol
Clin Oncol (R Coll Radiol)
Crit Rev Oncog
Curr Opin Oncol

Chapter 7 - The National Library of Medicine

A Perspective On The National Library of Medicine

Genes Chromosomes Cancer
Head Neck
J Pediatr Oncol Nurs
Leuk Lymphoma
IARC Monogr Eval Carcinog Risks Hum
Klin Onkol
Mol Carcinog
Acta Oncol
Cancer Detect Prev Suppl
Hematol Oncol Clin North Am
In Vivo
Leukemia
Oncogene
Oncology (Williston Park)
Int J Biol Markers
J Cancer Educ
Pediatr Hematol Oncol
Strahlenther Onkol
Eur J Surg Oncol
Int J Hyperthermia
Lung Cancer
Semin Oncol Nurs
J Environ Pathol Toxicol Oncol
J Assoc Pediatr Oncol Nurses
Leuk Lymphoma
IARC Monogr Eval Carcinog Risks Hum
Klin Onkol
Mol Carcinog
Acta Oncol
Hematol Oncol Clin North Am
In Vivo
Leukemia
Oncogene
Oncology (Williston Park)
Int J Biol Markers
J Cancer Educ
Pediatr Hematol Oncol
Strahlenther Onkol
Eur J Surg Oncol
Int J Hyperthermia
Lung Cancer
Semin Oncol Nurs
J Environ Pathol Toxicol Oncol
Tumour Biol
Cancer Invest
Clin Exp Metastasis
Crit Rev Oncol Hematol
Hematol Oncol
J Clin Oncol
J Neurooncol
J Psychosoc Oncol
Radiother Oncol
Am J Clin Oncol
Cancer Immunol Immunother
Cancer Metastasis Rev
J Exp Clin Cancer Res
J Egypt Natl Canc Inst
Med Pediatr Oncol Suppl
Anticancer Res
Breast Cancer Res Treat
Cancer Treat Res
Carcinogenesis
Eur J Gynaecol Oncol
IARC Sci Publ
J Cancer Res Clin Oncol
Zhonghua Zhong Liu Za Zhi
Cancer Chemother Pharmacol
Cancer Nurs
Nutr Cancer
Onkologie
Leuk Res
Oncol Nurs Forum
Curr Probl Cancer
Cancer Lett
Int J Radiat Oncol Biol Phys
Cancer Treat Rev
Gan To Kagaku Ryoho
Radiat Environ Biophys
Semin Oncol
Gynecol Oncol
Jpn J Clin Oncol
J Surg Oncol
Front Radiat Ther Oncol
Oncology
Bull Cancer
Int J Cancer
Recent Results Cancer Res
Indian J Cancer
J Radiat Res
Prog Exp Tumor Res
Magy Onkol
Neoplasma
Vopr Onkol
Adv Cancer Res
CA Cancer J Clin
Cancer
Br J Cancer
Cancer Res
J Natl Cancer Inst
Tumori
NEPHROLOGY (42) includes Dialysis And Hemodialysis
Nat Rev Nephrol
Arab J Nephrol Transplant
Iran J Kidney Dis
Clin J Am Soc Nephrol
J Ren Care
Nephrol Ther
Adv Chronic Kidney Dis
Nephron Clin Pract
Nephron Exp Nephrol

Nephron Physiol
BMC Nephrol
Hemodial Int
Nephrol Nurs J
Am J Physiol Renal Physiol
Clin Exp Nephrol
Kidney Blood Press Res
Nephrology (Carlton)
Saudi J Kidney Dis Transpl
Arch Ital Urol Androl
Curr Opin Nephrol Hypertens
J Ren Nutr
J Am Soc Nephrol

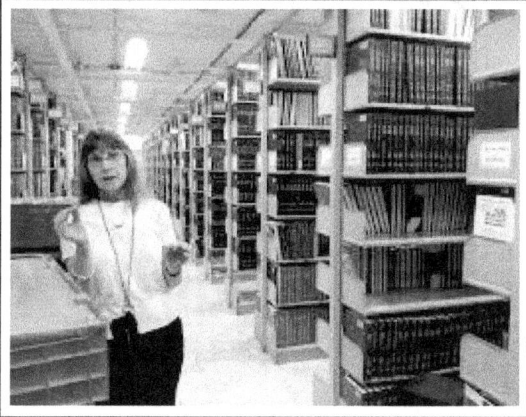

Stacks of the present library.

J Nephrol
Perit Dial Int
Semin Dial
Nephrol News Issues
Pediatr Nephrol
Ren Fail
Nephrol Dial Transplant
Adv Perit Dial
G Ital Nefrol
Minerva Urol Nefrol
Am J Kidney Dis
Am J Nephrol
Nefrologia
Semin Nephrol
J Bras Nefrol
Contrib Nephrol
Clin Nephrol
Kidney Int
Int Urol Nephrol
Nihon Jinzo Gakkai Shi
NEUROLOGY (295) includes Neurological Diseases And The Neurosciences
Amyotroph Lateral Scler Frontotemporal Degener
JAMA Neurol
Appl Neuropsychol Adult
Appl Neuropsychol Child
Neurodiagn J
Brain Connect
Dev Cogn Neurosci
Geriatr Psychol Neuropsychiatr Vieil
J Parkinsons Dis
ACS Chem Neurosci
Clin Neuroradiol
Cogn Neurosci
ASN Neuro
Curr Top Behav Neurosci
J Neurointerv Surg
Nat Rev Neurol
CNS Neurosci Ther
Brain Nerve
Can J Neurosci Nurs
Dev Neurobiol
Dev Neurorehabil
Front Neural Circuits
J Neuropsychol
Neurotherapeutics
Cent Nerv Syst Agents Med Chem
CNS Neurol Disord Drug Targets
Comput Intell Neurosci
J Neuroimmune Pharmacol
Mol Neurodegener
Neural Dev
Neuroradiol J
Recent Pat CNS Drug Discov

Soc Cogn Affect Neurosci
Soc Neurosci
Alzheimers Dement
Front Neurol Neurosci
J Clin Sleep Med
J Opioid Manag
Mol Pain
Neurosci Bull
Clin EEG Neurosci
Curr Alzheimer Res
Curr Neurovasc Res
J Neural Eng
J Neuroeng Rehabil

J Neuroinflammation
Neurodegener Dis
Neurocrit Care
Neuron Glia Biol
Purinergic Signal
Rev Neurol Dis
Am J Med Genet B Neuropsychiatr Genet
Cogn Behav Neurol
J Neurol Phys Ther
Auton Autacoid Pharmacol
J Integr Neurosci
J Pain Palliat Care Pharmacother
Lancet Neurol
Neurosignals
Neuroinformatics
Neuromolecular Med
BMC Neurol
Cogn Affect Behav Neurosci
Curr Pain Headache Rep
Curr Protoc Neurosci
Expert Rev Neurother
J Comp Physiol A Neuroethol Sens Neural Behav Physiol
Otol Neurotol
Pain Pract
Pract Neurol
Am J Alzheimers Dis Other Demen
Auton Neurosci
BMC Neurosci
Curr Neurol Neurosci Rep
Epilepsy Behav
J Headache Pain
J Musculoskelet Neuronal Interact
J Pain
Nat Rev Neurosci
Neurol Sci
Pain Manag Nurs
Pain Med
Sleep Med
Suppl Clin Neurophysiol
Clin Neurophysiol
Dialogues Clin Neurosci
Epileptic Disord
J Clin Neuromuscul Dis
Neuro Oncol
Neuropsychopharmacol Hung
Neurorehabil Neural Repair
Neurotox Res
Pain Physician
Int J Neuropsychopharmacol
J Alzheimers Dis
J ECT
Nat Neurosci
Neural Plast
Neuromodulation

Nutr Neurosci
Reg Anesth Pain Med
Dement Geriatr Cogn Disord
Eur J Paediatr Neurol
Eur J Pain
Motor Control
Neurogenetics
Sleep Med Rev
Acta Neurol Taiwan
CNS Spectr
J Neural Transm
J Peripher Nerv Syst
Laterality
Neuropsychol Dev Cogn B Aging Neuropsychol Cogn
Neurosciences (Riyadh)
Pain Res Manag
Spinal Cord
Stress
Child Neuropsychol
Dyslexia
Interv Neuroradiol
Invert Neurosci
J Neurovirol
J Spinal Cord Med
J Int Neuropsychol Soc
Mult Scler
Neurobiol Learn Mem
Neurocase
Neurologist
Neuroscientist
Parkinsonism Relat Disord
Psychiatry Clin Neurosci
CNS Drugs
Continuum (Minneap Minn)
Eur J Neurol
Folia Neuropathol
J Clin Neurosci
J Comput Neurosci
J Neuroophthalmol
Learn Mem
Neurobiol Dis
Neurogastroenterol Motil
Neuroimmunomodulation
Semin Pediatr Neurol
Curr Opin Neurol
J Orofac Pain
Neuropathology
Zh Nevrol Psikhiatr Im S S Korsakova
J Hist Neurosci
Seizure
Clin Auton Res
Curr Opin Neurobiol
J Neuroimaging
J Psychiatry Neurosci
Neuroimaging Clin N Am
Neuromuscul Disord
Neuropsychol Rehabil
NeuroRehabilitation
Cogn Neuropsychiatry
Eur Arch Psychiatry Clin Neurosci
Mol Cell Neurosci
Network
Neuropsychol Rev
Neuroreport
Agri
Eur J Neurosci
J Cogn Neurosci
J Mol Neurosci
J Neuroendocrinol
J Neuropsychiatry Clin Neurosci
Restor Neurol Neurosci
Behav Neurol
Glia
J Chem Neuroanat
J Geriatr Psychiatry Neurol
J Neurotrauma
Neural Netw
Neuron
Neurophysiol Clin
Somatosens Mot Res
Vis Neurosci
Alzheimer Dis Assoc Disord
Clin Neuropsychol
Epilepsy Res
Mol Neurobiol
Neuropsychology
Neuropsychopharmacology
Neurotoxicol Teratol
Schmerz
Synapse
Arch Clin Neuropsychol
Funct Neurol
J Child Neurol
J Neurosci Nurs
J Pain Symptom Manage
Mov Disord
Neurologia
Neuropsychiatr
Rev Neurosci
Childs Nerv Syst
Clin J Pain
Dev Neuropsychol
J Clin Exp Neuropsychol
Neurosci Res Suppl
Pediatr Neurol
Cogn Neuropsychol
J Clin Neurophysiol
Neurosci Res
Behav Neurosci
Int J Dev Neurosci

A Perspective On The National Library of Medicine

J Neurooncol
J Neurogenet
Neurol Clin
Ann Dyslexia
Clin Neuropathol
J Neuroimmunol Suppl
Neuroepidemiology
Neurourol Urodyn
Cell Mol Neurobiol
Cephalalgia
Fortschr Neurol Psychiatr
J Neuroimmunol
J Neurosci
Semin Neurol
AJNR Am J Neuroradiol
Neurobiol Aging
Neurochem Int
Neuropediatrics
Neuropeptides
J Neurosci Methods
Neuro Endocrinol Lett
Neurol Res
Neurotoxicology
Annu Rev Neurosci
Behav Brain Sci
Dev Neurosci
Muscle Nerve
Neurosci Biobehav Rev
Neurosci Lett Suppl
Trends Neurosci
Ann Neurol
J Neuroradiol
Neurochem Res
Neuroscience
Biol Cybern
J Neurosci Res
Neuropathol Appl Neurobiol
Neuropsychobiology
Neurosci Lett
Pain
Psychoneuroendocrinology
Can J Neurol Sci
Clin Neurol Neurosurg
J Neural Transm Suppl
J Neurol
Prog Neurobiol
Electromyogr Clin Neurophysiol
Rev Neurol
Acta Neurobiol Exp (Wars)
Acta Neurol Belg
Int J Neurosci
Neuropharmacology
Neuroradiology
Front Neuroendocrinol
Eur Neurol
Handb Clin Neurol
Neurol Neurochir Pol
Neuroendocrinology
Cortex
J Neurol Sci
Neurol India
Neuropsychologia
Acta Neurol Scand Suppl
Dev Med Child Neurol
Acta Neurol Scand
Acta Neuropathol
Headache
Rinsho Shinkeigaku
Exp Neurol
Int Rev Neurobiol
Neurol Med Chir (Tokyo)
J Neurochem
Ideggyogy Sz
Neurology
Zh Vyssh Nerv Deiat Im I P Pavlova
J Neurol Neurosurg Psychiatry
Arq Neuropsiquiatr
J Neuropathol Exp Neurol
J Neurophysiol
Seishin Shinkeigaku Zasshi
Nervenarzt
J Comp Neurol
Epilepsia
Rev Neurol (Paris)
Brain
J Nerv Ment Dis
NEUROSUGERY (30)
J Neurol Surg A Cent Eur Neurosurg
World Neurosurg
J Neurosurg Pediatr
J Neurosurg Spine
Neurosurg Focus
Acta Neurochir Suppl
Neurosurg Clin N Am
Pediatr Neurosurg
J Neurosurg Anesthesiol
Stereotact Funct Neurosurg
Turk Neurosurg
Br J Neurosurg
J Neurosci Nurs
J Reconstr Microsurg
Neurosurg Rev
Neurosurgery
Zh Vopr Neirokhir Im N N Burdenko
Adv Tech Stand Neurosurg
Clin Neurol Neurosurg
J Neurosurg Sci
No Shinkei Geka
Neurol Neurochir Pol
Prog Neurol Surg

Neurol Med Chir (Tokyo)
Neurochirurgie
Clin Neurosurg
Acta Neurochir (Wien)
J Neurol Neurosurg Psychiatry
J Neurosurg
Neurocirugia (Astur)

Radiats Biol Radioecol
Solid State Nucl Magn Reson
J Biomol NMR
NMR Biomed
Ann Nucl Med
IEEE Trans Ultrason Ferroelectr Freq Control
Physiol Chem Phys Med NMR

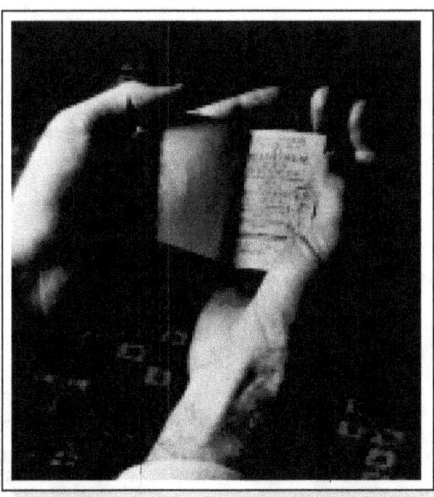

The Smallest Medical Book in the Library
&
The Largest Medical Book in the Library

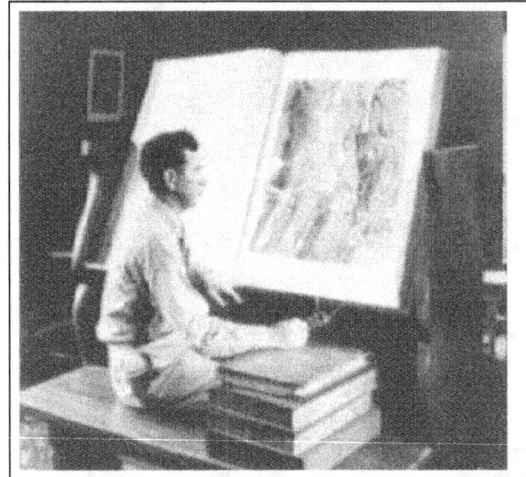

NUCLEAR MEDICINE (27) includes Radioisotopes - see
also Diagnostic Imaging; Radiology; Radiotherapy
Rev Esp Med Nucl Imagen Mol
Curr Radiopharm
Biomol NMR Assign
Hell J Nucl Med
Q J Nucl Med Mol Imaging
Eur J Nucl Med Mol Imaging
Nucl Med Rev Cent East Eur
Appl Radiat Isot
Nucl Med Biol

Radiat Prot Dosimetry
Nucl Med Commun
Clin Nucl Med
Nuklearmedizin
Rofo
J Nucl Med Technol
Semin Nucl Med
Prog Nucl Magn Reson Spectrosc
Kaku Igaku
J Nucl Med
Health Phys

NURSING (254)
J Nurses Prof Dev
J Am Assoc Nurse Pract
Int J Nurs Knowl
ORNAC J
Workplace Health Saf
Nurs Child Young People
Adv NPs PAs
Int Emerg Nurs
J Korean Acad Nurs
Midwives
NASN Sch Nurse
Res Gerontol Nurs
Can J Neurosci Nurs
Nurs Womens Health
ONS Connect
Prof Case Manag
AACN Adv Crit Care
Adv Emerg Nurs J
Int J Older People Nurs
J Perioper Pract
J Ren Care
Women Birth
Australas Emerg Nurs J
Complement Ther Clin Pract
J Forensic Nurs
Int J Nurs Educ Scholarsh
Jpn J Nurs Sci
Worldviews Evid Based Nurs
Nurs Leadersh (Tor Ont)
Perspect Infirm
Comput Inform Nurs
Eur J Cardiovasc Nurs
Int J Ment Health Nurs
J Spec Pediatr Nurs
J Fam Health Care
Nurs Educ Perspect
Res Theory Nurs Pract
J Infus Nurs
J Nurs Res
Ment Health Today
Nurse Educ Pract
Adv Skin Wound Care
Dynamics
J Midwifery Womens Health
J Nurs Scholarsh
Nephrol Nurs J
Nurs Law Regan Rep
Nurs Older People
Nurs Philos
Pain Manag Nurs
Policy Polit Nurs Pract
Prog Transplant
Assist Inferm Ric
Biol Res Nurs
Care Manag J
JONAS Healthc Law Ethics Regul
Nurs Health Sci
Alta RN
Community Pract
Eur J Oncol Nurs
Evid Based Nurs
Pract Midwife
Clin J Oncol Nurs
J Child Health Care
Midwifery Today Int Midwife
Journal ACITN.
CANNT J
J Addict Nurs
J Perianesth Nurs
Nurs Crit Care
Online J Issues Nurs
Soins Gerontol
Int J Nurs Pract
Int J Palliat Nurs
J Fam Nurs
J Am Psychiatr Nurses Assoc
Kai tiaki.
Nurs N Z
Soins Pediatr Pueric
Collegian
Creat Nurs
J Child Adolesc Psychiatr Nurs
J Cult Divers
J Psychiatr Ment Health Nurs
J Trauma Nurs
J Wound Ostomy Continence Nurs
Nurs Ethics
Nurs Inq
Nurs Manag (Harrow)
Pflege Z
S C Nurse
Aust Nurs J
Director
J Nurs Manag
J Nurs Meas
Nurse Res
Nurs Hist Rev
Pflege Aktuell
Rev Lat Am Enfermagem
Windows Time
Am J Crit Care
Aust Crit Care
Aust J Rural Health
Br J Nurs
Clin Nurs Res
Contemp Nurse
Emerg Nurse
Intensive Crit Care Nurs
J Clin Nurs

Chapter 7 - The National Library of Medicine

A Perspective On The National Library of Medicine

J Wound Care
Medsurg Nurs
Revue canadienne de nursing oncologique.
Can Oncol Nurs J
Enferm Clin
Eur J Cancer Care (Engl)
J Nurs Care Qual
J Sch Nurs
J Tissue Viability
Nurse Author Ed
ORL Head Neck Nurs
ABNF J
Br J Community Nurs
J Vasc Nurs
Tenn Nurse
Journal canadien en soins infirmiers cardio-vasculaires.
Can J Cardiovasc Nurs
Crit Care Nurs Clin North Am
Gastroenterol Nurs
J Pediatr Oncol Nurs
J Assoc Nurses AIDS Care
J Transcult Nurs
Appl Nurs Res
Revue canadienne de recherche en sciences infirmières.
Can J Nurs Res
Enferm Intensiva
Infect Control Hosp Epidemiol
Nurs Sci Q
Pflege
Urol Nurs
Arch Psychiatr Nurs
Clin Nurse Spec
Crit Care Nurs Q
J Pediatr Health Care
J Perinat Neonatal Nurs
Nephrol News Issues
Nurs Stand
Scand J Caring Sci
Holist Nurs Pract
J Cardiovasc Nurs
J Natl Black Nurses Assoc
J Neurosci Nurs
J Pediatr Nurs
Nutr Clin Pract
Colo Nurse
J Hum Lact
J Obstet Gynecol Neonatal Nurs
J Prof Nurs
Midwifery
Nurs Prax N Z
Rech Soins Infirm
Semin Oncol Nurs
Health Care Women Int
J Christ Nurs
J Community Health Nurs
Public Health Nurs
Annu Rev Nurs Res
Aust J Adv Nurs
Home Healthc Nurse
J Holist Nurs
Ky Nurse
Nurs Econ
Orthop Nurs
Patient Educ Couns
Plast Surg Nurs
Dimens Crit Care Nurs
Kinderkrankenschwester
Qld Nurse
Beginnings
J Psychosoc Nurs Ment Health Serv
Neonatal Netw
Nurse Educ Today
Nurs Manage
Rehabil Nurs
Crit Care Nurse
Geriatr Nurs
Issues
Krankenpfl J
Ostomy Wound Manage
Soins Psychiatr
Krankenpfl Soins Infirm
Rev Gaucha Enferm
West J Nurs Res
ANS Adv Nurs Sci
Aust Health Rev
Cancer Nurs
Curationis
Issues Ment Health Nurs
N J Nurse
Res Nurs Health
Rev Enferm
Oncol Nurs Forum
Perspectives
Insight
Issues Compr Pediatr Nurs
J Adv Nurs
MCN Am J Matern Child Nurs
Nurse Educ
Nurs Adm Q
Diabetes Educ
J Emerg Nurs
J Gerontol Nurs
Nurse Pract
Pediatr Nurs
AANA J
Tex Nurs
Am Nurse
J Nurs Adm
Nursing
Rev Infirm

J Contin Educ Nurs
J N Y State Nurses Assoc
Prof Inferm
Commun Nurs Res
Imprint
Rev-Esc Enferm USP
Nurs Clin North Am
AORN J
Int J Nurs Stud
J Pract Nurs
Perspect Psychiatr Care
J Nurs Educ
Nurs Forum
Soins
Fla Nurse
Rev Bras Enferm
Hu Li Za Zhi

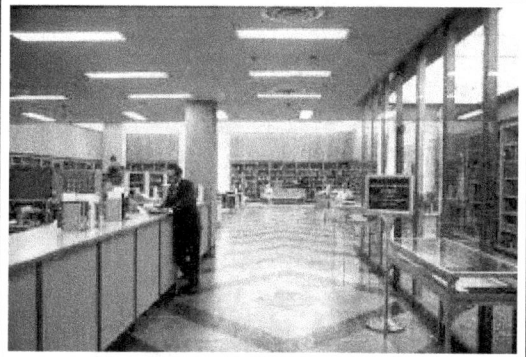

The Reading Room for the History of Medicine

Int Nurs Rev
Nurs Outlook
Servir
Nurs Res
Ahot Beyisrael
Ala Nurse
Nebr Nurse
Pa Nurse
Kans Nurse
Tar Heel Nurse
Miss RN
J Sch Health
Oreg Nurse
Mo Nurse
Prairie Rose
Ohio Nurses Rev
Mich Nurse
Okla Nurse
Can Nurse
Nurs J India
Nurs Times
Am J Nurs
School Nurse News
NUTRITIONAL SCIENCES (92) Includes Food, Animal Nutrition, And Vitamins
J Acad Nutr Diet
J Nutr Gerontol Geriatr
Nestle Nutr Inst Workshop Ser
Adv Nutr
Annu Rev Food Sci Technol
Food Funct
Food Environ Virol
Nutrients
Recent Pat Food Nutr Agric
Food Addit Contam Part A Chem Anal Control Expo Risk Assess
Food Addit Contam Part B Surveill
J Nutrigenet Nutrigenomics
Appl Physiol Nutr Metab
Breastfeed Med
Obesity (Silver Spring)
J Diet Suppl
Matern Child Nutr
Arch Anim Nutr
Foodborne Pathog Dis
Int J Behav Nutr Phys Act
Mol Nutr Food Res
Acta Sci Pol Technol Aliment
J Nutr Educ Behav
Nutr J
J Anim Physiol Anim Nutr (Berl)
Eat Behav
Int J Sport Nutr Exerc Metab

Food Drug Law J
Int J Food Sci Nutr
J Ren Nutr
Minerva Gastroenterol Dietol
Nutr Metab Cardiovasc Dis
J Nutr Biochem
Adv Food Nutr Res
Eur J Clin Nutr
J Hum Nutr Diet
Nutr Res Rev
Nutrition
Plant Foods Hum Nutr
Nutr Hosp
Nutr Clin Pract
Food Microbiol
Int J Food Microbiol
Breastfeed Rev
Clin Nutr
Food Chem Toxicol
J Pediatr Gastroenterol Nutr
J Am Coll Nutr
Nutr Health
Ann Nutr Metab
Annu Rev Nutr
Nutr Res
Appetite
Crit Rev Food Sci Nutr
Biol Trace Elem Res
Food Nutr Bull
Nutr Cancer
Adv Nutr Res
FAO Food Nutr Pap
J Food Prot
JPEN J Parenter Enteral Nutr
Meat Sci
Food Chem
J Nutr Sci Vitaminol (Tokyo)
Ecol Food Nutr
Int J Vitam Nutr Res
Arch Latinoam Nutr
J Food Sci
World Rev Nutr Diet
Am J Clin Nutr
J Agric Food Chem
J Sci Food Agric
Br J Nutr
Proc Nutr Soc
Vitam Horm
Nutr Rev
Vopr Pitan
J Nutr

O

OBSTETRICS (53) includes Midwifery - see also Gynecology; Perinatology; Women's Health
J Pregnancy
Sex Reprod Healthc
Midwives
Nurs Womens Health
Best Pract Res Clin Obstet Gynecol
BMC Pregnancy Childbirth
J Obstet Gynaecol Can
BJOG
Gynecol Obstet Fertil
J Midwifery Womens Health
Pract Midwife
J Am Coll Surg
Hypertens Pregnancy
Infect Dis Obstet Gynecol
Womens Health Data Book
Int J Obstet Anesth
Ultrasound Obstet Gynecol
Fetal Diagn Ther
Womens Health Issues
Curr Opin Obstet Gynecol
Arch Gynecol Obstet
Obstet Gynecol Clin North Am
J Hum Lact
J Obstet Gynecol Neonatal Nurs
Midwifery
Birth
J Psychosom Obstet Gynaecol
Prenat Diagn
J Obstet Gynaecol
Placenta
Rev Bras Ginecol Obstet
Gynecol Obstet Invest
Women Health
Eur J Obstet Gynecol Reprod Biol
J Gynecol Obstet Biol Reprod (Paris)
Int J Gynaecol Obstet
Akush Ginekol (Sofiia)
Aust N Z J Obstet Gynaecol
Clin Obstet Gynecol
Obstet Gynecol
Zhonghua Fu Chan Ke Za Zhi
Ginecol Obstet Mex
Obstet Gynecol Surv
Rozhl Chir
Am J Obstet Gynecol
OCCUPATIONAL MEDICINE (33)
Workplace Health Saf
Int J Occup Environ Med
Arch Environ Occup Health
J Occup Environ Hyg
Arch Prev Riesgos Labor
G Ital Med Lav Ergon
J Occup Health Psychol
J Occup Health
Int J Occup Environ Health
Int J Occup Saf Ergon
J Agric Saf Health
J Occup Environ Med
Sangyo Eiseigaku Zasshi
Int J Occup Med Environ Health
J Agromedicine
Occup Environ Med
Med Tr Prom Ekol
Occup Med (Lond)
New Solut
Work
Med Probl Perform Art
Toxicol Ind Health
Zhonghua Lao Dong Wei Sheng Zhi Ye Bing Za Zhi
Am J Ind Med
J UOEH
Occup Health Saf
Int Arch Occup Environ Health
Scand J Work Environ Health
Ind Health
Ann Occup Hyg
Arh Hig Rada Toksikol
Med Lav
EBRI Issue Brief
OPHTHALMOLOGY (78) includes Optics
JAMA Ophthalmol
Multisens Res
Ophthalmic Surg Lasers Imaging Retina
Binocul Vis Strabolog Q Simms Romano
Eye Sci
Nepal J Ophthalmol
Acta Ophthalmol Suppl (Oxf)
Acta Ophthalmol
Cutan Ocul Toxicol
Eye Contact Lens
Ocul Surf
BMC Ophthalmol
J Vis
Clin Experiment Ophthalmol
Vet Ophthalmol
J AAPOS
Opt Express
J Biomed Opt
Cesk Slov Oftalmol
Digit J Ophthalmol
J Ocul Pharmacol Ther
J Refract Surg
Mol Vis
J Neuroophthalmol

Chapter 7 - The National Library of Medicine

A Perspective On The National Library of Medicine

Ophthalmic Epidemiol
Ophthalmic Genet
Prog Retin Eye Res
J Opt Soc Am A Opt Image Sci Vis
Middle East Afr J Ophthalmol
Ocul Immunol Inflamm
Strabismus
J Glaucoma
Ophthalmologe
Eur J Ophthalmol
Curr Opin Ophthalmol
Oftalmologia
Vis Neurosci
Eye (Lond)
Korean J Ophthalmol
J Cataract Refract Surg
Semin Ophthalmol
Ophthal Plast Reconstr Surg
Cornea
Graefes Arch Clin Exp Ophthalmol
Orbit
Curr Eye Res
Dev Ophthalmol
Ophthalmic Physiol Opt
Retina
Int Ophthalmol
J Fr Ophtalmol
J Pediatr Ophthalmol Strabismus
Ophthalmology
Invest Ophthalmol Vis Sci
Opt Lett
Arch Soc Esp Oftalmol
Indian J Ophthalmol
Ophthalmic Res
Can J Ophthalmol
Klin Monbl Augenheilkd
Appl Opt
Exp Eye Res
Int Ophthalmol Clin
Vision Res
Jpn J Ophthalmol
Surv Ophthalmol
Am Orthopt J
Zhonghua Yan Ke Za Zhi
Arq Bras Oftalmol
Doc Ophthalmol
Ophthalmologica
Vestn Oftalmol
Klin Oczna
Br J Ophthalmol
Nihon Ganka Gakkai Zasshi
Bull Soc Belge Ophtalmol
Am J Ophthalmol
Trans Am Ophthalmol Soc
OPTOMETRY (6)
Optometry
Cont Lens Anterior Eye
Hindsight
Optom Vis Sci
Clin Exp Optom
Ophthalmic Physiol Opt
ORTHODONTICS (13)
Pol Orthop Traumatol
Orthodontics (Chic.)
Dental Press J Orthod
Int Orthod
Int J Orthod Milwaukee
Orthod Craniofac Res
J Orthod
J Orofac Orthop
Am J Orthod Dentofacial Orthop
Eur J Orthod
J Clin Orthod
Aust Orthod J
Angle Orthod
ORTHOPEDICS (77) includes Bone Diseases And Orthope-
dic Surgery
Bone Joint J
Bull Hosp Jt Dis (2013)
Musculoskelet Surg
Clin Orthop Surg
Orthop Surg
Orthop Traumatol Surg Res
Foot Ankle Spec
Rev Esp Cir Ortop Traumatol
Z Orthop Unfall
Arch Osteoporos
J Orthop Surg Res
Acta Orthop Suppl
Acta Orthop
Eklem Hastalik Cerrahisi
Head Face Med
Curr Osteoporos Rep
J Surg Orthop Adv
Musculoskeletal Care
Acta Ortop Mex
J Knee Surg
J Spinal Disord Tech
Spine J
BMC Musculoskelet Disord
J Musculoskelet Neuronal Interact
J Orthop Traumatol
Ortop Traumatol Rehabil
J Clin Densitom
Semin Musculoskelet Radiol
Foot Ankle Clin
Foot Ankle Surg
J Orthop Sci
Am J Orthop (Belle Mead NJ)
Eur J Orthop Surg Traumatol

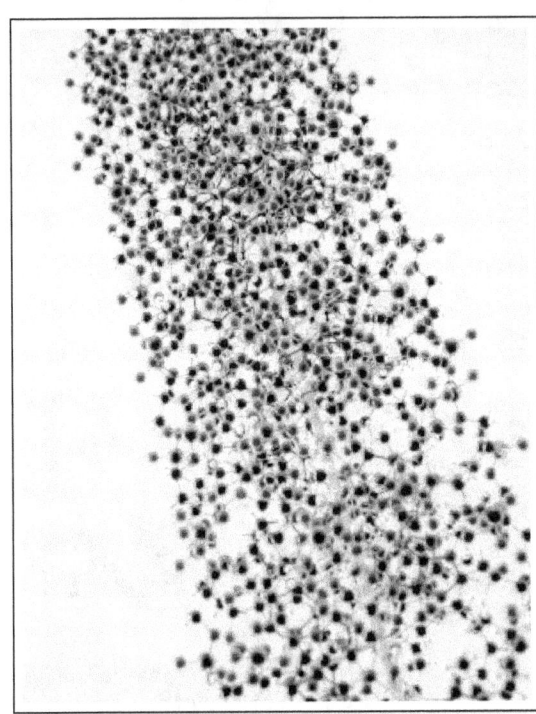

DNA model. Among the medical art/models of the Library is this DNA sculpture. It is huge and is suspended from the ceiling of the Reading Room, Building 38. It was originally placed in the library as part of an exhibit entitled: "The Genetic Code ... and How It Works," (1969). DNA is the physical "blue-print" of life. It contains information that can be translated into messenger molecule, RNA (ribonucleic acid), which in turn makes the specific amino acid sequence in functional proteins. Decoding the human DNA and manipulating its expression with chemicals such as "transcription factors" will be one of the principle technologies of medicine in the near future. The Human Genome Project is deciphering the sequences of DNA that make humans. The Library maintains the Gene Bank of this information, making the codes available to anyone in the world for research purposes.

J Clin Rheumatol
Foot Ankle Int
Knee
Gait Posture
J Foot Ankle Surg
J Orthop Surg (Hong Kong)
J Am Acad Orthop Surg
Osteoarthritis Cartilage
Sports Med Arthrosc
Eur Spine J
J Pediatr Orthop B
J Shoulder Elbow Surg
Foot (Edinb)
Hip Int
Osteoporos Int
Arch Orthop Trauma Surg
Oper Orthop Traumatol
Vet Comp Orthop Traumatol
J Orthop Trauma
Sportverletz Sportschaden
Zhongguo Gu Shang
J Arthroplasty
J Bone Miner Res
Arthroscopy
Bone
Hand Clin
J Orthop Res
Orthop Nurs
Iowa Orthop J
J Pediatr Orthop
J Orthop Sports Phys Ther
Orthopedics
Int Orthop
Prosthet Orthot Int
Skeletal Radiol
Spine (Phila Pa 1976)
Orthopade
Orthop Clin North Am
Clin Orthop Relat Res
Acta Orthop Traumatol Turc
Acta Chir Orthop Traumatol Cech
J Bone Joint Surg Am
Acta Orthop Belg
Instr Course Lect
OSTEOPATHIC MEDICINE (1)
J Am Osteopath Assoc
OTOLARYNGOLOGY (44) includes Rhinology - see also
Audiology
JAMA Otolaryngol Head Neck Surg
Int Forum Allergy Rhinol
Eur Ann Otorhinolaryngol Head Neck Dis
Am J Rhinol Allergy
J Otolaryngol Head Neck Surg
Lin Chung Er Bi Yan Hou Tou Jing Wai Ke Za Zhi
B-ENT
Clin Otolaryngol
Zhonghua Er Bi Yan Hou Tou Jing Wai Ke Za Zhi
Otol Neurotol
Braz J Otorhinolaryngol
J Assoc Res Otolaryngol
Curr Opin Otolaryngol Head Neck Surg
J Vestib Res
Kulak Burun Bogaz Ihtis Derg
ORL Head Neck Nurs
Eur Arch Otorhinolaryngol
Laryngorhinootologie
J Voice
Rhinol Suppl
Acta Otorhinolaryngol Ital
Otolaryngol Head Neck Surg
Am J Otolaryngol
Int J Pediatr Otorhinolaryngol
J Laryngol Otol Suppl
Ear Nose Throat J
An Otorrinolaringol Ibero Am
Auris Nasus Larynx
ORL J Otorhinolaryngol Relat Spec
Ann Otol Rhinol Laryngol Suppl
Rhinology
Adv Otorhinolaryngol
Otolaryngol Clin North Am
Acta Otorrinolaringol Esp
HNO
Nihon Jibiinkoka Gakkai Kaiho
Otolaryngol Pol
Vestn Otorinolaringol
J Laryngol Otol
Acta Otolaryngol Suppl
Acta Otolaryngol
Ann Otol Rhinol Laryngol
Laryngoscope
Rev Laryngol Otol Rhinol (Bord)

P

PAIN see Psychophysiology
PARASITOLOGY (34) includes Protozoology - see also
Tropical Medicine
Ann Parasitol
Ticks Tick Borne Dis
Parasit Vectors
Foodborne Pathog Dis
J Vector Borne Dis
Trends Parasitol
Parasitol Int
Parasite
J Eukaryot Microbiol
Korean J Parasitol

97

Chapter 7 - The National Library of Medicine

A Perspective On The National Library of Medicine

Acta Parasitol
Rev Bras Parasitol Vet
Bacteriol Virusol Parazitol Epidemiol
Zhongguo Xue Xi Chong Bing Fang Zhi Za Zhi
Parasitol Res
Zhongguo Ji Sheng Chong Xue Yu Ji Sheng Chong Bing Za Zhi
Exp Appl Acarol
Trop Biomed
Mol Biochem Parasitol
Parasite Immunol
Syst Parasitol
Turkiye Parazitol Derg
Vet Parasitol
Int J Parasitol
J Egypt Soc Parasitol
Parazitologiia
Folia Parasitol (Praha)
Adv Parasitol
Exp Parasitol
Med Parazitol (Mosk)
J Helminthol
J Parasitol
Mem Inst Oswaldo Cruz
Parasitology
PATHOLOGY (83) includes Pathologic Anatomy and Histopathology
Cell Oncol (Dordr)
Anal Cell Pathol (Amst)
Int J Clin Exp Pathol
Head Neck Pathol
Semin Immunopathol
Annu Rev Pathol
Diagn Pathol
Forensic Sci Med Pathol
Med Mol Morphol
Fetal Pediatr Pathol
Clin Physiol Funct Imaging
J Clin Exp Hematop
Pediatr Dev Pathol
Ann Diagn Pathol
Brain Tumor Pathol
Anat Pathol
Inflamm Res
Pathol Oncol Res
Adv Anat Pathol
Folia Neuropathol
Pathol Int
Pol J Pathol
Res Commun Mol Pathol Pharmacol
Virchows Arch
Int J Surg Pathol
Neuropathology
Cardiovasc Pathol
Diagn Mol Pathol
Exp Toxicol Pathol
Mediators Inflamm
Brain Pathol
Cytopathology
Endocr Pathol
Int J Exp Pathol
Pathobiology
J Oral Pathol Med
APMIS
APMIS Suppl
Int J Immunopathol Pharmacol
J Submicrosc Cytol Pathol
Mod Pathol
Histol Histopathol
Diagn Cytopathol
Turk Patoloji Derg
J Environ Pathol Toxicol Oncol
Semin Diagn Pathol
Clin Neuropathol
Int J Gynecol Pathol
Ann Pathol
Am J Forensic Med Pathol
Ultrastruct Pathol
Am J Dermatopathol
Calcif Tissue Int
Pathologe
Malays J Pathol
Pathol Res Pract
Toxicol Pathol
Am J Surg Pathol
Histopathology
Vet Clin Pathol
Arch Pathol Lab Med
Indian J Pathol Microbiol
Inflammation
Neuropathol Appl Neurobiol
J Cutan Pathol
Vet Pathol
Hum Pathol
J Pathol
Monogr Clin Cytol
Pathol Biol (Paris)
Pathology
Cesk Patol
J Comp Pathol
Exp Mol Pathol
Zhonghua Bing Li Xue Za Zhi
Rinsho Byori
Lab Invest
J Clin Pathol
Arkh Patol
J Neuropathol Exp Neurol
Am J Clin Pathol
Am J Pathol
Pathologica

PEDIATRICS (158) includes Adolescence and Child Development - see also Perinatology
JAMA Pediatr
Appl Neuropsychol Child
Paediatr Int Child Health
Pediatr Obes
Nestle Nutr Inst Workshop Ser
Nurs Child Young People
Child Obes
Horm Res Paediatr
World J Pediatr Congenit Heart Surg
Acad Pediatr
Ital J Pediatr

Arch Dis Child Educ Pract Ed
Fetal Pediatr Pathol
Pediatr Blood Cancer
Pediatr Emerg Med Pract
Semin Fetal Neonatal Med
An Pediatr (Barc)
J Dent Child (Chic)
Pediatr Endocrinol Rev
J Spec Pediatr Nurs
J Clin Child Adolesc Psychol
BMC Pediatr
Curr Probl Pediatr Adolesc Health Care
Eur J Paediatr Dent

Pediatr Transplant
Child Maltreat
Clin Child Psychol Psychiatry
J Pediatr Adolesc Gynecol
Z Kinder Jugendpsychiatr Psychother
Inj Prev
J Pediatr Endocrinol Metab
J Pediatr Hematol Oncol
Soins Pediatr Pueric
Arch Pediatr
J Child Adolesc Psychiatr Nurs
Semin Pediatr Neurol
Acta Paediatr Suppl
Acta Paediatr
Child Adolesc Psychiatr Clin N Am
Eur Child Adolesc Psychiatry
J Pediatr Orthop B
Semin Pediatr Surg
Cardiol Young
Eur J Pediatr Surg
Future Child
Int J Paediatr Dent
J Adolesc Health
Paediatr Anaesth
J Child Adolesc Psychopharmacol
J Clin Pediatr Dent
J Paediatr Child Health
Pediatr Allergy Immunol
Pediatr Neurosurg
Curr Opin Pediatr
J Pediatr Oncol Nurs
Pediatr Exerc Sci
Pediatr Phys Ther
Arch Dis Child Fetal Neonatal Ed
Cir Pediatr
J Pediatr Health Care
J Am Acad Child Adolesc Psychiatry
Paediatr Perinat Epidemiol
Pediatr Infect Dis J
Pediatr Nephrol
Pediatr Pulmonol Suppl
J Child Neurol
J Pediatr Nurs
Pediatr Hematol Oncol
Pediatr Surg Int
Childs Nerv Syst
Int J Adolesc Med Health
Pediatr Emerg Care
Pediatr Neurol
Pediatr Pulmonol
Br J Dev Psychol
Child Health Alert
Pediatr Dermatol
Rev Paul Pediatr
J Pediatr Gastroenterol Nutr
Med Pediatr Oncol Suppl
J Pediatr Orthop
J Dev Behav Pediatr
J Trop Pediatr
Neuropediatrics
Phys Occup Ther Pediatr
Brain Dev
Int J Pediatr Otorhinolaryngol
J Autism Dev Disord
Pediatr Med Chir
Pediatr Cardiol
Pediatr Dent
Pediatr Rev
Infant Behav Dev
J Adolesc
J Pediatr Ophthalmol Strabismus
Child Abuse Negl
Early Hum Dev
Issues Compr Pediatr Nurs
J Pediatr Psychol
Child Care Health Dev
Eur J Pediatr
Pediatr Nurs
J Abnorm Child Psychol
Pediatr Radiol
J Youth Adolesc
Klin Padiatr
Pediatr Ann
Child Psychiatry Hum Dev
Dev Psychol
No To Hattatsu
Dev Psychobiol
Pediatr Res
J Pediatr Surg
Indian Pediatr
J Exp Child Psychol
Adv Child Dev Behav
Clin Pediatr (Phila)
Dev Med Child Neurol
Turk J Pediatr
Pediatr Clin North Am
Prax Kinderpsychol Kinderpsychiatr
Zhonghua Er Ke Za Zhi
Minerva Pediatr
Child Welfare
Pediatrics
Psychoanal Study Child
Adv Pediatr
Monogr Soc Res Child Dev
J Pediatr (Rio J)
Indian J Pediatr
J Pediatr
Arch Argent Pediatr
Child Dev
Arch Dis Child

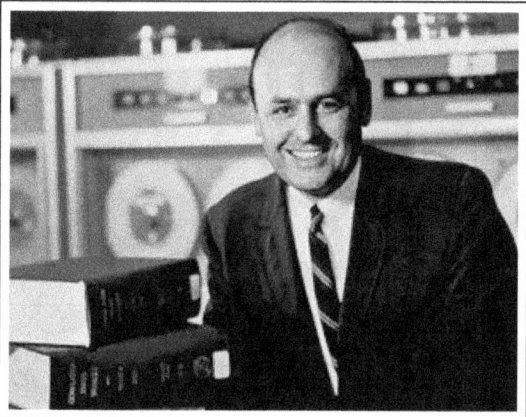

Martin M. Cummings, M.D. - Director of the Library (1964 to 1983). Under his twenty years of tenure, the Library's mission was broadened as a health information resource, emerging as a leader in the computer age, becoming a major biomedical communications center, and transforming the Library into the most advanced scientific library in the world. A major achievement was the planning and construction of the Lister Hill Center building which houses the research and development component of the library.

J Clin Res Pediatr Endocrinol
J Neurosurg Pediatr
J Pediatr Rehabil Med
Pediatr Neonatol
Adolesc Med State Art Rev
Dev Neurorehabil
Pediatr Endocrinol Diabetes Metab
Eur Arch Paediatr Dent
Evid Based Child Health
J Pediatr Urol
World J Pediatr
Afr J Paediatr Surg

Paediatr Respir Rev
Pediatr Crit Care Med
Paediatr Drugs
Pediatr Int
Zhongguo Dang Dai Er Ke Za Zhi
Clin Child Fam Psychol Rev
New Dir Child Adolesc Dev
Pediatr Dev Pathol
Eur J Paediatr Neurol
J AAPOS
J Child Health Care
Med Wieku Rozwoj

A Perspective On The National Library of Medicine

PERINATOLOGY - includes Neonatology
Neonatology
Nurs Womens Health
Complement Ther Clin Pract
Matern Child Nutr
Semin Fetal Neonatal Med
J Matern Fetal Neonatal Med
Adv Neonatal Care
Matern Child Health J
Z Geburtshilfe Neonatol
Fetal Diagn Ther
Arch Dis Child Fetal Neonatal Ed
J Perinat Neonatal Nurs
Paediatr Perinat Epidemiol
J Obstet Gynecol Neonatal Nurs
J Perinatol
Am J Perinatol
Neonatal Netw
Early Hum Dev
Semin Perinatol
Clin Perinatol
J Perinat Med
PHARMACOLOGY (200) see also Anti-Bacterial Agents;
Drug Therapy; Psychopharmacology; Toxicology
Drug Res (Stuttg)
BMC Pharmacol Toxicol
J Popul Ther Clin Pharmacol
Drug Test Anal
Pharmeur Bio Sci Notes
Curr Mol Pharmacol
Curr Radiopharm
Int J Comput Biol Drug Des
Drug Des Devel Ther
Drug Discov Ther
Drug Metab Lett
Expert Rev Clin Pharmacol
Recent Pat Drug Deliv Formul
Recent Pat Endocr Metab Immune Drug Discov
Recent Pat Inflamm Allergy Drug Discov
Antiinflamm Antiallergy Agents Med Chem
Cardiovasc Hematol Agents Med Chem
Cent Nerv Syst Agents Med Chem
Chem Biol Drug Des
ChemMedChem
Curr Clin Pharmacol
Curr Drug Saf
Expert Opin Drug Discov
J Neuroimmune Pharmacol
Mol Diagn Ther
Nat Prod Commun
Recent Pat Anticancer Drug Discov
Recent Pat Antiinfect Drug Discov
Recent Pat Cardiovasc Drug Discov
Recent Pat CNS Drug Discov
Curr Comput Aided Drug Des
Pharmacogenet Genomics
Pharmacol Rep
AAPS J
Basic Clin Pharmacol Toxicol
Curr Drug Deliv
Curr Drug Discov Technol
Drug Discov Today Technol
Expert Opin Drug Deliv
Mol Pharm
Q J Nucl Med Mol Imaging
Skin Pharmacol Physiol
Curr Vasc Pharmacol
J Pharmacol Sci
Mar Drugs
Profiles Drug Subst Excip Relat Methodol
Assay Drug Dev Technol
Auton Autacoid Pharmacol
Drug Metab Pharmacokinet
Expert Opin Drug Saf
Nat Rev Drug Discov
Pharm Stat
Vascul Pharmacol
Curr Opin Pharmacol
Curr Protoc Pharmacol
Expert Rev Pharmacoecon Outcomes Res
Int Immunopharmacol
J Pharmacokinet Pharmacodyn
Pharmacogenomics J
AAPS PharmSciTech
Acta Pharmacol Sin
Comp Biochem Physiol C Toxicol Pharmacol
Curr Pharm Biotechnol
Pharmacogenomics
Drugs R D
Expert Opin Pharmacother
J Pharm Pharm Sci
Pharm Biol
Value Health
Eur Rev Med Pharmacol Sci
Pulm Pharmacol Ther
Cancer Biother Radiopharm
Drug Discov Today
Environ Toxicol Pharmacol
J Cardiovasc Pharmacol Ther
Pharm Dev Technol
Clin Drug Investig
Curr Pharm Des
J Ocul Pharmacol Ther
Ceska Slov Farm
CNS Drugs
Int J Clin Pharmacol Ther
PDA J Pharm Sci Technol
Res Commun Mol Pathol Pharmacol
Biol Pharm Bull
Drug Deliv

Eur J Pharm Sci
J Drug Target
Acta Pharm
Ann Pharmacother
Eksp Klin Farmakol
Food Drug Law J
J Pharmacol Toxicol Methods
Pharmacoeconomics
Prescrire Int
Cell Physiol Biochem
Eur J Pharm Biopharm
Inflammopharmacology
J Biopharm Stat

J Physiol Pharmacol
Adv Pharmacol
J Basic Clin Physiol Pharmacol
Behav Pharmacol
Pharmacol Res
Zhongguo Zhong Yao Za Zhi
Drug Metabol Drug Interact
Drug News Perspect
Int J Immunopathol Pharmacol
Magnes Res
Pak J Pharm Sci
Adv Drug Deliv Rev
Aliment Pharmacol Ther
Fundam Clin Pharmacol
Immunopharmacol Immunotoxicol

J Control Release
Pharm Res
Invest New Drugs
J Pharm Biomed Anal
Int J Clin Pharmacol Res
Med Res Rev
Regul Toxicol Pharmacol
Biopharm Drug Dispos
J Cardiovasc Pharmacol
J Ethnopharmacol
J Nat Prod
Pharmacol Ther
Trends Pharmacol Sci

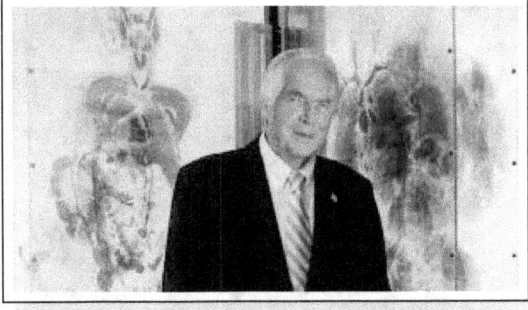

Donald A. B. Lindberg, M.D. - Director of the Library (1984 to the present). Dr. Lindberg is a specialist in medical informatics, and from 1992-1995 he served in a concurrent position as the founding Director of the National Coordination Office for High Performance Computing and Communications (HPCC) in the Office of Science and Technology Policy. He is author of three books: The Computer and Medical Care; Computers in Life Science Research; and The Growth of Medical Information Systems in the United States. He has written several book chapters, and more than 200 articles and reports.

Arch Pharm Res
Handb Exp Pharmacol
Int J Pharm
J Vet Pharmacol Ther
Drug Dev Ind Pharm
Annu Rev Pharmacol Toxicol
Clin Pharmacokinet
Eur J Drug Metab Pharmacokinet
Br J Clin Pharmacol
Clin Exp Pharmacol Physiol
Rev Physiol Biochem Pharmacol
Drug Metab Dispos
J Clin Pharmacol
Pharmacol Biochem Behav
Drug Metab Rev

Naunyn Schmiedebergs Arch Pharmacol
Drugs
Eur J Clin Pharmacol
Neuropharmacology
Chem Biol Interact
Indian J Pharmacol
Br J Pharmacol
Pharmacology
Prog Drug Res
Eur J Pharmacol
Mol Pharmacol
Can J Physiol Pharmacol
Drug Ther Bull
J Pharm Sci
Prog Med Chem
Clin Pharmacol Ther
Med Lett Drugs Ther
Toxicol Appl Pharmacol
Biochem Pharmacol
Chem Pharm Bull (Tokyo)
Proc West Pharmacol Soc
Indian J Physiol Pharmacol
Patol Fiziol Eksp Ter
Acta Pharm Hung
Yao Xue Xue Bao
J Pharm Pharmacol
Pharmacol Rev
Nihon Yakurigaku Zasshi
Ann Pharm Fr
Acta Pol Pharm
J Pharmacol Exp Ther
Boll Chim Farm
Yakugaku Zasshi
PHARMACY (36)
Int J Clin Pharm
Future Med Chem
Res Social Adm Pharm
J Am Pharm Assoc (2003)
Profiles Drug Subst Excip Relat Methodol
J Pharm Pharm Sci
Pharm Biol
Int J Pharm Compd
Pharm Hist Aust
Pharm Dev Technol
Am J Health Syst Pharm
J Manag Care Pharm
J Oncol Pharm Pract
Ceska Slov Farm
Int J Pharm Pract
Farm Hosp
J Pharm Pract
J Clin Pharm Ther
Consult Pharm
J Microencapsul
Veroff Schweiz Ges Gesch Pharm
Drug Dev Ind Pharm
Arch Pharm (Weinheim)
Pharm Hist (Lond)
Yakushigaku Zasshi
Pharm Hist
Theriaca
Yao Xue Xue Bao
Bull Cercle Benelux Hist Pharm
J Pharm Pharmacol
Pharmazie
Ann Pharm Fr
Am J Pharm Educ
Rev Hist Pharm (Paris)
J Pharm Belg
Yakugaku Zasshi
PHOTOGRAPHY (1)
J Vis Commun Med
PHYSICAL AND REHABILITATION MEDICINE (62)
includes Occupational Therapy
Braz J Phys Ther
J Physiother
Ann Phys Rehabil Med
PM R
Disabil Health J
Eur J Phys Rehabil Med
J Pediatr Rehabil Med
Dev Neurorehabil
J Cardiopulm Rehabil Prev
Disabil Rehabil Assist Technol
J Neuroeng Rehabil
J Neurol Phys Ther
J Rehabil Med Suppl
J Soc Work Disabil Rehabil
IEEE Trans Neural Syst Rehabil Eng
J Geriatr Phys Ther
J Rehabil Med
Phys Ther Sport
Neurorehabil Neural Repair
Ortop Traumatol Rehabil
J Dance Med Sci
J Bodyw Mov Ther
Physiother Res Int
J Spinal Cord Med
Man Ther
Occup Ther Int
Scand J Occup Ther
Top Stroke Rehabil
Disabil Rehabil
J Sport Rehabil
Qual Life Res
J Back Musculoskelet Rehabil
J Occup Rehabil
Neuropsychol Rehabil
NeuroRehabilitation
Torture

Chapter 7 - The National Library of Medicine

A Perspective On The National Library of Medicine

IEEE Int Conf Rehabil Robot
Phys Med Rehabil Clin N Am
Physiother Theory Pract
Assist Technol
Pediatr Phys Ther
Am J Phys Med Rehabil
Rehab Manag
Clin Rehabil
J Hand Ther
J Head Trauma Rehabil
J Rehabil Res Dev
Occup Ther Health Care
Rehabil Nurs
Phys Occup Ther Pediatr
J Orthop Sports Phys Ther
Int J Rehabil Res
Rehabil Psychol
Phys Ther
Aust Occup Ther J
Rehabilitation (Stuttg)
Vopr Kurortol Fizioter Lech Fiz Kult
Arch Phys Med Rehabil
Physiotherapy
Am J Occup Ther
Can J Occup Ther
Trans Am Clin Climatol Assoc
PHYSIOLOGY (120) includes Muscles - see also Psychophysiology
Compr Physiol
Food Funct
Sci Signal
J Exp Zool A Ecol Genet Physiol
Acta Physiol (Oxf)
Appl Physiol Nutr Metab
Int J Sports Physiol Perform
J Physiol Sci
Obesity (Silver Spring)
Physiology (Bethesda)
Rejuvenation Res
Skin Pharmacol Physiol
Musculoskeletal Care
Clin Physiol Funct Imaging
Electromagn Biol Med
Sports Biomech
BMC Physiol
Eur J Sport Sci
Exp Biol Med (Maywood)
J Anim Physiol Anim Nutr (Berl)
Phys Rev E Stat Nonlin Soft Matter Phys
BMC Musculoskelet Disord
Eur J Appl Physiol
J Musculoskelet Neuronal Interact
J Renin Angiotensin Aldosterone Syst
Suppl Clin Neurophysiol
Traffic
Acta Bioeng Biomech
Europace
J Clin Neuromuscul Dis
Physiol Biochem Zool
Comp Biochem Physiol A Mol Integr Physiol
J Physiol Biochem
Acta Myol
Am J Physiol Renal Physiol
Comput Methods Biomech Biomed Engin
Ross Fiziol Zh Im I M Sechenova
Semin Musculoskelet Radiol
J Neural Transm
Arch Physiol Biochem
J Clin Rheumatol
J Recept Signal Transduct Res
Fiziol Zh
Int MS J
J Gravit Physiol
J Appl Biomech
J Strength Cond Res
Physiol Meas
Rom J Physiol
Undersea Hyperb Med
J Physiol Paris
J Back Musculoskelet Rehabil
J Electromyogr Kinesiol
J Physiol Pharmacol
J Smooth Muscle Res
J Tissue Viability
Physiol Res
Exp Physiol
Herzschrittmacherther Elektrophysiol
J Basic Clin Physiol Pharmacol
J Cardiovasc Electrophysiol
Adv Physiol Educ
Am J Physiol Lung Cell Mol Physiol
Neurophysiol Clin
FASEB J
Clin Biomech (Bristol, Avon)
J Biol Rhythms
J Appl Physiol (1985)
Zhongguo Ying Yong Sheng Li Xue Za Zhi
Adapt Phys Activ Q
Chronobiol Int
J Clin Neurophysiol
J Comp Physiol B
Acta Physiol Hung
Arch Insect Biochem Physiol
Niger J Physiol Sci
Gen Physiol Biophys
Hum Mov Sci
Am J Physiol Endocrinol Metab
Am J Physiol Gastrointest Liver Physiol
Int J Orofacial Myology
J Muscle Res Cell Motil

Neurobiol Aging
Placenta
Muscle Nerve

Pacing Clin Electrophysiol
Am J Physiol Cell Physiol
Am J Physiol Heart Circ Physiol

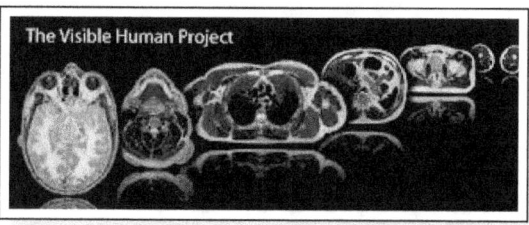

The Visible Human Project is an outgrowth of the NLM's 1986 Long-Range Plan. It is the creation of complete, anatomically detailed, library of three-dimensional representations of the normal male and female human bodies. Acquisition of the images of a representative male and female cadaver was done by advanced computer tomography (CT) and magnetic resonance (MR) technologies. The male was sectioned at one millimeter intervals, the female at intervals of one-third of a millimeter. The long-term goal of the Project is "to produce a system of knowledge structures that will transparently link visual knowledge forms to symbolic knowledge formats such as the names of body parts." Below is a section through the Visible Human Male - thorax, including heart (with muscular left ventricle), lungs, spinal column, major vessels, musculature (from Thorax data subset). Download a file of scans from the project at: http://www.nlm.nih.gov/research/visible/photos.html

Am J Physiol Regul Integr Comp Physiol
Proc Jpn Acad Ser B Phys Biol Sci
Biol Cybern
Fiziol Cheloveka
Clin Exp Pharmacol Physiol
J Neural Transm Suppl
Rev Physiol Biochem Pharmacol
Life Sci
Electromyogr Clin Neurophysiol
Usp Fiziol Nauk
J Mot Behav
J Biomech
Pflugers Arch
J Cell Physiol
Physiol Behav
Zh Evol Biokhim Fiziol
Can J Physiol Pharmacol
Chin J Physiol
Indian J Physiol Pharmacol
Patol Fiziol Eksp Ter
Physiologist
Sheng Li Ke Xue Jin Zhan
Sheng Li Xue Bao
Cesk Fysiol
Annu Rev Physiol
J Neurophysiol
Nihon Seirigaku Zasshi
Plant Physiol
Physiol Rev
J Gen Physiol
Harvey Lect
J Physiol
PODIATRY (3)
Foot Ankle Spec
Clin Podiatr Med Surg
J Am Podiatr Med Assoc
PRIMARY HEALTH CARE (32) includes Family Practice
J Prim Care Community Health
J Prim Health Care
J Am Board Fam Med
Ann Fam Med
FP Essent
Qual Prim Care
Inform Prim Care
J Fam Health Care
Aust J Prim Health
Educ Prim Care
BMC Fam Pract
Prim Care Diabetes
Prim Care Respir J
Prim Health Care Res Dev
Fam Syst Health
Semergen
Eur J Gen Pract
Fam Pract Manag
Br J Gen Pract
Occas Pap R Coll Gen Pract
Scand J Prim Health Care Suppl
Fam Pract
Aten Primaria
Scand J Prim Health Care
Fam Med
J Fam Pract
Prim Care
Aust Fam Physician
Am Fam Physician
Can Fam Physician
Fam Process
Practitioner
PSYCHIATRY (168) includes Mental Deficiency, Psycho-analysis, and Psychosomatic Medicine - see also Substance-Related Disorders
JAMA Psychiatry
Psychodyn Psychiatry
Epidemiol Psychiatr Sci
Geriatr Psychol Neuropsychiatr Vieil
Transl Psychiatry
East Asian Arch Psychiatry
Am J Intellect Dev Disabil
Asia Pac Psychiatry
Asian J Psychiatr
Atten Defic Hyperact Disord
Autism Res
Dev Disabil Res Rev
Rev Psiquiatr Salud Ment
Afr J Psychiatry (Johannesbg)
Clin Schizophr Relat Psychoses
Early Interv Psychiatry
Intellect Dev Disabil
Alzheimers Dement
J Intellect Disabil
Am J Med Genet B Neuropsychiatr Genet
Cogn Behav Neurol
Psychol Psychother
BMC Psychiatry
New Dir Youth Dev
J Psychiatr Pract
World J Biol Psychiatry
Actas Esp Psiquiatr
Bipolar Disord
Curr Psychiatry Rep
Nord J Psychiatry
Rev Bras Psiquiatr
Z Psychosom Med Psychother
Autism
Dement Geriatr Cogn Disord
Depress Anxiety
Int J Psychiatry Clin Pract
J Am Acad Psychiatry Law
Transcult Psychiatry

100

A Perspective On The National Library of Medicine

Clin Child Psychol Psychiatry
CNS Spectr
J Appl Res Intellect Disabil
J Atten Disord
J Intellect Dev Disabil
Mol Psychiatry
Z Kinder Jugendpsychiatr Psychother
J Am Psychiatr Nurses Assoc
Neurocase
Neuroscientist
Psychiatr Rehabil J
Psychiatr Serv
Psychiatry Clin Neurosci
Sex Abuse
J Child Adolesc Psychiatr Nurs
J Psychiatr Ment Health Nurs
Am J Geriatr Psychiatry
Behav Cogn Psychother
Clin Psychol Psychother
Downs Syndr Res Pract
Harv Rev Psychiatry
Zh Nevrol Psikhiatr Im S S Korsakova
Child Adolesc Psychiatr Clin N Am
Eur Child Adolesc Psychiatry
J Child Sex Abus
J Intellect Disabil Res
J Ment Health
Australas Psychiatry
Eur Psychiatry
Int J Methods Psychiatr Res
J Psychiatry Neurosci
Psychother Res
Cogn Neuropsychiatry
Eur Arch Psychiatry Clin Neurosci
Hist Psychiatry
Psychiatr Genet
Psychiatrike
Turk Psikiyatri Derg
Vertex
Acad Psychiatry
Ann Clin Psychiatry
Dev Psychopathol
Int Psychogeriatr
Int Rev Psychiatry
J Neuropsychiatry Clin Neurosci
Psychiatr Danub
Behav Med
Br J Psychiatry Suppl
Curr Opin Psychiatry
J Geriatr Psychiatry Neurol
Schizophr Res
Soc Psychiatry Psychiatr Epidemiol
Alzheimer Dis Assoc Disord
Arch Psychiatr Nurs
J Anxiety Disord
J Pers Disord
J Am Acad Child Adolesc Psychiatry
Res Dev Disabil
Int J Geriatr Psychiatry
Neuropsychiatr
Psychiatr Hung
Pharmacopsychiatry
Psychopathology
J Psychosom Obstet Gynaecol
Prog Neuropsychopharmacol Biol Psychiatry
Fortschr Neurol Psychiatr
Isr J Psychiatry Relat Sci
Psychother Psychosom Med Psychol
Soins Psychiatr
Can J Psychiatry
Gen Hosp Psychiatry
J Affect Disord
J Autism Dev Disord
J Marital Fam Ther
Psychiatry Res
Int J Law Psychiatry
J Clin Psychiatry
Psychiatr Clin North Am
Behav Modif
Cult Med Psychiatry
Sante Ment Que
Suicide Life Threat Behav
Neuropsychobiology
Psychoneuroendocrinology
J Sex Marital Ther
Psychiatr Prax
Int J Psychiatry Med
J Abnorm Child Psychol
Tijdschr Psychiatr
Arch Sex Behav
Hastings Cent Rep
J Pers Assess
Child Psychiatry Hum Dev
J Behav Ther Exp Psychiatry
Biol Psychiatry
Schizophr Bull
Adv Psychosom Med
Aust N Z J Psychiatry
Psychiatr Pol
Psychother Psychosom
Br J Psychiatry
Perspect Psychiatr Care
Psychoanal Rev
Acta Psychiatr Scand Suppl
Acta Psychiatr Scand
J Psychiatr Res
Compr Psychiatry
J Child Psychol Psychiatry
Psychosomatics
Riv Psichiatr

J Psychosom Res
Int J Soc Psychiatry
J Am Psychoanal Assoc
Prax Kinderpsychol Kinderpsychiatr
Int J Group Psychother
Am J Psychother
Psychoanal Study Child
J Neurol Neurosurg Psychiatry
Arq Neuropsiquiatr
Am J Psychoanal
Psychosom Med
Psychiatry
Bull Menninger Clin
Seishin Shinkeigaku Zasshi
Psychoanal Q
Am J Orthopsychiatry
Psychiatr Q
Am J Psychiatry
Int J Psychoanal
J Nerv Ment Dis
PSYCHOLOGY (178) includes Human Engineering, Hypnosis, Mental Health, Mental Processes, and Personality- see also Behavioral Sciences
Appl Neuropsychol Adult
Appl Neuropsychol Child
Geriatr Psychol Neuropsychiatr Vieil
Cogn Neurosci
Cyberpsychol Behav Soc Netw
Personal Disord
Appl Psychol Health Well Being
Atten Percept Psychophys
Top Cogn Sci
IEEE Trans Haptics
Rev Psiquiatr Salud Ment
Integr Psychol Behav Sci
J Neuropsychol
Neth J Psychol
Q J Exp Psychol (Hove)
Annu Rev Clin Psychol
Body Image
Psychol Serv
Cogn Behav Neurol
Evol Psychol
Exp Psychol
Int J Ment Health Nurs
J Clin Child Adolesc Psychol
J Pastoral Care Counsel
Psychol Psychother
Emotion
Ment Health Today
New Dir Youth Dev
Psychogeriatrics
Stress Health
Cogn Process
Am Indian Alsk Native Ment Health Res
Cultur Divers Ethnic Minor Psychol
Int J Emerg Ment Health
Arch Womens Ment Health
Clin Child Fam Psychol Rev
Dev Sci
Evid Based Ment Health
Hist Psychol
J Ment Health Policy Econ
Span J Psychol
Aging Ment Health
Autism
Nonlinear Dynamics Psychol Life Sci
Pers Soc Psychol Rev
Trends Cogn Sci
Br J Health Psychol
Clin Child Psychol Psychiatry
Fam Syst Health
J Health Psychol
J Occup Health Psychol
Neuropsychol Dev Cogn B Aging Neuropsychol Cogn
Psychol Methods
Psychol Health Med
Child Neuropsychol
Int J Occup Saf Ergon
J Exp Psychol Appl
J Int Neuropsychol Soc
J Gerontol B Psychol Sci Soc Sci
Neurocase
Assessment
J Clin Psychol Med Settings
J Psychiatr Ment Health Nurs
Psychon Bull Rev
Can J Exp Psychol
Clin Psychol Psychother
Memory
Anxiety Stress Coping
Conscious Cogn
J Ment Health
Psychooncology
Crim Behav Ment Health
Neuropsychol Rehabil
Psychother Res
Harv Ment Health Lett
J Gambl Stud
Neuropsychol Rev
Psychol Sci
Sch Psychol Q
Dev Psychopathol
Psicothema
Psychol Assess
Adm Policy Ment Health
J Sport Exerc Psychol
J Trauma Stress
Luzif Amor
Clin Neuropsychol

Cogn Emot
J Fam Psychol
J Pers Disord
Neuropsychology
Psychol Health
Psychol Addict Behav
Arch Clin Neuropsychol
Psychol Aging
Violence Vict
Death Stud
Dev Neuropsychol
J Clin Exp Neuropsychol
Cogn Neuropsychol
Br J Dev Psychol
J Comp Psychol
J Psychosoc Oncol
Can J Commun Ment Health
Health Psychol
J Exp Psychol Learn Mem Cogn
Br J Clin Psychol
Br J Soc Psychol
Clin Psychol Rev
J Psychosoc Nurs Ment Health Serv
J Marital Fam Ther
Behav Brain Sci
Issues Ment Health Nurs
Cogn Sci
J Pediatr Psychol
J Psycholtist
Sante Ment Que
J Exp Psychol Anim Behav Process
J Exp Psychol Gen
J Exp Psychol Hum Percept Perform
Pers Soc Psychol Bull
J Child Lang
Psychol Res
Am J Community Psychol
J Abnorm Child Psychol
Mem Cognit
Cognition
J Hum Ergol (Tokyo)
J Youth Adolesc
Perception
Rehabil Psychol
J Pers Assess
J Psycholinguist Res
Cogn Psychol
Psychol Med
Appl Ergon
Dev Psychol
J Consult Clin Psychol
J Learn Disabil
Int J Psychol
Br J Math Stat Psychol
Community Ment Health J
J Abnorm Psychol
J Pers Soc Psychol
J Exp Child Psychol
J Sch Psychol
Neuropsychologia
Psychotherapy (Chic)
Fam Process
J Relig Health
J Child Psychol Psychiatry
Scand J Psychol
Int J Clin Exp Hypn
Am J Clin Hypn
Hum Factors
Ergonomics
J Anal Psychol
Percept Mot Skills
Psychol Rep
J Couns Psychol
J Genet Psychol
Br J Psychol
Prax Kinderpsychol Kinderpsychiatr
Annu Rev Psychol
Am J Psychol
J Clin Psychol
J Pers
Acta Psychol (Amst)
J Psychol
Br J Educ Psychol
Am J Orthopsychiatry
J Soc Psychol
J Gen Psychol
Shinrigaku Kenkyu
J Appl Psychol
Psychol Bull
Psychol Rev
Am J Psychol
PSYCHOPHARMACOLOGY (21)
Harm Reduct J
Neuropsychopharmacol Hung
Nord J Psychiatry
Int J Neuropsychopharmacol
Essent Psychopharmacol
Nihon Shinkei Seishin Yakurigaku Zasshi
Exp Clin Psychopharmacol
Eur Neuropsychopharmacol
J Child Adolesc Psychopharmacol
J Psychopharmacol
Neuropsychopharmacology
Hum Psychopharmacol
Int Clin Psychopharmacol
Pharmacopsychiatry
Prog Neuropsychopharmacol Biol Psychiatry
J Clin Psychopharmacol
J Psychoactive Drugs
Clin Neuropharmacol

Psychopharmacology (Berl)
Pharmacol Biochem Behav
Psychopharmacol Bull
PSYCHOPHYSIOLOGY (53) includes Sleep Research
Multisens Res
BMJ Support Palliat Care
Dev Cogn Neurosci
Atten Percept Psychophys
Q J Exp Psychol (Hove)
J Clin Sleep Med
J Opioid Manag
Mol Pain
Behav Sleep Med
J Pain Palliat Care Pharmacother
Curr Pain Headache Rep
Pain Pract
J Headache Pain
J Pain
Pain Manag Nurs
Pain Med
Sleep Med
Suppl Clin Neurophysiol
Clin Neurophysiol
Pain Physician
Z Psychosom Med Psychother
Reg Anesth Pain Med
Appl Psychophysiol Biofeedback
Eur J Pain
Motor Control
Sleep Med Rev
Audiol Neurootol
Pain Res Manag
Sleep Breath
J Orofac Pain
Conscious Cogn
J Sleep Res
Anasthesiol Intensivmed Notfallmed Schmerzther
Agri
Somatosens Mot Res
Brain Behav Immun
Schmerz
J Pain Symptom Manage
Clin J Pain
Int J Psychophysiol
Brain Cogn
Cephalalgia
Sleep
Pain
Brain Lang
Biol Psychol
Perception
Biol Psychiatry
Dev Psychobiol
Physiol Behav
Psychophysiology
Headache
Percept Mot Skills
PUBLIC HEALTH (199) includes Community Health, Preventive Medicine, Public Health Policy, and Hygiene - see also Communicable Diseases; Environmental Health; Health Services; Health Services Research; Social Medicine, Statistics as Topic
Hawaii J Med Public Health
Med Sante Trop
Pathog Glob Health
J Epidemiol Glob Health
Western Pac Surveill Response J
Glob Health Promot
Glob J Health Sci
Int Health
J Environ Public Health
J Prim Care Community Health
Perspect Public Health
Disabil Health J
Emerg Health Threats J
Glob Health Action
J Infect Public Health
Popul Health Manag
Public Health Genomics
Am J Mens Health
Disaster Med Public Health Prep
Int J Public Health
J Health Life Sci Law
NCHS Data Brief
Prog Community Health Partnersh
Soc Work Public Health
Zoonoses Public Health
Dtsch Arztebl Int
Glob Public Health
Health Econ Policy Law
Int J Qual Stud Health Well-being
J Immigr Minor Health
World Health Popul
Global Health
Healthc Policy
Int J Prison Health
Issue Brief George Wash Univ Natl Health Policy Forum
J Res Health Sci
Salud Colect
East Afr J Public Health
HIV AIDS Policy Law Rev
Int J Environ Res Public Health
J Prev Med Public Health
J Public Health (Oxf)
Postepy Hig Med Dosw (Online)
Prev Chronic Dis
Health Qual Life Outcomes
Health Res Policy Syst
Appl Health Econ Health Policy
Int J Equity Health

Chapter 7 - The National Library of Medicine

A Perspective On The National Library of Medicine

MMWR Surveill Summ
Rev Peru Med Exp Salud Publica
Synth Proj Res Synth Rep
BMC Int Health Hum Rights
BMC Public Health
Eur J Health Econ
Policy Brief George Wash Univ Cent Health Serv Res Policy
Rural Remote Health
Yale J Health Policy Law Ethics
Health Promot Pract
Hisp Health Care Int
Int J Hyg Environ Health
J Health Popul Nutr
Policy Polit Nurs Pract
Bundesgesundheitsblatt Gesundheitsforschung
Gesundheitsschutz
Health Stat Q
MEDICC Rev
Nicotine Tob Res
Policy Anal Brief H Ser
Probl Sotsialnoi Gig Zdravookhranenniiai Istor Med
Rev Salud Publica (Bogota)
Scand J Public Health
Ethiop J Health Sci
Health Expect
Issue Brief (Mass Health Policy Forum)
Issue Brief George Wash Univ Cent Health Serv Res Policy
J Ment Health Policy Econ
J Urban Health
Policy Anal Brief W Ser
Public Health Nutr
Rev Esp Sanid Penit
An Sist Sanit Navar
Health Educ Behav
Kokuritsu Iyakuhin Shokuhin Eisei Kenkyusho Hokoku
Rev Panam Salud Publica
Rural Policy Brief
Adv Health Sci Educ Theory Pract
Aust N Z J Public Health
Cien Saude Colet
Environ Health Prev Med
Ethn Health
J Health Commun
J Health Serv Res Policy
J Prev Interv Community
Trop Med Int Health
Health Place
J Public Health Manag Pract
Rev Esp Salud Publica
Eur J Health Law
Health Hum Rights
Hist Cienc Saude Manguinhos
J Correct Health Care
J Med Screen
J Travel Med
Pac Health Dialog
Policy Brief UCLA Cent Health Policy Res
Cent Eur J Public Health
Health Care Anal
Health Law J
Ann Health Law
Aust J Rural Health
Cornell J Law Public Policy
Dev Health Econ Public Policy
Gesundheitswesen
Ethn Dis
Eur J Cancer Prev
Eur J Public Health
Health Matrix Clevel
Health Promot J Austr
Health Promot Int
N S W Public Health Bull
Ann Ig
Health Rep
Int J Drug Policy
J Aging Soc Policy
J Prev Med Hyg
MMWR Recomm Rep
Vital Health Stat 21
Sante Publique
Asia Pac J Public Health
Gac Sanit
AIDS Policy Law
AIDS Public Policy J
Am J Health Promot
Health Policy Plan
Health Serv J
J Law Health
Milbank Q
Am J Prev Med
Cad Saude Publica
J Rural Health
Community Dent Health
Health Policy
J Community Health Nurs
Public Health Nurs
Vital Health Stat 5
J Health Adm Educ
Vital Health Stat 3
Health Aff (Millwood)
Int Q Community Health Educ
J Policy Anal Manage
J Prim Prev
Annu Rev Public Health
J Public Health Policy
J Epidemiol Community Health
Popul Rep L
Fam Community Health
Vital Health Stat 23
J Health Polit Policy Law

MMWR Morb Mortal Wkly Rep
Rev Epidemiol Sante Publique
J Community Health
Probl Khig
Public Health Rep
Prev Med
Am J Public Health
Southeast Asian J Trop Med Public Health
Rev Saude Publica
Vital Health Stat 13
Ann Ist Super Sanita
J Public Health Dent
Vital Health Stat 4
Vital Health Stat 20
Demography
Vital Health Stat 11
Vital Health Stat 1
Vital Health Stat 10
Vital Health Stat 2
Cah Sociol Demogr Med
Shokuhin Eiseigaku Zasshi
Salud Publica Mex
Indian J Public Health
Arch Inst Pasteur Madagascar
Nihon Koshu Eisei Zasshi
Rocz Panstw Zakl Hig
World Health Organ Tech Rep Ser
Bull World Health Organ
Nihon Eiseigaku Zasshi
Ig Sanita Pubbl
Can J Public Health
Consum Rep
Gig Sanit
J Egypt Public Health Assoc
Arch Inst Pasteur Tunis
Trans R Soc Trop Med Hyg
Int J Health Geogr
Issue Brief Health Policy Track Serv
Issues Brief (Alan Guttmacher Inst)
Policy Brief Commonw Fund
Public Health
PULMONARY MEDICINE (81) includes Respiratory Tract Diseases, Thoracic Diseases, and Pulmonary Tuberculosis
Ann Am Thorac Soc
Respir Investig
J Bronchology Interv Pulmonol
Tuberk Biolezni Legkih
J Aerosol Med Pulm Drug Deliv
Clin Respir J
Expert Rev Respir Med
Gen Thorac Cardiovasc Surg
J Breath Res
J Cardiopulm Rehabil Prev
Ther Adv Respir Dis
Int J Chron Obstruct Pulmon Dis
J Cardiothorac Surg
J Thorac Oncol
Chron Respir Dis
COPD
J Bras Pneumol
Thorac Surg Clin
Multimed Man Cardiothorac Surg
Interact Cardiovasc Thorac Surg
J Cyst Fibros
Respir Physiol Neurobiol
BMC Pulm Med
Curr Allergy Asthma Rep
Tuberculosis (Edinb)
Heart Lung Circ
Paediatr Respir Rev
Prim Care Respir J
Respir Res
Clin Lung Cancer
Semin Thorac Cardiovasc Surg Pediatr Card Surg Annu
Zhongguo Fei Ai Za Zhi
Int J Tuberc Lung Dis
Pulm Pharmacol Ther
Allergy Asthma Proc
Respirology
Sarcoidosis Vasc Diffuse Lung Dis
Sleep Breath
Ann Allergy Asthma Immunol
Ann Thorac Cardiovasc Surg
Curr Opin Pulm Med
Rev Port Pneumol
Am J Respir Crit Care Med
Can Respir J
Semin Respir Crit Care Med
Asian Cardiovasc Thorac Ann
Monaldi Arch Chest Dis
Eur Respir Rev
J Cardiothorac Vasc Anesth
J Heart Lung Transplant
Pneumonol Alergol Pol
Pneumologia
Am J Physiol Lung Cell Mol Physiol
Pneumologie
Respir Med
Semin Thorac Cardiovasc Surg
Eur Respir J
Eur J Cardiothorac Surg
Pediatr Pulmonol Suppl
Zhonghua Jie He Hu Hu Xi Za Zhi
J Thorac Imaging
Pediatr Pulmonol
Rev Pneumol Clin
Rev Mal Respir
J Asthma
Clin Chest Med

Exp Lung Res
Thorac Cardiovasc Surg
Indian J Chest Dis Allied Sci
Lung
Heart Lung
Respir Care
Chest
Respiration
Ann Thorac Surg
Arch Bronconeumol
J Thorac Cardiovasc Surg
Tuberk Toraks
Kyobu Geka
Thorax
Kekkaku

Q

None

R

RADIOLOGY (65) includes Radiography - see also Diagnostic Imaging; Nuclear Medicine; Radiotherapy
Diagn Interv Imaging
Clin Neuroradiol
Jpn J Radiol
J Med Imaging Radiat Oncol
Radiol Phys Technol
J Cardiovasc Comput Tomogr
J Radiol Case Rep
Int J Comput Assist Radiol Surg
Neuroradiol J
Diagn Interv Radiol
Acta Radiol Suppl (Stockholm)
J Am Coll Radiol
J ICRU
Korean J Radiol
JBR-BTR
Tech Vasc Interv Radiol
Semin Musculoskelet Radiol
Interv Neuroradiol
Acad Radiol
Emerg Radiol
J Synchrotron Radiat
Vet Radiol Ultrasound
Eur Radiol
Semin Radiat Oncol
J Vasc Interv Radiol
BJR Suppl
J Xray Sci Technol
Int J Radiat Biol
J Digit Imaging
J Radiol Prot
Acta Radiol
Can Assoc Radiol J
Lasers Med Sci
Surg Radiol Anat
Eur J Radiol
Radiographics
AJNR Am J Neuroradiol
Cardiovasc Intervent Radiol
Radiol Manage
J Comput Assist Tomogr
AJR Am J Roentgenol
Curr Probl Diagn Radiol
J Neuroradiol
Skeletal Radiol
Int J Radiat Oncol Biol Phys
Rofo
Radiat Environ Biophys
Pediatr Radiol
Dentomaxillofac Radiol
Neuroradiology
Invest Radiol
Semin Roentgenol
Radiol Clin North Am
Radiol Technol
Rontgenpraxis
Radiologe
Clin Radiol
J Radiat Res
Radiologia
Radiat Res
Nihon Hoshasen Gijutsu Gakkai Zasshi
Br J Radiol
Radiology
Vestn Rentgenol Radiol
Radiol Med
RADIOTHERAPY (17) see also Nuclear Medicine; Radiology
Jpn J Radiol
Curr Radiopharm
Radiat Oncol
Q J Nucl Med Mol Imaging
Brachytherapy
J ICRU
Cancer Radiother
Cancer Biother Radiopharm
Med Dosim
Strahlenther Onkol
Radiother Oncol
Int J Radiat Oncol Biol Phys
Radiat Environ Biophys
Pediatr Radiol

Front Radiat Ther Oncol
Vestn Rentgenol Radiol
Z Med Phys
REPRODUCTIVE MEDICINE (48) includes Andrology, Fertility, and Sterility - see also Family Planning Services; Gynecology; Obstetrics
Andrology
Sex Reprod Healthc
Int Perspect Sex Reprod Health
Syst Biol Reprod Med
Reprod Sci
Soc Reprod Fertil Suppl
J Sex Med
Reprod Health
Reprod Biol Endocrinol
J Fam Plann Reprod Health Care
Reprod Abstr Ser
Reproduction
Reprod Biol
Reprod Biomed Online
Semin Reprod Med
Asian J Androl
Hum Fertil (Camb)
Hum Reprod Genet Ethics
Afr J Reprod Health
Int J Fertil Womens Med
Eur J Contracept Reprod Health Care
Hum Reprod Update
Mol Hum Reprod
Zhonghua Nan Ke Xue
Arch Ital Urol Androl
Reprod Health Matters
J Assist Reprod Genet
J Reprod Dev
Reprod Domest Anim
Am J Reprod Immunol
Int J Impot Res
Reprod Fertil Dev
Mol Reprod Dev
Reprod Toxicol
Hum Reprod
J Anim Breed Genet
J Reprod Immunol
Anim Reprod Sci
Andrologia
Theriogenology
Eur J Obstet Gynecol Reprod Biol
J Gynecol Obstet Biol Reprod (Paris)
Contraception
Theor Popul Biol
Biol Reprod
J Reprod Med
J Sex Res
Fertil Steril
RHEUMATOLOGY (32) includes Arthritis
Bull Hosp Jt Dis (2013)
Arthritis Care Res (Hoboken)
Nat Rev Rheumatol
Int J Rheum Dis
Reumatol Clin
Arthritis Res Ther
Best Pract Res Clin Rheumatol
Joint Bone Spine
Mod Rheumatol
Curr Rheumatol Rep
Rheumatology (Oxford)
J Clin Rheumatol
Osteoarthritis Cartilage
Lupus
Curr Opin Rheumatol
Rheum Dis Clin North Am
Clin Exp Rheumatol
Clin Rheumatol
Rheumatol Int
J Rheumatol Suppl
J Rheumatol
Z Rheumatol
Acta Reumatol Port
Scand J Rheumatol Suppl
Connect Tissue Res
Scand J Rheumatol
Semin Arthritis Rheum
Arthritis Rheum
Rev Bras Reumatol
Reumatizam
Reumatismo
Ann Rheum Dis

S

SCIENCE (45) includes Medical and Life Sciences; most of these Journals are Selectively Indexed
Sci Rep
Nat Commun
Sci China Life Sci
Sci Transl Med
Sci Signal
CBE Life Sci Educ
Nat Protoc
PLoS One
Nat Mater
J Philos Sci Law
Prev Sci
ScientificWorldJournal
Early Sci Med
Neuere Med Wiss Quellen Stud
Hist Cienc Saude Manguinhos
Public Underst Sci

102

A Perspective On The National Library of Medicine

Chaos
EXS
Sci Context
Nuncius
Kos
Sci Can
Politics Life Sci
Clin Sci (Lond)
Ber Wiss
Stud Hist Philos Sci
Hist Sci Med
Organon
Br J Hist Sci
Hist Sci
Physis Riv Int Stor Sci
Kwart Hist Nauki Tech
Endeavour
Kagakushi Kenkyu
Ann Sci
Osiris
An Acad Bras Cienc
Sci Prog
Proc Natl Acad Sci U S A
Naturwissenschaften
Science
Ann N Y Acad Sci
Nature
Am Nat
Sci Am
SEXUALLY TRANSMITTED DISEASES (12) see also
Acquired Immunodeficiency Syndrome; Dermatology
Sex Health
Sex Transm Infect
AIDS Patient Care STDS
Acta Dermatovenerol Alp Panonica Adriat
J Eur Acad Dermatol Venereol
G Ital Dermatol Venereol
Ann Dermatol Venereol
Sex Transm Dis
Indian J Dermatol Venereol Leprol
Acta Derm Venereol Suppl (Stockh)
Acta Derm Venereol
Actas Dermosifiliogr
SOCIAL MEDICINE (9)
Salud Colect
Attach Hum Dev
Scand J Public Health
Med Confl Surviv
Health Soc Care Community
Milbank Q
Rev Med Inst Mex Seguro Soc
Soc Sci Med
Cult Med Psychiatry
SOCIAL SCIENCES (50) includes Sociology and Ethnology
Biodemography Soc Biol
Can Rev Sociol
J Immigr Minor Health
Soc Cogn Affect Neurosci
Soc Neurosci
J Ethnobiol Ethnomed
J Soc Work End Life Palliat Care
J Evid Based Soc Work
SAHARA J
Econ Hum Biol
J Ethn Subst Abuse
J Soc Work Disabl Rehabil
Adv Life Course Res
Cultur Divers Ethnic Minor Psychol
Cult Health Sex
Stud Hist Philos Biol Biomed Sci
Pers Soc Psychol Rev
Ethn Health
J Gerontol B Psychol Sci Soc Sci
Health Hum Rights
J Cult Divers
Health Soc Care Community
Ethn Dis
Torture
Hum Nat
J Transcult Nurs
Soc Psychiatry Psychiatr Epidemiol
J Interpers Violence
J Natl Black Nurses Assoc
J Psychosoc Oncol
Med Anthropol Q
Soc Sci Med
J Ethnopharmacol
Sociol Health Illn
J Gerontol Soc Work
Cult Med Psychiatry
Med Anthropol
Health Soc Work
Soc Stud Sci
Soc Work Health Care
Soc Sci Res
Rev Law Soc Change
J Biosoc Sci
AJS
Fam Process
Cah Sociol Demogr Med
J Relig Health
Soc Work
Br J Sociol
Anthropol Anz
SPEECH-LANGUAGE PATHOLOGY (18) includes
Communicative and Language Disorders
J Soc Bras Fonoaudiol
Int J Speech Lang Pathol
Int J Lang Commun Disord
J Speech Lang Hear Res

Logoped Phoniatr Vocol
Folia Phoniatr Logop
Am J Speech Lang Pathol
Clin Linguist Phon
Augment Altern Commun
Semin Speech Lang
S Afr J Commun Disord
Brain Lang
J Fluency Disord
Lang Speech Hear Serv Sch
J Commun Disord
Lang Speech
Phonetica
J Acoust Soc Am
SPORTS MEDICINE (38)
Appl Physiol Nutr Metab
Diving Hyperb Med
Int J Sports Physiol Perform
Int J Behav Nutr Phys Act
J Phys Act Health
Res Sports Med
Curr Sports Med Rep
Sports Biomech
Eur J Sport Sci
Int J Sport Nutr Exerc Metab
Phys Ther Sport
J Sci Med Sport
J Dance Med Sci
J Appl Biomech
Knee Surg Sports Traumatol Arthrosc
Sports Med Arthrosc
Undersea Hyperb Med
J Athl Train
J Sport Rehabil
Clin J Sport Med
Scand J Med Sci Sports
Pediatr Exerc Sci
J Sport Exerc Psychol
Sportverletz Sportschaden
Adapt Phys Activ Q
Med Sport Sci
Sports Med
J Sports Sci
Clin Sports Med
Int J Sports Med
Med Sci Sports Exerc
Res Q Exerc Sport
J Orthop Sports Phys Ther
Am J Sports Med
Exerc Sport Sci Rev
Phys Sportsmed
Br J Sports Med
J Sports Med Phys Fitness
STATISTICS AS TOPIC (41) includes Biometry, Demography, Mathematics, and Risk Factors - see also Vital Statistics
Int j numer method biomed eng
Healthy People Stat Notes
Natl Health Stat Report
NCHS Data Brief
Int J Biostat
Pharm Stat
Stat Appl Genet Mol Biol
Phys Rev E Stat Nonlin Soft Matter Phys
Biostatistics
J Appl Meas
Health Stat Q
Philos Trans A Math Phys Eng Sci
Health Care Financ Rev Stat Suppl
Lifetime Data Anal
Evol Comput
Annu Stat Suppl Soc Secur Bull
Stat Methods Med Res
J Biopharm Stat
Health Rep
Vital Health Stat 21
Vital Health Stat 5
Vital Health Stat 3
Stat Med
Risk Anal
Biom J
Vital Health Stat 23
Bull Math Biol
Math Biosci
Vital Health Stat 13
Br J Math Stat Psychol
Vital Health Stat 4
Vital Health Stat 20
Demography
Vital Health Stat 11
Vital Health Stat 1
Vital Health Stat 10
Vital Health Stat 2
Cah Sociol Demogr Med
Biometrics
Wkly Epidemiol Rec
SUBSTANCE-RELATED DISORDERS (38) includes
Alcoholism, Drug Addiction, and Drug Abuse - see also
Psychiatry; Psychology
Alcohol Res
J Stud Alcohol Drugs Suppl
Curr Drug Abuse Rev
Addict Sci Clin Pract
J Addict Med
J Stud Alcohol Drugs
Subst Abuse Treat Prev Policy
J Opioid Manag
Harm Reduct J
Issue Brief (George Wash Univ Med Cent Ensuring Solut
Alcohol Probl)

J Ethn Subst Abuse
Addict Biol
J Addict Nurs
Nihon Arukoru Yakubutsu Igakkai Zasshi
Subst Use Misuse
Eur Addict Res
Addiction
Am J Addict
Tob Control
J Addict Dis
Drug Alcohol Rev
Adicciones
Int J Drug Policy
Alcohol Alcohol Suppl
Psychol Addict Behav
Alcohol
J Subst Abuse Treat
Alcohol Alcohol
Recent Dev Alcohol
J Psychoactive Drugs
Subst Abus
Alcohol Clin Exp Res
NIDA Res Monogr
Addict Behav
Drug Alcohol Depend
Am J Drug Alcohol Abuse
J Drug Educ
Bull Narc
SURGERY SEE GENERAL SURGERY

T

TECHNOLOGY (37) see also Biomedical Engineering;
Biotechnology; Nanotechnology
Adv Healthc Mater
Annu Rev Food Sci Technol
Mater Sci Eng C Mater Biol Appl
Radiol Phys Technol
Int J Med Robot
NIH Consens State Sci Statements
Ont Health Technol Assess Ser
Sensors (Basel)
Dev Biol (Basel)
ScientificWorldJournal
Evid Rep Technol Assess (Full Rep)
J Capill Electrophor Microchip Technol
Value Health
Health Technol Assess
Br J Biomed Sci
Technol Health Care
Bioresour Technol
Biotech Histochem
J Long Term Eff Med Implants
Stud Health Technol Inform
Surg Technol Int
Biologicals
Environ Technol
IEEE Int Conf Rehabil Robot
Assist Technol
Clin Lab Sci
Zhongguo Yi Liao Qi Xie Za Zhi
J Clin Lab Anal
Int J Technol Assess Health Care
Stand News
J Med Eng Technol
Health Devices
J Extra Corpor Technol
Med Tekh
NTM
Technol Cult
Kwart Hist Nauki Tech
TERATOLOGY (5) includes Abnormalities
Birth Defects Res A Clin Mol Teratol
Birth Defects Res B Dev Reprod Toxicol
Birth Defects Res C Embryo Today
Clin Dysmorphol
Congenit Anom (Kyoto)
THERAPEUTICS (97) see also Complementary Therapies;
Drug Therapy; Radiotherapy
Hum Gene Ther Clin Dev
Hum Gene Ther Methods
BMJ Support Palliat Care
Stem Cells Transl Med
Theranostics
Cardiovasc Interv Ther
Stem Cell Res Ther
Ther Deliv
Immunotherapy
Cardiovasc Ther
CNS Neurosci Ther
Curr Opin Support Palliat Care
Ther Adv Cardiovasc Dis
Ther Adv Respir Dis
Curr Stem Cell Res Ther
Rev Recent Clin Trials
Trials
Contemp Clin Trials
EuroIntervention
J Cancer Res Ther
J Soc Work End Life Palliat Care
Nephrol Ther
Clin Trials
Expert Rev Med Devices
Photodiagnosis Photodyn Ther
Expert Rev Cardiovasc Ther
Palliat Support Care
Cancer Biol Ther
Cogn Behav Ther

Integr Cancer Ther
Psychol Psychother
Technol Cancer Res Treat
Curr Gene Ther
Expert Opin Biol Ther
Expert Opin Ther Targets
Expert Rev Anticancer Ther
Expert Rev Neurother
Hemodial Int
HIV Clin Trials
Mol Ther
Cytotherapy
Diabetes Technol Ther
J ECT
J HIV Ther
J Palliat Med
BioDrugs
J Immunother
Cancer Biother Radiopharm
J Bodyw Mov Ther
Minim Invasive Ther Allied Technol
Am J Ther
Cancer Gene Ther
Expert Opin Ther Pat
Gene Ther
GMHC Treat Issues
Clin Psychol Psychother
Qual Life Res
Gastrointest Endosc Clin N Am
Psychother Res
Am J Hosp Palliat Care
BETA
Hum Gene Ther
Int J Risk Saf Med
Lasers Surg Med Suppl
TreatmentUpdate
J Clin Pharm Ther
Palliat Med
J Pain Symptom Manage
Int J Hyperthermia
J Palliat Care
Adv Ther
Cancer Immunol Immunother
Cancer Treat Res
Lasers Surg Med
J Marital Fam Ther
Pharmacol Ther
J Vet Pharmacol Ther
Clin Ther
Int J Offender Ther Comp Criminol
Behav Ther
J Behav Ther Exp Psychiatry
Endoscopy
Gastrointest Endosc
Psychother Psychosom
Behav Res Ther
Psychotherapy (Chic)
Ther Umsch
Int J Clin Exp Hypn
Med Lett Drugs Ther
Am J Clin Hypn
Patol Fiziol Eksp Ter
Am Orthopt J
Clin Ter
Int J Group Psychother
Am J Psychother
Therapie
Ter Arkh
TOXICOLOGY (88) includes Pesticides, Poisoning, and
Xenobiotics
BMC Pharmacol Toxicol
NTP Monogr
Toxins (Basel)
ChemSusChem
Rep Carcinog Backgr Doc
Nanotoxicology
Clin Toxicol (Phila)
Cutan Ocul Toxicol
Expert Opin Drug Metab Toxicol
J Med Toxicol
Natl Toxicol Program Genet Modif Model Rep
Basic Clin Pharmacol Toxicol
J Immunotoxicol
Part Fibre Toxicol
Birth Defects Res B Dev Reprod Toxicol
Toxicol Mech Methods
Cardiovasc Toxicol
Comp Biochem Physiol C Toxicol Pharmacol
Pest Manag Sci
Rep Carcinog
Curr Protoc Toxicol
Environ Toxicol
J Biochem Mol Toxicol
J Environ Sci Health A Tox Hazard Subst Environ Eng
J Toxicol Environ Health A
J Toxicol Environ Health B Crit Rev
Toxicol Sci
Eur Rev Med Pharmacol Sci
Int J Toxicol
Environ Toxicol Pharmacol
Environ Sci Pollut Res Int
Ecotoxicology
Exp Toxicol Pathol
J Pharmacol Toxicol Methods
Toxic Rep Ser
Water Environ Res
J Environ Sci Health C Environ Carcinog Ecotoxicol Rev
Drug Saf
Environ Technol
Hum Exp Toxicol

Chapter 7 - The National Library of Medicine

A Perspective On The National Library of Medicine

Inhal Toxicol
Waste Manag
Chem Res Toxicol
IARC Monogr Eval Carcinog Risks Hum
Chudoku Kenkyu
Immunopharmacol Immunotoxicol
Neurotoxicol Teratol
Reprod Toxicol
Rev Environ Contam Toxicol
Toxicol In Vitro
J Contam Hydrol
Toxicol Ind Health
Cell Biol Toxicol
J Environ Pathol Toxicol Oncol
Waste Manag Res
Environ Toxicol Chem
Food Chem Toxicol
Natl Toxicol Program Tech Rep Ser
Aquat Toxicol
J Appl Toxicol
Regul Toxicol Pharmacol
Water Sci Technol
Crit Rev Toxicol
J Environ Biol
Neurotoxicology
Environ Int
Mar Environ Res
Toxicol Pathol
Drug Chem Toxicol
Ecotoxicol Environ Saf
J Anal Toxicol
Toxicol Lett
Annu Rev Pharmacol Toxicol
Environ Manage
J Environ Sci Health B
J Toxicol Sci
Arch Toxicol
Arch Environ Contam Toxicol
Toxicology
Ambio
Xenobiotica
Arch Med Sadowej Kryminol
Water Res
Bull Environ Contam Toxicol
Ground Water
Toxicon
Toxicol Appl Pharmacol
Arh Hig Rada Toksikol
TRANSPLANTATION (28) - includes Artificial Organs
Chimerism
Exp Clin Transplant
Am J Transplant
Cell Tissue Bank
Liver Transpl
Prog Transplant
Transpl Infect Dis
Pediatr Transplant
Ann Transplant
Biol Blood Marrow Transplant
Saudi J Kidney Dis Transpl
Xenotransplantation
Transpl Immunol
ASAIO J
Cell Transplant
J Heart Lung Transplant
Curr Opin Organ Transplant
Transpl Int
Clin Transplant
Transplant Rev (Orlando)
Bone Marrow Transplant
Clin Transpl
Nephrol Dial Transplant
Int J Artif Organs
Artif Organs
Immunol Rev
Transplant Proc
Transplantation
TRAUMATOLOGY (46) includes Wounds, Injuries, and Accidents
J Trauma Acute Care Surg
Pol J Orthop Traumatol
Chronic Dis Inj Can
J Inj Violence Res
Orthop Traumatol Surg Res
PM R
Ann Adv Automot Med
Rev Esp Cir Ortop Traumatol
Scand J Trauma Resusc Emerg Med
J Hand Surg Eur Vol
Z Orthop Unfall
J Burn Care Res
Int J Inj Contr Saf Promot
Int Wound J
Ulus Travma Acil Cerrahi Derg
Int J Low Extrem Wounds
Traffic Inj Prev
Dent Traumatol
J Orthop Traumatol
J Trauma Dissociation
Stapp Car Crash J
Trauma Violence Abuse
Zhonghua Shao Shang Za Zhi
Ortop Traumatol Rehabil
Chin J Traumatol
Eur J Orthop Surg Traumatol
Inj Prev
Violence Against Women
J Trauma Nurs
Knee Surg Sports Traumatol Arthrosc
Emerg Nurse

Torture
Arch Orthop Trauma Surg
Burns
Oper Orthop Traumatol
J Neurotrauma
Vet Comp Orthop Traumatol
J Orthop Trauma
Zhongguo Gu Shang
J Head Trauma Rehabil
Unfallchirurg
J Hand Surg Am
Accid Anal Prev
Injury
Acta Orthop Traumatol Turc
Acta Chir Orthop Traumatol Cech
TROPICAL MEDICINE (38) includes Leprosy and Malaria - see also Parasitology
Med Sante Trop
Paediatr Int Child Health
Asian Pac J Trop Biomed
Int Health
Asian Pac J Trop Med
Parasit Vectors
PLoS Negl Trop Dis
J Vector Borne Dis
Malar J
Int Marit Health
Nihon Hansenbyo Gakkai Zasshi
Trop Med Int Health
Bull Soc Pathol Exot
J Am Mosq Control Assoc
Indian J Lepr
Trop Biomed
J Trop Pediatr
Trop Gastroenterol
Dakar Med
Odontostomatol Trop
Afr J Med Med Sci
Indian J Dermatol Venereol Leprol
Trop Doct
Southeast Asian J Trop Med Public Health
Trop Anim Health Prod
Rev Soc Bras Med Trop
Rev Cubana Med Trop
Ann Acad Med Stetin
Ethiop Med J
Rev Inst Med Trop Sao Paulo
Cent Afr J Med
Rev Biol Trop
Am J Trop Med Hyg
Acta Trop
East Afr Med J
Lepr Rev
Trans R Soc Trop Med Hyg
Mem Inst Oswaldo Cruz

U

UROLOGIA (44) see also Nephrology
Andrology
Scand J Urol
Urolithiasis
Female Pelvic Med Reconstr Surg
Int Urogynecol J
Nat Rev Urol
Clin Genitourin Cancer
J Pediatr Urol
J Sex Med
Urol J
Int Braz J Urol
BMC Urol
Curr Urol Rep
Asian J Androl
BJU Int
Urologiia
Prostate Cancer Prostatic Dis
Urol Oncol
Can J Urol
Int J Urol
Arch Ital Urol Androl
Curr Opin Urol
Prog Urol
Int J Impot Res
Urol Nurs
J Endourol
Minerva Urol Nefrol
World J Urol
Neurourol Urodyn
Prostate
Actas Urol Esp
Eur Urol
Aktuelle Urol
Andrologia
Urol Clin North Am
Urology
Int Urol Nephrol
Urologe A
Hinyokika Kiyo
Urol Int
Arch Esp Urol
Urologia
Nihon Hinyokika Gakkai Zasshi
J Urol

V

VASCULAR DISEASES (131) includes Blood Circulation, Hypertension, and Thrombosis
Eur J Prev Cardiol
J Am Heart Assoc
Cardiovasc Interv Ther
Methodist Debakey Cardiovasc J
Arch Cardiovasc Dis
Cardiovasc Ther
Circ Arrhythm Electrophysiol
Circ Cardiovasc Genet
Circ Cardiovasc Imaging
Circ Cardiovasc Interv
Circ Cardiovasc Qual Outcomes
Circ Heart Fail
JACC Cardiovasc Imaging
JACC Cardiovasc Interv
J Cardiovasc Transl Res
Cardiovasc J Afr
Gen Thorac Cardiovasc Surg
J Cardiovasc Comput Tomogr
J Am Soc Hypertens
Ther Adv Cardiovasc Dis
Cardiovasc Hematol Agents Med Chem
Cardiovasc Hematol Disord Drug Targets
Int J Stroke
J Cardiovasc Med (Hagerstown)
Recent Pat Cardiovasc Drug Discov
Cardiovasc Revasc Med
Curr Hypertens Rev
EuroIntervention
Innovations (Phila)
Vasc Health Risk Manag
Curr Neurovasc Res
Diab Vasc Dis Res
Vascular
Cardiovasc Ultrasound
Curr Vasc Pharmacol
Expert Rev Cardiovasc Ther
Cardiovasc Diabetol
Circ J
Eur J Cardiovasc Nurs
Interact Cardiovasc Thorac Surg
Vasc Endovascular Surg
Vascul Pharmacol
Am J Cardiovasc Drugs
BMC Cardiovasc Disord
Cardiovasc Eng
Cardiovasc Toxicol
Perspect Vasc Surg Endovasc Ther
Atheroscler Suppl
Heart Lung Circ
J Endovasc Ther
J Vasc Access
Rev Cardiovasc Med
Curr Atheroscler Rep
Curr Hypertens Rep
J Clin Hypertens (Greenwich)
J Cardiovasc Magn Reson
Semin Thorac Cardiovasc Surg Pediatr Card Surg Annu
Tech Vasc Interv Radiol
Clin Hemorheol Microcirc
Scand Cardiovasc J
Timely Top Med Cardiovasc Dis
Blood Press Monit
J Cardiovasc Pharmacol Ther
Sarcoidosis Vasc Diffuse Lung Dis
Vasc Med
Ann Thorac Cardiovasc Surg
Arterioscler Thromb Vasc Biol
Clin Appl Thromb Hemost
Eur J Vasc Endovasc Surg
J Atheroscler Thromb
J Thromb Thrombolysis
Microcirculation
Shock
Top Stroke Rehabil
Asian Cardiovasc Thorac Ann
Cardiol Rev
Clin Exp Hypertens
Hypertens Pregnancy
Blood Press
Cardiovasc Pathol
Curr Opin Nephrol Hypertens
High Blood Press Cardiovasc Prev
Hypertens Res
J Vasc Res
Rev Port Cir Cardiotorac Vasc
Cardiol Young
Cerebrovasc Dis
J Stroke Cerebrovasc Dis
Nutr Metab Cardiovasc Dis
Trends Cardiovasc Med
Blood Coagul Fibrinolysis
Coron Artery Dis
J Cardiovasc Electrophysiol
J Vasc Interv Radiol
J Vasc Nurs
Clin Investig Arterioscler
Semin Thorac Cardiovasc Surg
Am J Hypertens
Semin Vasc Surg
Cardiovasc Drugs Ther
J Hum Hypertens
Ann Vasc Surg
J Cardiovasc Nurs
Phlebology
Rev Bras Cir Cardiovasc
J Vasc Surg
J Hypertens Suppl
J Hypertens

Int Angiol
J Cereb Blood Flow Metab
Cardiovasc Intervent Radiol
Hypertension
Thorac Cardiovasc Surg
J Mal Vasc
Thromb Haemost
Semin Thromb Hemost
Zhonghua Xin Xue Guan Bing Za Zhi
Thromb Res
Vasa
Atherosclerosis
Stroke
Ann Cardiol Angeiol (Paris)
Microvasc Res
Cardiovasc Res
J Cardiovasc Surg (Torino)
J Thorac Cardiovasc Surg
Prog Cardiovasc Dis
Circ Res
Minerva Cardioangiol
Angiology
Circulation
VETERINARY MEDICINE (100) includes Dairy and Poultry Science - see also Laboratory Animal Science
Top Companion Anim Med
Transbound Emerg Dis
Animal
Zoonoses Public Health
Compend Contin Educ Vet
BMC Vet Res
Arch Anim Nutr
Learn Behav
Vet Comp Oncol
J Anim Physiol Anim Nutr (Berl)
J Vet Emerg Crit Care (San Antonio)
Vector Borne Zoonotic Dis
Anim Health Res Rev
J Vet Sci
Vet Anaesth Analg
Anim Sci J
J Feline Med Surg
J Vet Cardiol
Anim Cogn
J Appl Anim Welf Sci
Med Mycol
Pol J Vet Sci
Vet Clin North Am Exot Anim Pract
Vet Ophthalmol
Tierarztl Prax Ausg G Grosstiere Nutztiere
Tierarztl Prax Ausg K Kleintiere Heimtiere
Vet J
J Avian Med Surg
Vet Res
Rev Bras Parasitol Vet
Vet Radiol Ultrasound
J Vet Med Sci
Jt Meet Abstr Am Dairy Sci Assoc
Reprod Domest Anim
Argos
J Aquat Anim Health
J Vet Diagn Invest
J Zoo Wildl Med
Vet Dermatol
J Vet Dent
Vet Comp Orthop Traumatol
J Vet Intern Med
Med Vet Entomol
Can J Vet Res
J Anim Breed Genet
Dis Aquat Organ
Vet Clin North Am Equine Pract
Vet Clin North Am Food Anim Pract
Domest Anim Endocrinol
Acta Vet Hung
Equine Vet J Suppl
Prev Vet Med
Rev Sci Tech
Vet Herit
Dongwuxue Yanjiu
Vet Res Commun
Vet Clin North Am Small Anim Pract
Vet Immunol Immunopathol
Vet Q
Anim Reprod Sci
Comp Immunol Microbiol Infect Dis
J Vet Pharmacol Ther
Vet Surg
Vet Clin Pathol
Hist Med Vet
Vet Microbiol
Vet Parasitol
J Vet Med Educ
Theriogenology
Anat Histol Embryol
Avian Pathol
J S Afr Vet Assoc
Dtsch Tierarztl Wochenschr
Vet Pathol
J Wildl Dis
Trop Anim Health Prod
Equine Vet J
J Am Anim Hosp Assoc
J Comp Pathol
Br Poult Sci
Can Vet J
J Small Anim Pract
Res Vet Sci
Acta Vet Scand
Avian Dis

Chapter 7 - The National Library of Medicine

A Perspective On The National Library of Medicine

Jpn J Vet Res
Vet Ital
N Z Vet J
Onderstepoort J Vet Res
J Anim Sci
Am J Vet Res
Berl Munch Tierarztl Wochenschr
J Dairy Res
Aust Vet J
Poult Sci
J Dairy Sci
Tijdschr Diergeneeskd
J Am Vet Med Assoc
Vet Rec
Schweiz Arch Tierheilkd
VIROLOGY (33)
Curr Opin Virol
Top Antivir Med
Food Environ Virol
Viruses
Influenza Other Respir Viruses
Virol Sin
Retrovirology
Virol J
J Clin Virol
Antivir Ther
J Neurovirol
Arch Virol Suppl
Rev Med Virol
Antivir Chem Chemother
Bacteriol Virusol Parazitol Epidemiol
Viral Immunol
Virus Genes
Zhonghua Shi Yan He Lin Chuang Bing Du Xue Za Zhi
Bing Du Xue Bao
Virus Res
Mol Gen Mikrobiol Virusol
Antiviral Res
J Virol Methods
J Med Virol
Arch Virol
Intervirology
J Gen Virol
J Virol
Uirusu
Acta Virol
Vopr Virusol
Virology
Adv Virus Res
VITAL STATISTICS (17)
Natl Health Stat Report
MMWR Surveill Summ
Health Stat Q
Natl Vital Stat Rep
MMWR Recomm Rep
Vital Health Stat 21
Vital Health Stat 5
Vital Health Stat 3
Vital Health Stat 23
MMWR Morb Mortal Wkly Rep
Vital Health Stat 13
Vital Health Stat 4
Vital Health Stat 20
Vital Health Stat 11
Vital Health Stat 1
Vital Health Stat 10
Vital Health Stat 2

Fly (Austin)
J Exp Zool A Ecol Genet Physiol
Integr Zool
Insect Sci
WormBook
Zebrafish
J Exp Zool B Mol Dev Evol
Integr Comp Biol
J Insect Sci
Neotrop Entomol
Arthropod Struct Dev
Evol Dev
Physiol Biochem Zool
Zoology (Jena)
In Vitro Cell Dev Biol Anim
Insect Biochem Mol Biol
Insect Mol Biol
Fish Shellfish Immunol
Anim Biotechnol
Reprod Domest Anim
Med Vet Entomol
Anim Genet
Fish Physiol Biochem
J Anim Breed Genet
Exp Appl Acarol
Domest Anim Endocrinol
Zoolog Sci
Arch Insect Biochem Physiol
Zoo Biol
Am J Primatol
Dongwuxue Yanjiu
Anim Reprod Sci
J Fish Dis
Avian Pathol
Environ Entomol
J Med Primatol
J Fish Biol
J Invertebr Pathol
J Med Entomol
Folia Primatol (Basel)
J Insect Physiol
Primates
Annu Rev Entomol
J Anim Ecol
Bull Entomol Res
J Econ Entomol

W

WOMEN'S HEALTH (15) see also Gynecology; Obstetrics; Reproductive Medicine
Nurs Womens Health
Womens Health (Lond Engl)
Gend Med
J Womens Health (Larchmt)
BMC Womens Health
J Midwifery Womens Health
Arch Womens Ment Health
Int J Fertil Womens Med
Violence Against Women
Harv Womens Health Watch
Womens Health Data Book
Womens Health Issues
J Women Aging
Health Care Women Int
Women Health

X

None

Y

None

Z

ZOOLOGY (47) includes Entomology
Animal

105

Chapter 7 - The National Library of Medicine

Chapter 8
PubMed Search Engine and the MEDLINE Database

Here, you can move into researching the medical and scientific literature for the cancer of concern. In the previous, Chapter 7, a history of the National Library of Medicine (NLM) was given against a tableau of the names of the journals which are currently indexed - some 5,600 in all. To repeat, the information in those journals constitutes the MEDLINE database which is accessed via the PubMed Search engine, both of which are maintained by the NLM (National Library of Medicine). The database, MEDLINE, comprises more than 23 million citations of the biomedical literature; going back to 1900 with some 2,000 to 4,000 new articles being added to the database each day. Scientists throughout the world conduct investigations and then report them to professional societies which specialize in the subject matter (peers), who then review those report, make suggested corrections, and either accept or reject them for publication in their respective journals. This process of peer review is a kind of quality control, attempting to certify the relevance and accuracy of the reports (up to the time of publication). The staff librarians of the NLM (all highly trained and many of whom are medical doctors and scientists) read the reports and tag them with relevant Medical Subject Headings and Subheadings and, thereby, enable you to use the PubMed search engine to find ones that are relevant to your interests. This is a complex, powerful, and professional level database/program; and it takes a fair amount of instruction and experience to learn how to fully command it. Thus, we will provide only a generic search routine that everyone would use when approaching this resource, and we will leave more advance instruction to the materials that are provided at the site. This is intended for professional researchers; and you can skip this section of it is too difficult.

Expert Summary

- *Go to:*   http://www.PubMed.gov .
- *Select:*   The "**MeSH**" function from the pull-down menu.
- *Select:*   Type in the term for the cancer of interest and Select the formal term.
- *Select:*   Any "**Subheading**" desired or leave those unselected.
- *Select:*   "**Add to search builder**" button and note the command.
- *Select:*   The "**Search PubMed**" button.

For more detailed functions, see the following instructions.

Step 1 - Log-on to the site: http://www.PubMed.gov [1]

Go to the **drop-down menu** and select the **MeSH** link, which stands for the "**Me**dical **S**ubject **H**eading" function - a specialized dictionary of search terms.

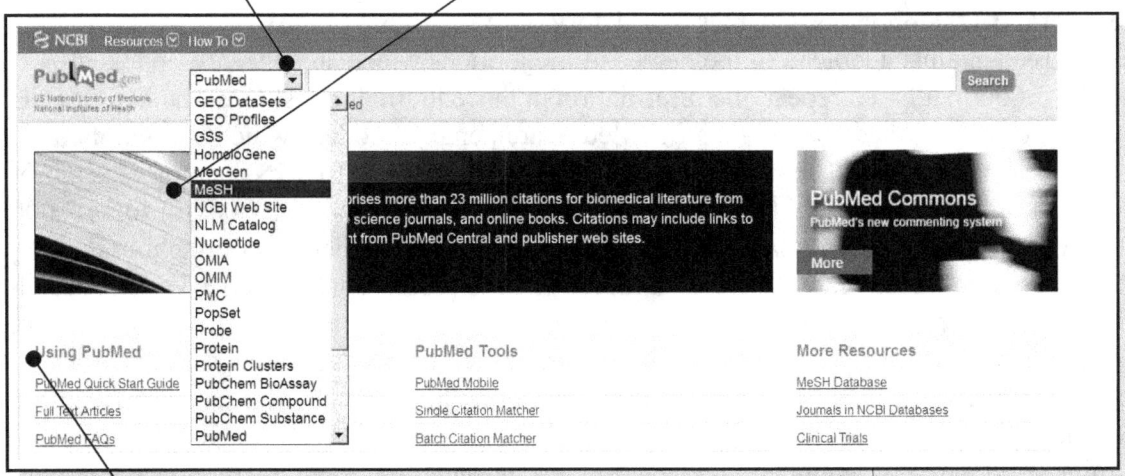

Note "**Using PubMed**" for links to detailed instructional materials.

In the **search box**, of the MeSH function, type in the specific type of cancer of interest.

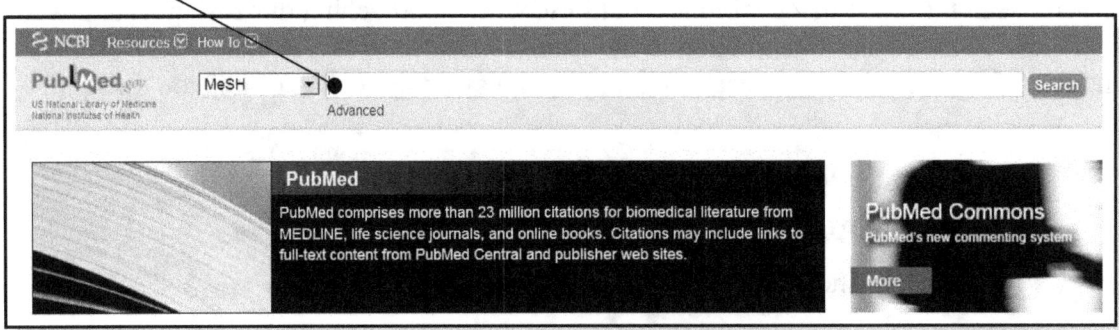

We will use as an example: "breast cancer". At first, this will be a little tricky because two terms are used for referencing cancer - both "cancer" (used in medicine) and "neoplasm" (the more scientific term). Further, it can be complicated by the "Auto-complete" function which tries to anticipate your command and displays options in advance so that you do not have to type in everything, many of which will not be relevant

---

1 Using the **PubMed.gov** URL, you will be directed to **ncbi.nlm.nih.gov/pubmed/** which stands for the various governmental agencies that are involved: i.e., "ncbi" = National Center for Biotechnology Information; "nlm" = National Library of Medicine; and "nih" = National Institutes of Health

Chapter 8 - PubMed Search Engine and the Medline Database

to you. Thus, when you type "breast", it will automatically jump to a long list of terms that are related to "breast", but only some of which are related to cancer.

Step 2 - When you type in the full term "**breast cancer**", you will be presented with a list of **52** terms, of which "**breast neoplasms**" is relevant to our purpose, here. Select that.

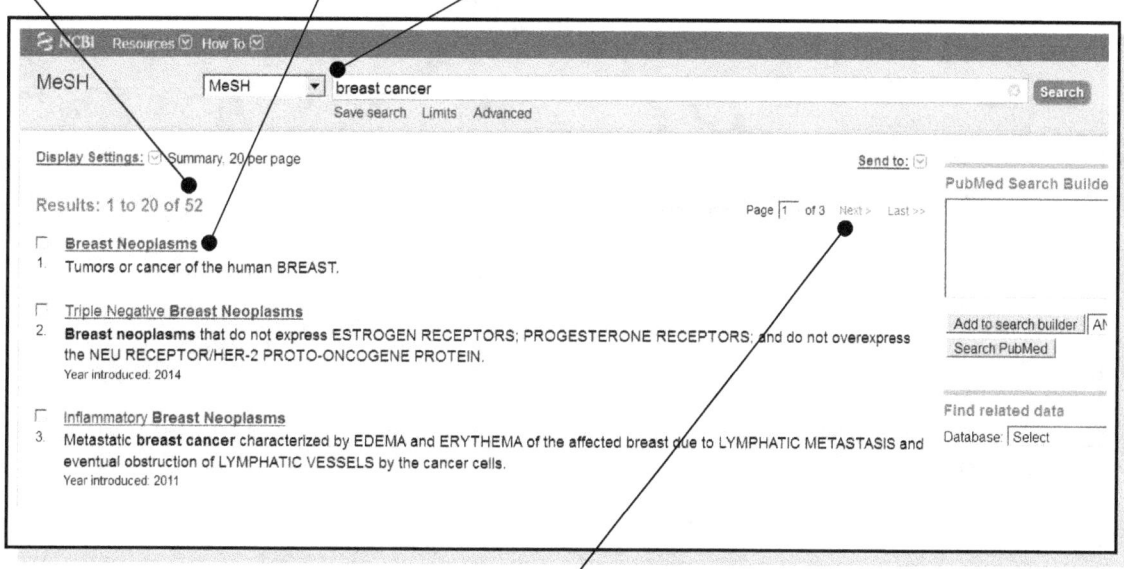

(**The** other, 51 terms are relevant to some aspect of "breast cancer"; and after you complete this initial, more general search, you may want to go back and review these, scrolling down and going through the additional **pages**.)

Step 3 - The MeSH search template. When you select "**breast neoplasms**", it will take you to the master search template for that **subject**. To perform the search on the subject, select the button called: "**Add to search builder**". The search term "**Breast Neoplasms [Mesh]**" will be added to the box. For this initial example, select the button: "**Search PubMed**".

This search, using "Breast Neoplasms" by itself and without any qualifiers or "subheadings", will perform the broadest search - encompassing all reports in which "Breast Neoplasms" is a principal topic of each citation; and they will be sorted in reverse chronological order - i.e., the most recent first.

Step 4 - The search results. The results screen has a variety of components. First, the **database** and **search term** are displayed; then, the **number of citations** (both the items on the page and the total number in the database) and the links to the **citations** are shown.

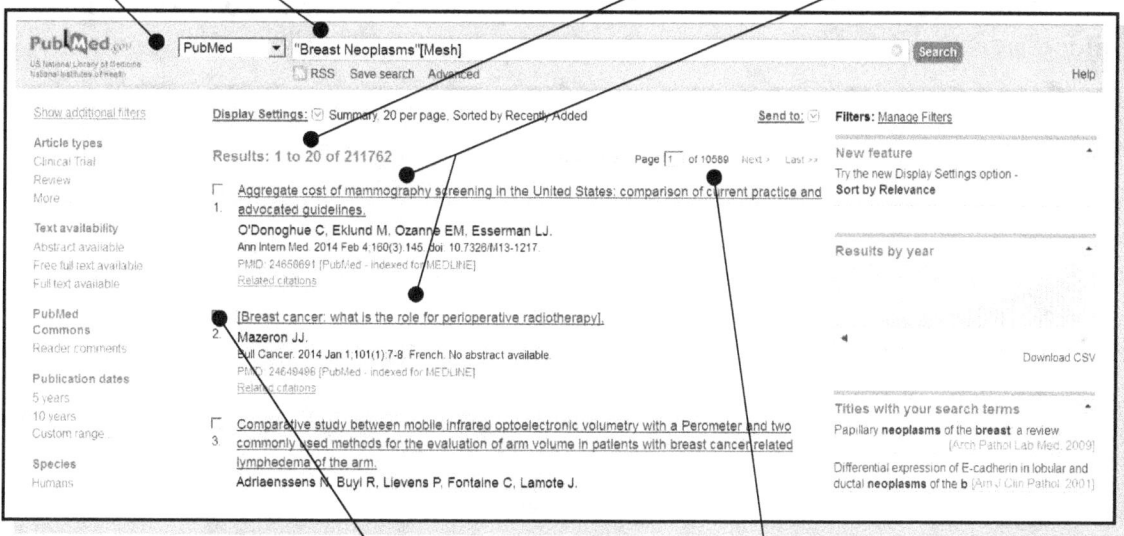

Scroll down to read the titles, and proceed to the subsequent **pages**. The one which you think might be of interest, select **adjacent box**.

Step 5 - The citation itself. The **components** of a citation are in bold font. Some citations have access to the **full text** (some of which are free while other require a fee) and you can also **Send [*the citation*] to** a File or E-mail.

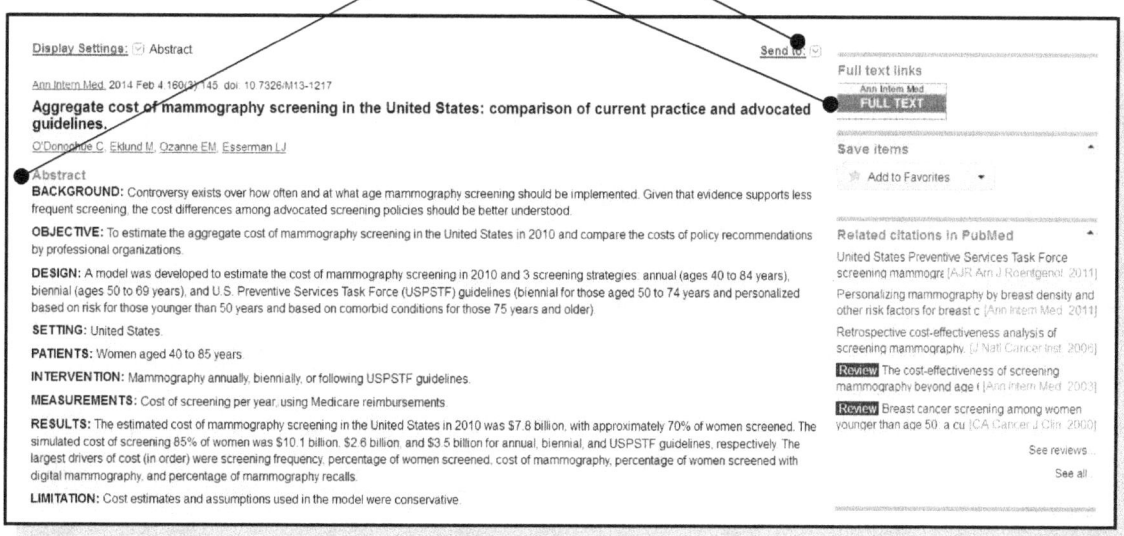

110

Step 6 - Defining your search more accurately. Return to "**Step 3 - The search template**". Note the "**Subheadings**" section and the various options for narrowing the retrieval. Select the desired Subheading - for example, "**therapy**". Use only one subheading at a time; otherwise, its seems to give aberrant results. Select the "**Add to search builder**" as discussed previously.

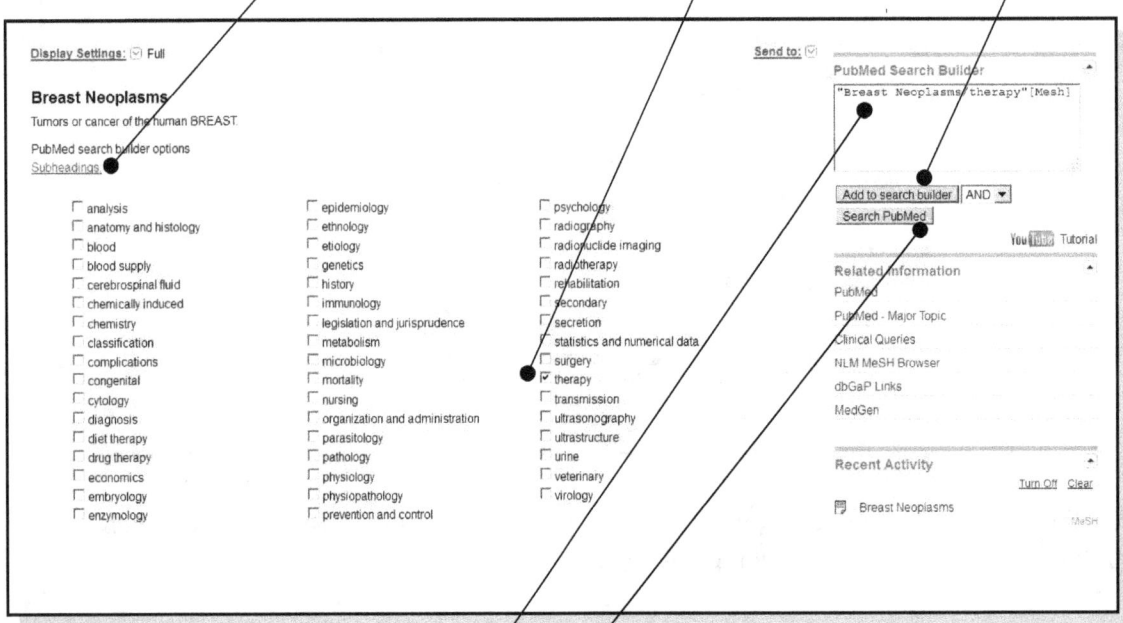

You will see that a command-line "**Breast Neoplasms/therapy[Mesh]**" has been entered into the box. Now, hit the "**Search PubMed**" button; and you will see a listing of citations related to that subject with the subheading.

The Subheadings for a search term are listed below with their definitions. The Subheadings in red are commonly relevant to cancer. These are not links. Search format is: "*cancer-type*/subheading"[Mesh] .

Subheadings	Definitions
/analysis	Used for the identification or quantitative determination of a substance or its constituents and metabolites; includes the analysis of air, water, or other environmental carrier. It excludes the chemical analysis of tissues, tumors, body fluids, organisms, and plants for which "chemistry" is used. The concept applies to both methodology and results. For analysis of substances in blood,

Chapter 8 - PubMed Search Engine and the Medline Database

Subheadings	Definitions
	cerebrospinal fluid, and urine the specific subheading designating the fluid is used. Year introduced: 1967.
/anatomy and histology	Used with organs, regions, and tissues for normal descriptive anatomy and histology, and for the normal anatomy and structure of animals and plants. Year introduced: 1966.
/blood	Used for the presence or analysis of substances in the blood; also for examination of, or changes in, the blood in disease states. It excludes serodiagnosis, for which the subheading "diagnosis" is used, and serology, for which "immunology" is used. Year introduced: 1967.
/blood supply	Used for arterial, capillary, and venous systems of an organ or region whenever the specific heading for the vessel does not exist. It includes blood flow through the organ. Year introduced: 1966.
/cerebrospinal fluid	Used for the presence or analysis of substances in the cerebrospinal fluid; also for examination of or changes in cerebrospinal fluid in disease states. Year introduced: 1967.
/chemically induced	Used for biological phenomena, diseases, syndromes, congenital abnormalities, or symptoms caused by endogenous or exogenous substances. Year introduced: 1967.
/chemistry	Used with chemicals, biological, and non-biological substances for their composition, structure, characterization, and properties; also used for the chemical composition or content of organs, tissue, tumors, body fluids, organisms, and plants. Excludes chemical analysis and determination of substances for which "analysis" is used; excludes synthesis for which "chemical synthesis" is used; excludes isolation and purification of substances for which "isolation and purification" is used. Year introduced: 1991.
/classification	Used for taxonomic or other systematic or hierarchical classification systems. Year introduced: 1966.
/complications	Used with diseases to indicate conditions that co-exist or follow, i.e., co-existing diseases, complications, or sequelae. Year introduced: 1966.
/congenital	Used with disease headings to indicate those conditions existing at, and usually before, birth. It excludes morphologic abnormalities and birth injuries, for which "abnormalities" and "injuries" are used. Year introduced: 1966.
/cytology	Used for cellular appearance of unicellular and multicellular organisms. Year introduced: 1967.

Subheadings	Definitions
/diagnosis	Used with diseases for all aspects of diagnosis, including examination, differential diagnosis and prognosis; excludes mass screening for which "prevention and control" is used. Excludes radiographic diagnosis for which "radiography" is used; excludes scintigraphic diagnosis for which "radionuclide imaging" is used; excludes ultrasonic diagnosis for which "ultrasonography" is used. Year introduced: 1966.
/diet therapy	Used with disease headings for dietary and nutritional management of the disease. The concept does not include vitamin or mineral supplements, for which "drug therapy" may be used. Year introduced: 1975.
/drug therapy	Used with disease headings for the treatment of disease by the administration of drugs, chemicals, and antibiotics. For diet therapy and radiotherapy, use specific subheadings. Excludes immunotherapy for which "therapy" is used. Year introduced: 1966.
/economics	Used for the economic aspects of any subject, as well as for all aspects of financial management. It includes the raising or providing of funds. Year introduced: 1978.
/embryology	Used with organs, regions, and animal headings for embryologic and fetal development. It is used also with diseases for embryologic factors contributing to postnatal disorders. Year introduced: 1966.
/enzymology	Used with organisms, except vertebrates, and with organs and tissues. It is also used with diseases for enzymes during the course of the disease, but excludes diagnostic enzyme tests, for which "diagnosis" is used. Year introduced: 1966
/epidemiology	Used with human and veterinary diseases for the distribution of disease, factors which cause disease, and the attributes of disease in defined populations; includes incidence, frequency, prevalence, endemic and epidemic outbreaks; also surveys and estimates of morbidity in geographic areas and in specified populations. Used also with geographical headings for the location of epidemiologic aspects of a disease. Excludes mortality for which "mortality" is used. Year introduced: 1989.
/ethnology	Used with diseases for ethnic, cultural, or anthropological aspects, and with geographic headings to indicate the place of origin of a group of people. Year introduced: 1975.
/etiology	Used with diseases for causative agents including microorganisms and includes environmental and social factors and personal habits as contributing factors. It includes pathogenesis. Year introduced: 1966.

Chapter 8 - PubMed Search Engine and the Medline Database

Subheadings	Definitions
/genetics	Used for mechanisms of heredity and the genetics of organisms, for the genetic basis of normal and pathologic states, and for the genetic aspects of endogenous chemicals. It includes biochemical and molecular influence on genetic material. Year introduced: 1978.
/history	Used for the historical aspects of any subject. It includes brief historical notes but excludes case histories. Year introduced: 1966
/immunology	Used for immunologic studies of tissues, organs, microorganisms, fungi, viruses, and animals. It includes immunologic aspects of diseases but not immunologic procedures used for diagnostic, preventive, or therapeutic purposes, for which "diagnosis", "prevention and control", or "therapy" are used. The concept is also used for chemicals as antigens or haptens. Year introduced: 1966
/legislation and jurisprudence	Used for laws, statutes, ordinances, or government regulations, as well as for legal controversy and court decisions. Year introduced: 1978
/metabolism	Used with organs, cells and subcellular fractions, organisms, and diseases for biochemical changes and metabolism. It is used also with drugs and chemicals for catabolic changes (breakdown of complex molecules into simpler ones). For anabolic processes (conversion of small molecules into large), BIOSYNTHESIS is used. For enzymology, pharmacokinetics, and secretion use the specific subheadings. Year introduced: 1966
/microbiology	Used with organs, animals, and higher plants and with diseases for microbiologic studies. For parasites, "parasitology" is used; for viruses, "virology" is used. Year introduced: 1967
/mortality	Used with human and veterinary diseases for mortality statistics. For deaths resulting from various procedures statistically but for a death resulting in a specific case, use FATAL OUTCOME, not /mortality. Year introduced: 1967
/nursing	Used with diseases for nursing care and techniques in their management. It includes the nursing role in diagnostic, therapeutic, and preventive procedures. Year introduced: 1966
/organization and administration	Used for administrative structure and management. Year introduced: 1978
/parasitology	Used with animals, higher plants, organs, and diseases for parasitic factors. In

114

Chapter 8 - PubMed Search Engine and the Medline Database

Subheadings	Definitions
	diseases, it is not used if the parasitic involvement is implicit in the diagnosis. Year introduced: 1975
/pathology	Used for organ, tissue, or cell structure in disease states. Year introduced: 1966.
/physiology	Used with organs, tissues, and cells of unicellular and multicellular organisms for normal function. It is used also with biochemical substances, endogenously produced, for their physiologic role. Year introduced: 1966
/physiopathology	Used with organs and diseases for disordered function in disease states. Year introduced: 1966
/prevention and control	Used with disease headings for increasing human or animal resistance against disease (e.g., immunization), for control of transmission agents, for prevention and control of environmental hazards, or for prevention and control of social factors leading to disease. It includes preventive measures in individual cases. Year introduced: 1966
/psychology	Used with non-psychiatric diseases, techniques, and named groups for psychologic, psychiatric, psychosomatic, psychosocial, behavioral, and emotional aspects, and with psychiatric disease for psychologic aspects; used also with animal terms for animal behavior and psychology. Year introduced: 1978
/radiography	Used with organs, regions, and diseases for x-ray examinations. It does not include radionuclide imaging for which "radionuclide imaging" is used. Year introduced: 1967.
/radionuclide imaging	Used for radionuclide imaging of any anatomical structure, or for the diagnosis of disease. Year introduced: 1978.
/radiotherapy	Used with disease headings for the therapeutic use of ionizing and nonionizing radiation. It includes the use of radioisotope therapy. Year introduced: 1966.
/rehabilitation	Used with diseases and surgical procedures for restoration of function of the individual. Year introduced: 1967.
/secondary	Used with neoplasms to indicate the secondary location to which the neoplastic process has metastasized. Year introduced: 1980. See also **Neoplasm Metastasis.**
/secretion	Used for the discharge across the cell membrane, into the extracellular space or ducts, of endogenous substances resulting from the activity of intact cells of glands, tissues, or organs. Year introduced: 1968

Subheadings	Definitions
/statistics and numerical data	Used with non-disease headings for the expression of numerical values which describe particular sets or groups of data. It excludes manpower distribution for which "manpower" is used and excludes supply or demand for which "supply and distribution" is used. Year introduced: 1989
/surgery	Used for operative procedures on organs, regions, or tissues in the treatment of diseases, including tissue section by lasers. It excludes transplantation, for which "transplantation" is used. Year introduced: 1966
/therapy	Used with diseases for therapeutic interventions except drug therapy, diet therapy, radiotherapy, and surgery, for which specific subheadings exist. The concept is also used for articles and books dealing with multiple therapies. Year introduced: 1966
/transmission	Used with diseases for studies of the modes of transmission. Year introduced: 1975.
/ultrasonography	Used with organs and regions for ultrasonic imaging and with diseases for ultrasonic diagnosis. Does not include ultrasonic therapy. Year introduced: 1991
/ultrastructure	Used with tissues and cells (including neoplasms) and microorganisms for microanatomic structures, generally below the size visible by light microscopy. Year introduced: 1975
/urine	Used for the presence or analysis of substances in the urine, and also for the examination of, or changes in, the urine in disease. Year introduced: 1967.
/veterinary	Used for naturally occurring diseases in animals, or for diagnostic, preventive, or therapeutic procedures used in veterinary medicine. Year introduced: 1966
/virology	Used with organs, animals, and higher plants and with diseases for virologic studies. For bacteria, rickettsia, and fungi, "microbiology" is used; for parasites, "parasitology" is used. Year introduced: 1995

Chapter 8 - PubMed Search Engine and the Medline Database

Step 7 - Additional display features. Going back to "**Step 4 - The search results**", there are additional features which warrant consideration. The "**Results by year**" gives you a graphical display of the number of citations in the database by year. You can see that, for "breast neoplasms", there is a steady increase in scientific reports each year - meaning that there is sustained and increasing work in this area. Again as you scroll through the citation titles, select the ones that appear to be of interest by checking the adjacent **box**. You can do this for any number of items including those on the subsequent pages. Then, select "**Display Settings**" and in that pull-down menu select the "Apply" button. All of the unselected items will be edited out, making it easier to consolidated your search.

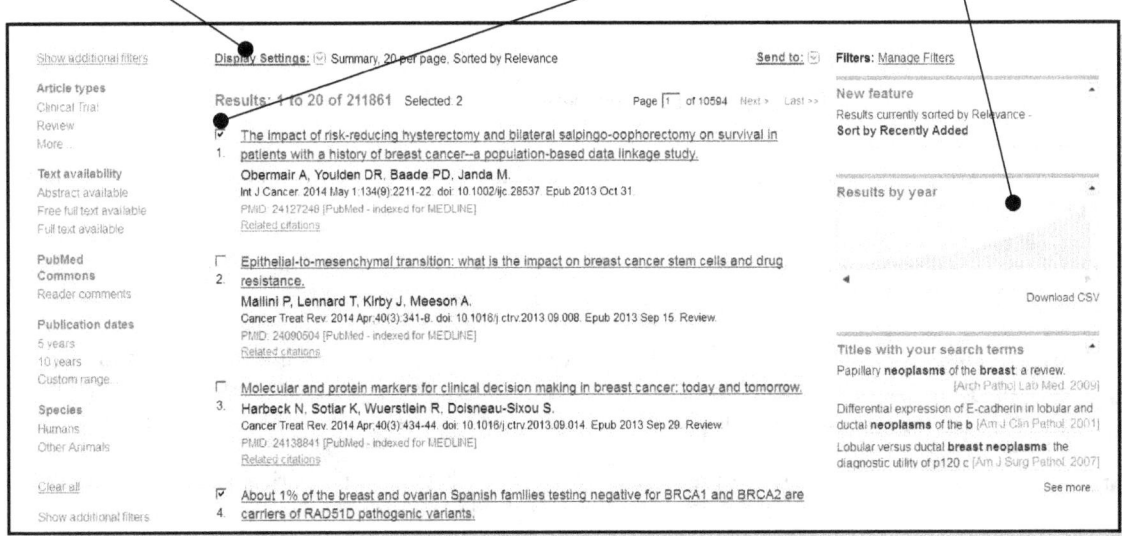

In the "**Display Settings**" menu, you can also retrieve your citations in a different "**Format**" - e.g., with the "**Abstract**" or Summary of the report or in the "**MEDLINE**" text format.

The default number of citations per page is 20; but you can display up to 200 **Items per page**; and although normally of little use, you can "**Sort by**" different ways.

(Note: at the time of this writing, the "Display Settings" link disappeared, which in correspondence with the technical staff appears to be a mistake. So, if you do not see it, then use the "Summary" and "20 per page" links if you want to make adjustments to the Display functions.)

Chapter 8 - PubMed Search Engine and the Medline Database

Step 8 - Searches which join two or more MeSH terms.
Using a modification of the previous procedures that were used in the "**Step 3 - The search template**", assume that you have selected the MeSH search term "**Breast Neoplasms**" and that you add the subheading "**/diagnosis**".   Select the "**Add to search builder**" button; and in the box, you will see the expanded command "**Breast Neoplasms/diagnosis"[Mesh]**". Do NOT Select the "Search PubMed" button at this point.   Next, type "**consensus**" in the MeSH search bar and **Search**.

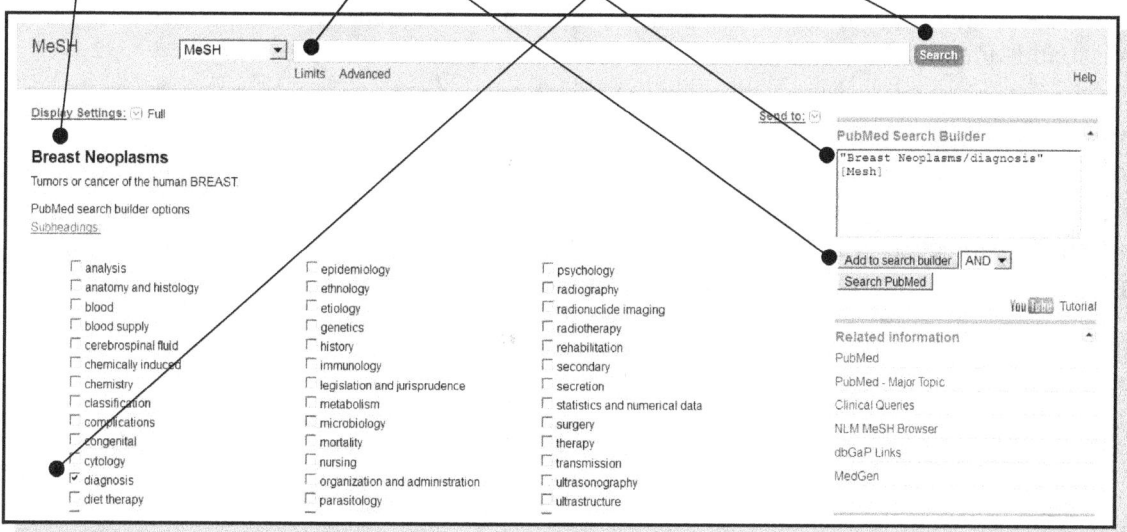

That will take you to various MeSH terms that contain "**consensus**".
Select "**Consensus**". From that page, use the "**Add to search builder**" button; and note the modified command: "**Breast Neoplasms/diagnosis"[Mesh]) AND "Consensus"[Mesh]**".

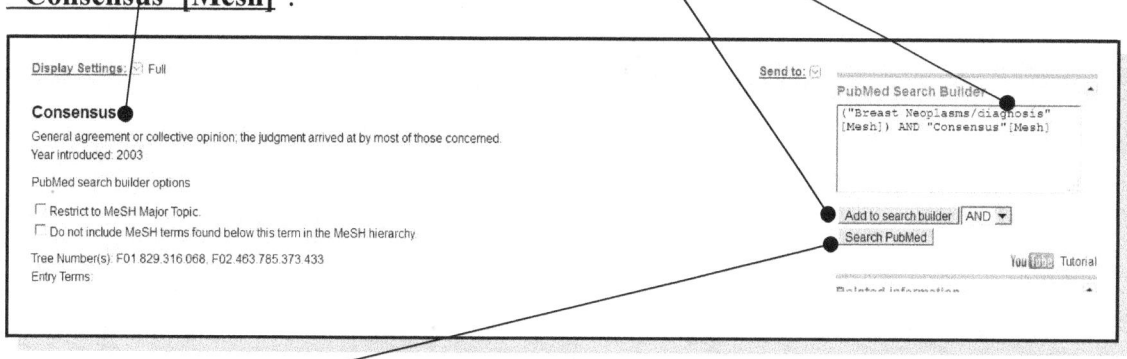

Now, Select the "**Search PubMed**" button, and it will take you to a listing of the citations. This will retrieve "Consensus" reports on the "Diagnosis" of "Breast Cancer".

Chapter 8 - PubMed Search Engine and the Medline Database

The procedures, thus far, seem a bit contorted, which is an "adverse effect" of using a graphical interface to structure an inquiry rather than a command line, which takes some training. In comparison, programs such as Google, Yahoo, and others simply allow you to type in what you think you want and, ostensibly, that will retrieve the specific type of information that is desired. However, in Google when you type in "breast cancer", you get over 271 million citations, which obviously is absurd. No one can meaningfully navigate through that number; the primary links are advertisements; and few are by peer reviewed scientists. Later, we will give some instructions on how to construct a search in a command-line.

Step 9 - Using the "Related citations" function.
When you find a specific citation that pertains very precisely to your interest, use the **Related citations in PubMed** function. This is a sophisticated routine which attempts to match the subjects in the article which you selected to other articles in the database and lists them below. This can save you an immense amount of work.

It flags those which are **Review** articles and allows you to **See reviews** or to **See all** the related articles.

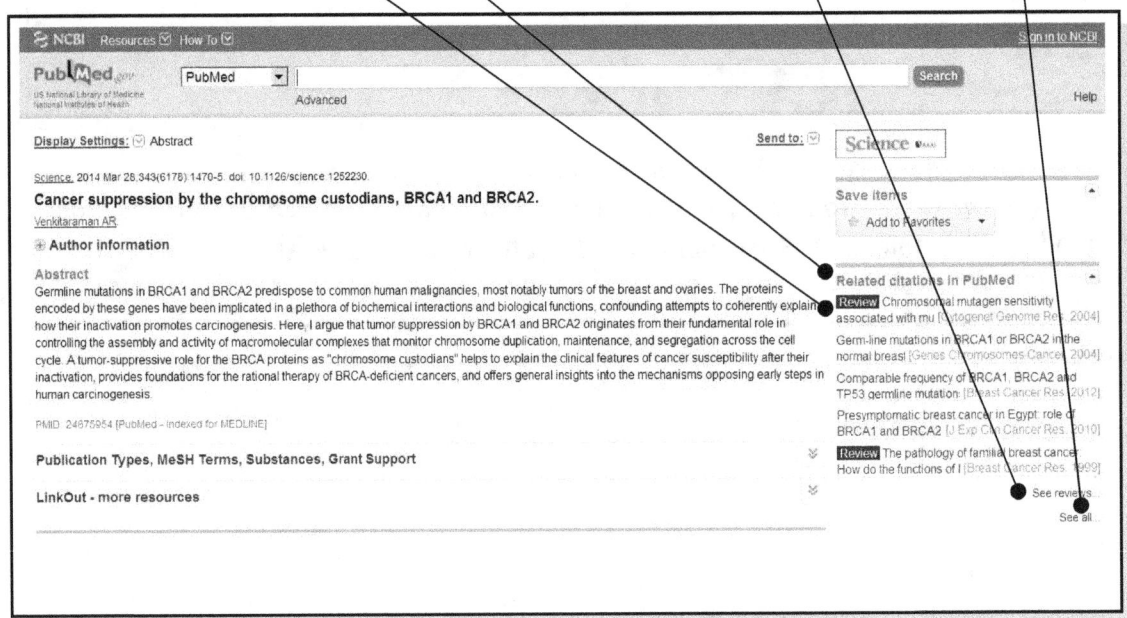

Chapter 8 - PubMed Search Engine and the Medline Database

Step 10 - Searches using the "command-line" rather than the Search Form.
Thus far, we have used the Search Form to compose the search commands. The Form approach is; but it attempts to enable one to structure a command by selection buttons and boxes and, therefore, obviating the knowledge of the command terms in advance and having to type them in, thereby avoiding mistakes. However, once one becomes familiar with the general syntax and learns how to find the exact search terms in the MeSH dictionary, then the search can be constructed directly as a command-line at the top of any page in the search box. For example, using the very first page in the program (or any page wherever you might be), make sure that you are being directed to the **PubMed** program, and then type in the **search box** the command which was used in previous, Step 8 - see below.

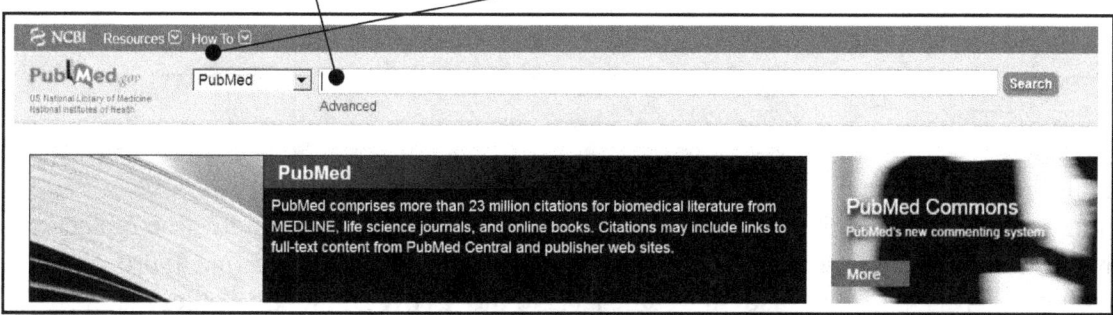

Build the command in segments - first: **"Breast Neoplasms/diagnosis"[Mesh]** and **send** it to verify that you get results. As you seen you get **103,632** citations.

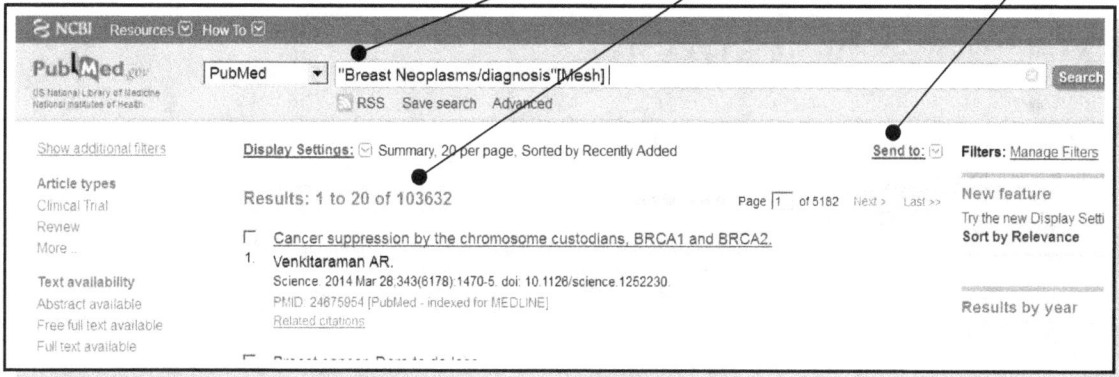

Chapter 8 - PubMed Search Engine and the Medline Database

Then, add the remainder of the terms **AND "Consensus"[Mesh]** to narrow the search. Now, you extract **31** citations that are relevant to your specific interest.

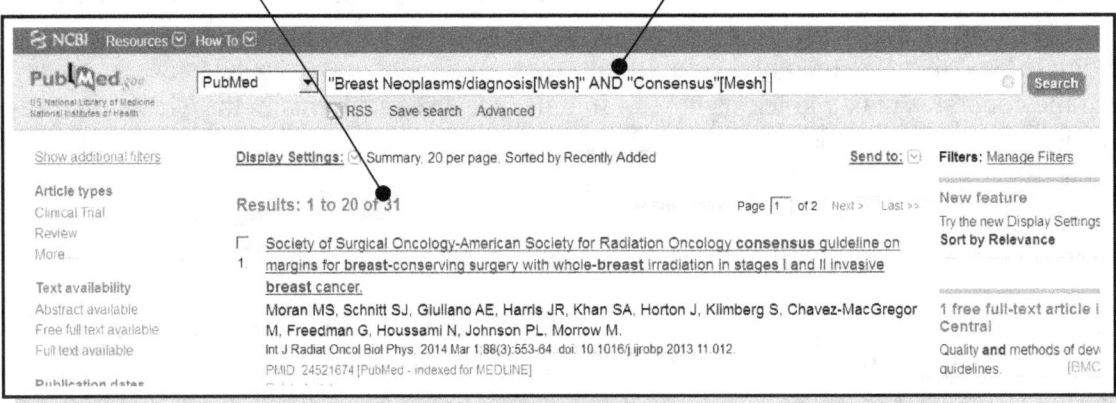

The following is some supporting and reference information. **B**elow are various command-line searches that are relevant to cancer. **T**he items in ***italics*** must be replace by what you find to be the proper term. **A**lso, when you use the command-line approach, the spelling of terms must be exactly the same as is in the MeSH Dictionary, otherwise you might get only a partial or null response. **T**he following searches are designed to answer the **question in the header** of each section

HAS THE PROPER DIAGNOSIS BEEN MADE?

"*cancer type*/Diagnosis"[MeSH]
Diagnosis [Subheading] is used with diseases for all aspects of diagnosis, including examination, differential diagnosis and prognosis; excludes mass screening for which "prevention and control" is used. Excludes radiographic diagnosis for which "radiography" is used; excludes scintigraphic diagnosis for which "radionuclide imaging" is used; excludes ultrasonic diagnosis for which "ultrasonography" is used. (Do not forget the slash "/".) Initially, to narrow the search, use the command for the **Publication Type** "Review" - i.e., "*neoplasm type*/**Diagnosis**" [Mesh] AND Review[ptyp]; and then by itself.

"Diagnostic Errors" [MeSH] AND *"the particular diagnostic technique"*[MeSH]
Diagnostic Errors refers to incorrect diagnoses after clinical examination or technical diagnostic procedures. (To find the specific diagnostic technicque use the MeSH

function as originally described in the beginning of this chapter; and ask your physician(s).)

"Sensitivity and Specificity"[MeSH] AND *"the diagnostic technique"*[MeSH]
Sensitivity and Specificity means binary classification measures to assess test results. Sensitivity or recall rate is the proportion of true positives. Specificity is the probability of correctly determining the absence of a condition. (From Last, Dictionary of Epidemiology, 2d ed) Year introduced: 1991

"False Negative Reactions"[MeSH] AND *"the diagnostic technique"*[MeSH]
False Negative Reactions are negative test results in subjects who possess the attribute for which the test is conducted. The labeling of diseased persons as healthy when screening in the detection of disease. (Last, A Dictionary of Epidemiology, 2d ed) Year introduced: 1973(1970)

"False Positive Reactions"[Mesh] AND *"the diagnostic technique"*[Mesh]
False Positive Reactions are positive test results in subjects who do not possess the attribute for which the test is conducted. The labeling of healthy persons as diseased when screening in the detection of disease. (Last, A Dictionary of Epidemiology, 2d ed) Year introduced: 1970(1968)

WHAT IS THE RESEARCH LITERATURE ON THE TREATMENT FOR THE PARTICULAR CANCER?

"cancer type/Therapy"[Mesh] AND Review[Publication Type]

Therapy [Subheading] - used with diseases for therapeutic interventions except drug therapy, diet therapy, radiotherapy, and surgery, for which specific subheadings exist. The concept is also used for articles and books dealing with multiple therapies. There are different sub-headings for specific modalities - see below. Again, do not forget the forward slash "/" with Subheadings.) Use initially with Review [Publication Type]. That will retrieve a articles or books published after a review of the published material on a subject. It may be comprehensive to various degrees and the time range of material scrutinized may be broad or narrow, but the reviews most often desired are reviews of the current literature. The textual material examined may be equally broad and can encompass, in medicine specifically, clinical material as well as experimental research or case reports. State-of-the-art reviews tend to address more current matters. A review of the literature must be differentiated from HISTORICAL ARTICLE on the same

> **WHAT IS THE RESEARCH LITERATURE ON THE TREATMENT FOR THE PARTICULAR CANCER?**

subject, but a review of historical literature is also within the scope of this publication type. Year introduced: 2008(1966)

"cancer type/Drug Therapy"[Mesh]   (*Self-explicit*)

"cancer type/Diet Therapy"[Mesh]   (*Self-explicit*)

"cancer type/Surgery"[Mesh]   (*Self-explicit*)

"cancer type/Radiotherapy"[Mesh]   (*"Radio" refers to radiation.*)

"cancer type/Rehabilitation"[Mesh]   (*Self-explicit*)

"Practice Guideline" [Publication Type] AND "cancer type"[Mesh]
Practice Guideline [Publication Type] - work consisting of a set of directions or principles to assist the health care practitioner with patient care decisions about appropriate diagnostic, therapeutic, or other clinical procedures for specific clinical circumstances. Practice guidelines may be developed by government agencies at any level, institutions, organizations such as professional societies or governing boards, or by the convening of expert panels. They can provide a foundation for assessing and evaluating the quality and effectiveness of health care in terms of measuring improved health, reduction of variation in services or procedures performed, and reduction of variation in outcomes of health care delivered. Year introduced: 2008(1992)

"Evidence-Based Medicine"[Mesh] AND "cancer type"[Mesh]
Evidence-Based Medicine - an approach of practicing medicine with the goal to improve and evaluate patient care. It requires the judicious integration of best research evidence with the patient's values to make decisions about medical care. This method is to help physicians make proper diagnosis, devise best testing plan, choose best treatment and methods of disease prevention, as well as develop guidelines for large groups of patients with the same disease. (from JAMA 296 (9), 2006) Year introduced: 1997

"Consensus Development Conference" [publication type] AND "cancer type"[Mesh]

WHAT IS THE RESEARCH LITERATURE ON THE TREATMENT FOR THE PARTICULAR CANCER?

Consensus Development Conference - a work that consists of summary statements representing the majority and current agreement of physicians, scientists, and other professionals meeting to reach a consensus on a selected subject. Year introduced: 2008(1991)

"Consensus Development Conferences as Topic"[Mesh] AND *"cancer type"*[Mesh]

Consensus Development Conferences as Topic - presentations of summary statements representing the majority agreement of physicians, scientists, and other professionals convening for the purpose of reaching a consensus--often with findings and recommendations--on a subject of interest. The Conference, consisting of participants representing the scientific and lay viewpoints, is a significant means of evaluating current medical thought and reflects the latest advances in research for the respective field being addressed. Year introduced: 2008(1987)

"Consensus Development Conference, NIH" [publication type] AND *"cancer type"*[Mesh]

Consensus Development Conference, NIH - work consisting of summary statements, from a conference sponsored by NIH, representing the majority of current opinion of physicians, scientists, and other professionals on a selected subject. Year introduced: 2008(2005)

TO WHAT EXTENT HAS THE TREATMENT DEMONSTRATED EFFICACY IN SCIENTIFIC TERMS?

"Randomized Controlled Trial" [publication type] AND *"cancer type"*[Mesh]

Randomized Controlled Trial - a clinical trial that involves at least one test treatment and one control treatment, concurrent enrollment and follow-up of the test- and control-treated groups, and in which the treatments to be administered are selected by a random process, such as the use of a random-numbers table. Treatment allocations using coin flips, odd-even numbers, patient social security numbers, days of the week, medical record numbers, or other such pseudo- or quasi-random processes, are not truly

TO WHAT EXTENT HAS THE TREATMENT DEMONSTRATED EFFICACY IN SCIENTIFIC TERMS?

randomized and a trial employing any of these techniques for patient assignment is designated simply a CONTROLLED CLINICAL TRIAL [PUBLICATION TYPE].

"Randomized Controlled Trials as Topic"[Mesh] AND *"cancer type"*[Mesh]

Randomized Controlled Trials as Topic - clinical trials that involve at least one test treatment and one control treatment, concurrent enrollment and follow-up of the test- and control-treated groups, and in which the treatments to be administered are selected by a random process, such as the use of a random-numbers table. Year introduced: 2008(1990)

"Controlled Clinical Trial" [Publication Type] AND *"cancer type"*[Mesh]

Controlled Clinical Trial - reports consisting of a clinical trial involving one or more test treatments, at least one control treatment, specified outcome measures for evaluating the studied intervention, and a bias-free method for assigning patients to the test treatment. The treatment may be drugs, devices, or procedures studied for diagnostic, therapeutic, or prophylactic effectiveness. Control measures include placebos, active medicine, no-treatment, dosage forms and regimens, historical comparisons, etc. When randomization using mathematical techniques, such as the use of a random numbers table, is employed to assign patients to test or control treatments, the trial is characterized as a RANDOMIZED CONTROLLED TRIAL. Year introduced: 2008(1995)

"Meta-Analysis" [Publication Type] AND *"cancer type"*[Mesh]

Meta-Analysis - works consisting of studies using a quantitative method of combining the results of independent studies (usually drawn from the published literature) and synthesizing summaries and conclusions which may be used to evaluate therapeutic effectiveness, plan new studies, etc. It is often an overview of clinical trials. It is usually called a meta-analysis by the author or sponsoring body and should be differentiated from reviews of literature. Year introduced: 2008(1993)

"Meta-Analysis as Topic"[Mesh] AND *"cancer type"*[Mesh]

Meta-Analysis as Topic - a quantitative method of combining the results of independent studies (usually drawn from the published literature) and synthesizing summaries and conclusions which may be used to evaluate therapeutic effectiveness, plan new

---

TO WHAT EXTENT HAS THE TREATMENT DEMONSTRATED EFFICACY IN SCIENTIFIC TERMS?

---

studies, etc., with application chiefly in the areas of research and medicine. Year introduced: 2008(1989)

WHAT ARE THE ADVERSE EFFECTS OF THE TREATMENT?

"the type of therapy"/Adverse Effects" [MeSH]

Adverse Effects [a subheading to a MeSH term] - used with drugs, chemicals, or biological agents in accepted dosage - or with physical agents or manufactured products in normal usage - when intended for diagnostic, therapeutic, prophylactic, or anesthetic purposes. It is used also for adverse effects or complications of diagnostic, therapeutic, prophylactic, anesthetic, surgical, or other procedures, but excludes contraindications for which "contraindications" is used. Year introduced: 1966

"the type of therapy/Contraindications"[MeSH]

Contraindications [a subheading to a MeSH term] - used with drugs, chemicals, and biological and physical agents in any disease or physical state that might render their use improper, undesirable, or inadvisable. Used also with contraindicated diagnostic, therapeutic, prophylactic, anesthetic, surgical or other procedures. Year introduced: 1991

DOES THE TREATMENT OFFER TANGIBLE BENEFITS TO THE PATIENT IN TERMS OF QUALITY OF LIVING AND LENGTH OF LIFE, OR IS IT CLOSE TO A ZERO SUM EQUATION, OR IS IT LIKELY TO BE A NET DETRIMENT?

"cancer type" [MeSH] AND "Disease-Free Survival"[Mesh]
or *"the therapy"* [MeSH] AND "Disease-Free Survival"[Mesh]

Disease-Free Survival - the period after successful treatment in which there is no appearance of the symptoms or effects of the disease. Year introduced: 1995

"treatment type"[MeSH] AND "Quality-Adjusted Life Years"[Mesh]
or *"cancer type"* [MeSH] AND "Quality-Adjusted Life Years"[Mesh]

Quality-Adjusted Life Years - a measurement index derived from a modification of

126

standard life-table procedures and designed to take account of the quality as well as the duration of survival. This index can be used in assessing the outcome of health care procedures or services. (BIOETHICS Thesaurus, 1994) Year introduced: 1996

"Outcome and Process Assessment (Health Care)"[Mesh] AND "*cancer type*"[Mesh]

Outcome and Process Assessment (Health Care) - evaluation procedures that focus on both the outcome or status (OUTCOMES ASSESSMENT) of the patient at the end of an episode of care - presence of symptoms, level of activity, and mortality; and the process (ASSESSMENT, PROCESS) - what is done for the patient diagnostically and therapeutically. Year introduced: 1979

WHAT MEASURES ARE USEFUL IN LIFE-STYLE MODIFICATION AND PHYSICAL CONDITIONING THAT MIGHT BE USED IN REPLACE OF OR IN SUPPORT OF CONVENTIONAL TREATMENTS?

"*cancer type/*prevention and control" [MeSH]

Prevention and control [Subheading] - used with disease headings for increasing human or animal resistance against disease (e.g., immunization), for control of transmission agents, for prevention and control of environmental hazards, or for prevention and control of social factors leading to disease. It includes preventive measures in individual cases. Year introduced: 1966

"Secondary Prevention"[Mesh] AND "*cancer type*"[Mesh]

Secondary Prevention - the prevention of recurrences or exacerbations of a disease or complications of its therapy. Year introduced: 2009

WHAT CLINICAL TRIALS ARE BEING REPORTED ON THE PARTICULAR TYPE OF CANCER AND WOULD PARTICIPATING IN AN EXPERIMENTAL TRIAL BE APPROPRIATE FOR THE PARTICULAR PATIENT?

"Controlled Clinical Trials as Topic"[Mesh] AND "*cancer type*" [Mesh]

Controlled Clinical Trials as Topic - clinical trials involving one or more test treatments, at least one control treatment, specified outcome measures for evaluating the

127

studied intervention, and a bias-free method for assigning patients to the test treatment. The treatment may be drugs, devices, or procedures studied for diagnostic, therapeutic, or prophylactic effectiveness. Control measures include placebos, active medicines, no-treatment, dosage forms and regimens, historical comparisons, etc. When randomization using mathematical techniques, such as the use of a random numbers table, is employed to assign patients to test or control treatments, the trials are characterized as RANDOMIZED CONTROLLED TRIALS AS TOPIC. Year introduced: 2008(1995)

"Controlled Clinical Trial" [Publication Type] AND "*cancer type*" [Mesh]

"Controlled Clinical Trial" [Publication Type] - work consisting of a clinical trial involving one or more test treatments, at least one control treatment, specified outcome measures for evaluating the studied intervention, and a bias-free method for assigning patients to the test treatment. The treatment may be drugs, devices, or procedures studied for diagnostic, therapeutic, or prophylactic effectiveness. Control measures include placebos, active medicine, no-treatment, dosage forms and regimens, historical comparisons, etc. When randomization using mathematical techniques, such as the use of a random numbers table, is employed to assign patients to test or control treatments, the trial is characterized as a RANDOMIZED CONTROLLED TRIAL. Year introduced: 2008(1995)

"Randomized Controlled Trials as Topic"[Mesh] AND "*cancer type*" [Mesh]

"Randomized Controlled Trials as Topic" - clinical trials that involve at least one test treatment and one control treatment, concurrent enrollment and follow-up of the test- and control-treated groups, and in which the treatments to be administered are selected by a random process, such as the use of a random-numbers table. Year introduced: 2008(1990)

"Clinical Trials, Phase I as Topic"[Mesh] AND "*cancer type*" [Mesh]

"Clinical Trials, Phase I as Topic" - studies performed to evaluate the safety of diagnostic, therapeutic, or prophylactic drugs, devices, or techniques in healthy subjects and to determine the safe dosage range (if appropriate). These tests also are used to determine pharmacologic and pharmacokinetic properties (toxicity, metabolism, absorption, elimination, and preferred route of administration). They involve a small number of persons and usually last about 1 year. This concept includes phase I studies conducted both in the U.S. and in other countries. Year introduced: 2008(1993)

"Clinical Trials, Phase II as Topic"[Mesh] AND "*cancer type*"[Mesh]

"Clinical Trials, Phase II as Topic" - studies that are usually controlled to assess the effectiveness and dosage (if appropriate) of diagnostic, therapeutic, or prophylactic drugs, devices, or techniques. These studies are performed on several hundred volunteers, including a limited number of patients with the target disease or disorder, and last about two years. This concept includes phase II studies conducted in both the U.S. and in other countries. Year introduced: 2008(1993)

"Clinical Trials, Phase III as Topic"[Mesh] AND "*cancer type*"[Mesh]

Clinical Trials, Phase III as Topic - comparative studies to verify the effectiveness of diagnostic, therapeutic, or prophylactic drugs, devices, or techniques determined in phase II studies. During these trials, patients are monitored closely by physicians to identify any adverse reactions from long-term use. These studies are performed on groups of patients large enough to identify clinically significant responses and usually last about three years. This concept includes phase III studies conducted in both the U.S. and in other countries. Year introduced: 2008(1993)

"Clinical Trials, Phase IV as Topic"[Mesh] AND "*cancer type*"[Mesh]

Clinical Trials, Phase III as Topic - planned post-marketing studies of diagnostic, therapeutic, or prophylactic drugs, devices, or techniques that have been approved for general sale. These studies are often conducted to obtain additional data about the safety and efficacy of a product. This concept includes phase IV studies conducted in both the U.S. and in other countries. Year introduced: 2008(1993)

RESEARCHING DRUGS

Researching a specific drug is done according to the same procedures as any other MeSH term; however special procedures may be required in order to find the correct chemical name for the drug. Drugs are commonly known by their trade names; but the research is usually reported according to the generic, chemical names. Thus, the trick is to find the right term. Try the usual routine by using the "**MeSH Browser**" link, entering the drug name, and selecting "**Go**". That may be sufficient, leading you to the proper term. If that is not successful, use the procedures in Chapter 4 Medline-Plus and the section entitled "Drugs & Supplements".

"*drug name*/Therapeutic Use"[MeSH]

Therapeutic Use - used with drugs, biological preparations, and physical agents for their use in the prophylaxis and treatment of disease. It includes veterinary use. For

RESEARCHING DRUGS

treatment or preventive use of drugs or physical agents in clinical or experimental human or animal disease.

"drug name/Administration & Dosage"[MeSH]

Administration & Dosage - used with drugs for dosage forms, routes of administration, frequency and duration of administration, quantity of medication, and the effects of these factors.

"drug name/Pharmacology"[MeSH]

Pharmacology - used with drugs and exogenously administered chemical substances for their effects on living tissues and organisms. It includes acceleration and inhibition of physiological and biochemical processes and other pharmacologic mechanisms of action. With exogenous chemicals only; includes "effect", "mechanism of action", "mode of action"; not for pharmacokinetics (= /pharmacokinetics); see also /adverse effects, /poisoning & /toxicity.

"drug name/Adverse Effects"[MeSH]

Adverse Effects - used with drugs, chemicals, or biological agents in accepted dosage - or with physical agents or manufactured products in normal usage - when intended for diagnostic, therapeutic, prophylactic, or anesthetic purposes. It is used also for adverse effects or complications of diagnostic, therapeutic, prophylactic, anesthetic, surgical, or other procedures, but excludes contraindications for which "contraindications" is used. Includes "injurious effects", "undesirable effects", "side effects" in normal use; for complications following various procedures; see also /poisoning & /toxicity.

"drug name/Contraindications"[MeSH]

Contraindications - used with drugs, chemicals, and biological and physical agents in any disease or physical state that might render their use improper, undesirable, or inadvisable. Used also with contraindicated diagnostic, therapeutic, prophylactic, anesthetic, surgical or other procedures. With substances or physical agents possibly rendering their use improper, undesirable, or inadvisable in the presence of existing conditions & with contraindicated procedures.

"drug name/Toxicity"[MeSH]

Toxicity - used with drugs and chemicals for experimental human and animal studies of their ill effects. It includes studies to determine the margin of safety or the reactions accompanying administration at various dose levels. It is used also for experimental

RESEARCHING DRUGS

studies of exposure to environmental agents. For experimental human & animal studies; includes margin of safety & experimental exposure to environmental agents; see also /adverse effects & /poisoning.

SUNDRY SEARCH STRATEGIES

"cancer type"[Mesh] AND "Prognosis" [Mesh]
or *"treatment type"*[Mesh] AND "Prognosis" [Mesh]
Prognosis - the prediction as to the probable outcome of a disease or disorder as indicated by the nature and symptoms of the case.

"cancer type"[Mesh] AND "Pathological Conditions, Signs and Symptoms"[Mesh]
Pathological Conditions, Signs and Symptoms - manifestations of disease and pathological conditions which may occur in various diseases and different organs.

"anatomical site"[Mesh] AND "Pathological Conditions, Signs and Symptoms" [Mesh]
This search might be useful in pre-clinical evaluation of a symptom(s). Examples might be correlating: "feet with numbness"; "chest with pain"; "stomach with burning". Experiment with different combinations.

"cancer type"[Mesh] AND "Disease Progression"[Mesh]
Disease Progression - the worsening of a disease over time. This concept is most often used for chronic and incurable diseases where the stage of the disease is an important determinant of therapy and prognosis.

"cancer type"[Mesh] AND "Recurrence"[Mesh]
Recurrence - the return of symptoms after a remission (diminution or abatement or lessening in severity) of a disease or after therapy. Relapse is often considered a synonym or in many texts as the return of manifestations of a disease after an interval of improvement. Recrudescence, also often a synonym for recurrence, differs from relapse in that a recrudescence occurs after days or weeks while a relapse occurs after weeks or months. The terms in the literature are not used as precisely as the dictionaries define them.

SUNDRY SEARCH STRATEGIES

"treatment type"[Mesh] AND "Iatrogenic Disease"[Mesh]

Iatrogenic Disease - any adverse condition in a patient occurring as the result of treatment by a physician, surgeon, or other health professional, especially infections acquired by the patient during the course of treatment.

"cancer type"[Mesh] AND "Severity of Illness Index"[Mesh]

Severity of Illness Index - levels of severity of illness within a diagnostic group which are established by various measurement criteria.

"cancer type"[Mesh] AND "Survival Rate"[Mesh]

Survival Rate - the proportion of survivors in a group, e.g., of patients, studied and followed over a period, or the proportion of persons in a specified group alive at the beginning of a time interval who survive to the end of the interval. It is often studied using life table methods.

"cancer type"[Mesh] AND "Prognosis"[Mesh]

Prognosis - prediction as to the probable outcome of a disease or disorder as indicated by the nature and symptoms of the case.

"cancer type"[Mesh] AND "Medical Futility"[Mesh]

Medical Futility - the absence of a useful purpose or useful result in a diagnostic procedure or therapeutic intervention. The situation of a patient whose condition will not be improved by treatment or instances in which treatment preserves permanent unconsciousness or cannot end dependence on intensive medical care.

"cancer type"[Mesh] AND "Disease-Free Survival"[Mesh] or *"treatment type"*[Mesh] AND "Disease-Free Survival"[Mesh]

Disease-Free Survival - period after successful treatment in which there is no appearance of the symptoms or effects of the disease.

"cancer type"[Mesh] AND "Karnofsky Performance Status"[Mesh] or "treatment type"[Mesh] AND "Karnofsky Performance Status"[Mesh]

Karnofsky Performance Status - a performance measure for rating the ability of a person to perform usual activities, evaluating a patient's progress after a therapeutic procedure, and determining a patient's suitability for therapy. It is used most commonly in the prognosis of cancer therapy, usually after chemotherapy and customarily

132

administered before and after therapy. It was named for Dr. David A. Karnofsky, an American specialist in cancer chemotherapy.

"cancer type"[Mesh] AND "Treatment Failure"[Mesh]

Treatment Failure - a measure of the quality of health care by assessment of unsuccessful results of management and procedures used in combating disease, in individual cases or series.

"cancer type"[Mesh] AND "Treatment Outcome"[Mesh]

Treatment Outcome - evaluation undertaken to assess the results or consequences of management and procedures used in combating disease in order to determine the efficacy, effectiveness, safety, practicability, etc., of these interventions in individual cases or series.

"cancer type"[Mesh] AND "Watchful Waiting"[Mesh]

Watchful Waiting - an approach in medicine in which the patient is monitored closely without medical treatment to evaluate the trend and course of a disease. Palliative and life-style modifications may be applied with the hope that restoration will occur without treatment.

"cancer type"[Mesh] AND "History of Medicine"[Mesh] or *"treatment type"*[Mesh] AND "History of Medicine"[Mesh] or *"diagnostic technique"*[Mesh] AND "History of Medicine"[Mesh]

History of Medicine - obtaining a historical perspective on a subject can be interesting and useful. To be more definitive, use one of the following MeSH terms:
"**History of Medicine, Modern [Mesh]**" (The from 1601 A.D. to the present)
"**History of Medicine, Early Modern [Mesh]**" (The from 1451 through 1600 A.D.)
"**History of Medicine, 20th Century [Mesh]**" (1900-1999)
"**History of Medicine, 19th Century [Mesh]**" (1800-1899)
"**History of Medicine, 18th Century [Mesh]**" (1700-1799)
"**History of Medicine, 17th Century [Mesh]**" (1600-1699)
"**History of Medicine, 16th Century [Mesh]**" (1500-1599)
"**History of Medicine, 15th Century [Mesh]**" (1400-1499).

A Glossary of MeSH terms for all types of cancer (neoplasms)

Abdominal Neoplasms

Adrenal Gland Neoplasms - Tumors or cancer of the ADRENAL GLANDS.

Adrenal Cortex Neoplasms - Tumors or cancers of the ADRENAL CORTEX. Year introduced: 1979(1975)1963-1967

Anal Gland Neoplasms - Tumors or cancer of the anal gland. Year introduced: 1968

Anus Neoplasms - Tumors or cancer of the ANAL CANAL.

Appendiceal Neoplasms - Tumors or cancer of the APPENDIX.

Bile Duct Neoplasms - Tumors or cancer of the BILE DUCTS.

Biliary Tract Neoplasms - Tumors or cancer in the BILIARY TRACT including the BILE DUCTS and the GALLBLADDER. Year introduced: 1980

Bone Neoplasms - Tumors or cancer located in bone tissue or specific BONES.

Bone Marrow Neoplasms - Neoplasms located in the bone marrow. They are differentiated from neoplasms composed of bone marrow cells, such as MULTIPLE MYELOMA. Most bone marrow neoplasms are metastatic. Year introduced: 1996

Brain Neoplasms - Neoplasms of the intracranial components of the central nervous system, including the cerebral hemispheres, basal ganglia, hypothalamus, thalamus, brain stem, and cerebellum. Brain neoplasms are subdivided into primary (originating from brain tissue) and secondary (i.e., metastatic) forms. Primary neoplasms are subdivided into benign and malignant forms. In general, brain tumors may also be classified by age of onset, histologic type, or presenting location in the brain.

Brain Stem Neoplasms - Benign and malignant intra-axial tumors of the MESENCEPHALON; PONS; or MEDULLA OBLONGATA of the BRAIN STEM. Primary and metastatic neoplasms may occur in this location. Clinical features include ATAXIA, cranial neuropathies (see CRANIAL NERVE DISEASES), NAUSEA, hemiparesis (see HEMIPLEGIA), and quadriparesis. Primary brain stem neoplasms are more frequent in children. Histologic subtypes include GLIOMA; HEMANGIOBLASTOMA; GANGLIOGLIOMA; and EPENDYMOMA. Year introduced: 2000

Breast Neoplasms - Tumors or cancer of the human BREAST.

Breast Neoplasms, Male - Any neoplasms of the male breast. These occur infrequently in males in developed countries, the incidence being about 1% of that in females. Year introduced: 1995

Bronchial Neoplasms - Tumors or cancer of the BRONCHI.

A Glossary of MeSH terms for all types of cancer (neoplasms)

Carcinoma - A malignant neoplasm made up of epithelial cells tending to infiltrate the surrounding tissues and give rise to metastases. It is a histological type of neoplasm but is often wrongly used as a synonym for "cancer." (From Dorland, 27th ed)

Carcinoma in Situ - A lesion with cytological characteristics associated with invasive carcinoma but the tumor cells are confined to the epithelium of origin, without invasion of the basement membrane. Year introduced: 1973

Cecal Neoplasms - Tumors or cancer of the CECUM.

Central Nervous System Neoplasms - Benign and malignant neoplastic processes that arise from or secondarily involve the brain, spinal cord, or meninges. Year introduced: 1992

Cerebellar Neoplasms - Primary or metastatic neoplasms of the CEREBELLUM. Tumors in this location frequently present with ATAXIA or signs of INTRACRANIAL HYPERTENSION due to obstruction of the fourth ventricle. Common primary cerebellar tumors include fibrillary ASTROCYTOMA and cerebellar HEMANGIOBLASTOMA. The cerebellum is a relatively common site for tumor metastases from the lung, breast, and other distant organs. (From Okazaki and Scheithauer, Atlas of Neuropathology, 1988, p86 and p141)

Cerebral Ventricle Neoplasms - Neoplasms located in the brain ventricles, including the two lateral, the third, and the fourth ventricle. Ventricular tumors may be primary (e.g., CHOROID PLEXUS NEOPLASMS and GLIOMA, SUBEPENDYMAL), metastasize from distant organs, or occur as extensions of locally invasive tumors from adjacent brain structures.

Cervical Intraepithelial Neoplasia - A malignancy arising in uterine cervical epithelium and confined thereto, representing a continuum of histological changes ranging from well-differentiated CIN 1 (formerly, mild dysplasia) to severe dysplasia/carcinoma in situ, CIN 3. The lesion arises at the squamocolumnar cell junction at the transformation zone of the endocervical canal, with a variable tendency to develop invasive epidermoid carcinoma, a tendency that is enhanced by concomitant human papillomaviral infection. (Segen, Dictionary of Modern Medicine, 1992) Year introduced: 1994

Choroid Neoplasms - Tumors of the choroid; most common intraocular tumors are malignant melanomas of the choroid. These usually occur after puberty and increase in incidence with advancing age. Most malignant melanomas of the uveal tract develop from benign melanomas (nevi).

Choroid Plexus Neoplasms - Benign or malignant tumors which arise from the choroid plexus of the ventricles of the brain. Papillomas (see PAPILLOMA, CHOROID PLEXUS) and carcinomas are the most common histologic subtypes, and tend to seed throughout the ventricular and subarachnoid spaces. Clinical features include headaches, ataxia and alterations of consciousness, primarily resulting from associated HYDROCEPHALUS. (From Devita et al.,

A Glossary of MeSH terms for all types of cancer (neoplasms)

Cancer: Principles and Practice of Oncology, 5th ed, p2072; J Neurosurg 1998 Mar;88(3):521-8) Year introduced: 1992

Colonic Neoplasms - Tumors or cancer of the COLON. Year introduced: 1964

Colorectal Neoplasms - Tumors or cancer of the COLON or the RECTUM or both. Risk factors for colorectal cancer include chronic ULCERATIVE COLITIS; FAMILIAL POLYPOSIS COLI; exposure to ASBESTOS; and irradiation of the CERVIX UTERI. Year introduced: 1989

Colorectal Neoplasms, Hereditary Nonpolyposis - A group of autosomal-dominant inherited diseases in which COLON CANCER arises in discrete adenomas. Unlike FAMILIAL POLYPOSIS COLI with hundreds of polyps, hereditary nonpolyposis colorectal neoplasms occur much later, in the fourth and fifth decades. HNPCC has been associated with germline mutations in mismatch repair (MMR) genes. It has been subdivided into Lynch syndrome I or site-specific colonic cancer, and LYNCH SYNDROME II which includes extracolonic cancer. Year introduced: 1987

Common Bile Duct Neoplasms -Tumor or cancer of the COMMON BILE DUCT including the AMPULLA OF VATER and the SPHINCTER OF ODDI. Year introduced: 1980

Conjunctival Neoplasms - Tumors or cancer of the CONJUNCTIVA. Year introduced: 1981

Cranial Nerve Neoplasms - Benign and malignant neoplasms that arise from one or more of the twelve cranial nerves. Year introduced: 1978

Digestive System Neoplasms - Tumors or cancer of the DIGESTIVE SYSTEM. Year introduced: 1980

Duodenal Neoplasms - Tumors or cancer of the DUODENUM.

Ear Neoplasms - Tumors or cancer of any part of the hearing and equilibrium system of the body (the EXTERNAL EAR, the MIDDLE EAR, and the INNER EAR). Year introduced: 1966

Endocrine Gland Neoplasms -Tumors or cancer of the ENDOCRINE GLANDS. Year introduced: 1992

Endometrial Neoplasms - Tumors or cancer of ENDOMETRIUM, the mucous lining of the UTERUS. These neoplasms can be benign or malignant. Their classification and grading are based on the various cell types and the percent of undifferentiated cells. Year introduced: 1992

Epidural Neoplasms - Neoplasms located in the space between the vertebral PERIOSTEUM and DURA MATER surrounding the SPINAL CORD. Tumors in this location are most often metastatic in origin and may cause neurologic deficits by mass effect on the spinal cord or nerve roots or by interfering with blood supply to the spinal cord. Year introduced: 1989

Esophageal Neoplasms - Tumors or cancer of the ESOPHAGUS.

A Glossary of MeSH terms for all types of cancer (neoplasms)

Eye Neoplasms - Tumors or cancer of the EYE.

Eyelid Neoplasms - Tumors of cancer of the EYELIDS. Year introduced: 1970

Facial Neoplasms

Fallopian Tube Neoplasms - Benign or malignant neoplasms of the FALLOPIAN TUBES. They are uncommon. If they develop, they may be located in the wall or within the lumen as a growth attached to the wall by a stalk.

Femoral Neoplasms

Gallbladder Neoplasms - Tumors or cancer of the gallbladder.

Gastrointestinal Stromal Tumors - All tumors in the GASTROINTESTINAL TRACT arising from mesenchymal cells (MESODERM) except those of smooth muscle cells (LEIOMYOMA) or Schwann cells (SCHWANNOMA). Year introduced: 2005

Gastrointestinal Neoplasms - Tumors or cancer of the GASTROINTESTINAL TRACT, from the MOUTH to the ANAL CANAL.

Genital Neoplasms, Male - Tumor or cancer of the MALE GENITALIA. Year introduced: 1978

Genital Neoplasms, Female - Tumor or cancer of the female reproductive tract (GENITALIA, FEMALE). Year introduced: 1979

Gestational Trophoblastic Disease - A group of diseases arising from pregnancy that are commonly associated with hyperplasia of trophoblasts (TROPHOBLAST) and markedly elevated human CHORIONIC GONADOTROPIN. They include HYDATIDIFORM MOLE, invasive mole (HYDATIDIFORM MOLE, INVASIVE), placental-site trophoblastic tumor (TROPHOBLASTIC TUMOR, PLACENTAL SITE), and CHORIOCARCINOMA. These neoplasms have varying propensities for invasion and spread. Year introduced: 2012 (2003)

Gingival Neoplasms - Year introduced: 1974(1971)

Head and Neck Neoplasms - Soft tissue tumors or cancer arising from the mucosal surfaces of the LIP; oral cavity; PHARYNX; LARYNX; and cervical esophagus. Other sites included are the NOSE and PARANASAL SINUSES; SALIVARY GLANDS; THYROID GLAND and PARATHYROID GLANDS; and MELANOMA and non-melanoma skin cancers of the head and neck. (from Holland et al., Cancer Medicine, 4th ed, p1651) Year introduced: 1976

Heart Neoplasms - Tumors in any part of the heart. They include primary cardiac tumors and metastatic tumors to the heart. Their interference with normal cardiac functions can cause a wide variety of symptoms including HEART FAILURE; CARDIAC ARRHYTHMIAS; or EMBOLISM.

A Glossary of MeSH terms for all types of cancer (neoplasms)

Hematologic Neoplasms - Neoplasms located in the blood and blood-forming tissue (the bone marrow and lymphatic tissue). The commonest forms are the various types of LEUKEMIA, of LYMPHOMA, and of the progressive, life-threatening forms of the MYELODYSPLASTIC SYNDROMES. Year introduced: 1997

Hypopharyngeal Neoplasms - Tumors or cancer of the HYPOPHARYNX. Year introduced: 1991(1985)

Hypothalamic Neoplasms - Benign and malignant tumors of the HYPOTHALAMUS. Pilocytic astrocytomas and hamartomas are relatively frequent histologic types. Neoplasms of the hypothalamus frequently originate from adjacent structures, including the OPTIC CHIASM, optic nerve (see OPTIC NERVE NEOPLASMS), and pituitary gland (see PITUITARY NEOPLASMS). Relatively frequent clinical manifestations include visual loss, developmental delay, macrocephaly, and precocious puberty. (From Devita et al., Cancer: Principles and Practice of Oncology, 5th ed, p2051) Year introduced: 1981

Ileal Neoplasms - Tumors or cancer in the ILEUM region of the small intestine (INTESTINE, SMALL). Year introduced: 1980

Inflammatory Breast Neoplasms - Metastatic breast cancer characterized by EDEMA and ERYTHEMA of the affected breast due to LYMPHATIC METASTASIS and eventual obstruction of LYMPHATIC VESSELS by the cancer cells. Year introduced: 2011

Infratentorial Neoplasms - Intracranial tumors originating in the region of the brain inferior to the tentorium cerebelli, which contains the cerebellum, fourth ventricle, cerebellopontine angle, brain stem, and related structures. Primary tumors of this region are more frequent in children, and may present with ATAXIA; CRANIAL NERVE DISEASES; vomiting; HEADACHE; HYDROCEPHALUS; or other signs of neurologic dysfunction. Relatively frequent histologic subtypes include TERATOMA; MEDULLOBLASTOMA; GLIOBLASTOMA; ASTROCY-TOMA; EPENDYMOMA; CRANIOPHARYNGIOMA; and choroid plexus papilloma (PAPIL-LOMA, CHOROID PLEXUS). Year introduced: 1989

Intestinal Neoplasms - Tumors or cancer of the INTESTINES.

Iris Neoplasms - Tumors of the iris characterized by increased pigmentation of melanocytes. Iris nevi are composed of proliferated melanocytes and are associated with neurofibromatosis and malignant melanoma of the choroid and ciliary body. Malignant melanoma of the iris often originates from preexisting nevi. Year introduced: 1990

Jaw Neoplasms - Cancers or tumors of the MAXILLA or MANDIBLE unspecified. For neoplasms of the maxilla, MAXILLARY NEOPLASMS is available and of the mandible, MANDIBULAR NEOPLASMS is available. Year introduced: 1967

Jejunal Neoplasms - Tumors or cancer in the JEJUNUM region of the small intestine (INTES-TINE, SMALL). Year introduced: 1980

A Glossary of MeSH terms for all types of cancer (neoplasms)

Kidney Neoplasms - Tumors or cancers of the KIDNEY.

Laryngeal Neoplasms - Cancers or tumors of the LARYNX or any of its parts: the GLOTTIS; EPIGLOTTIS; LARYNGEAL CARTILAGES; LARYNGEAL MUSCLES; and VOCAL CORDS.

Lip Neoplasms - Tumors or cancer of the LIP.

Liver Neoplasms, Experimental - Experimentally induced tumors of the LIVER. Year introduced: 1985

Liver Neoplasms - Tumors or cancer of the LIVER.

Lung Neoplasms - Tumors or cancer of the LUNG.

Mammary Neoplasms, Experimental - Experimentally induced mammary neoplasms in animals to provide a model for studying human BREAST NEOPLASMS.

Mammary Neoplasms, Animal - Tumors or cancer of the MAMMARY GLAND in animals (MAMMARY GLANDS, ANIMAL). Year introduced: 2004 (1990)

Mandibular Neoplasms - Tumors or cancer of the MANDIBLE.

Maxillary Sinus Neoplasms - Tumors or cancer of the MAXILLARY SINUS. They represent the majority of paranasal neoplasms. Year introduced: 1991(1984)

Maxillary Neoplasms - Cancer or tumors of the MAXILLA or upper jaw.

Mediastinal Neoplasms - Tumors or cancer of the MEDIASTINUM.

Meningeal Neoplasms - Benign and malignant neoplastic processes that arise from or secondarily involve the meningeal coverings of the brain and spinal cord. Year introduced: 1978

Mouth Neoplasms - Tumors or cancer of the MOUTH.

Multiple Endocrine Neoplasia Type 1 - A form of multiple endocrine neoplasia that is characterized by the combined occurrence of tumors in the PARATHYROID GLANDS, the PITUITARY GLAND, and the PANCREATIC ISLETS. The resulting clinical signs include HYPERPARATHYROIDISM; HYPERCALCEMIA; HYPERPROLACTINEMIA; CUSHING DISEASE; GASTRINOMA; and ZOLLINGER-ELLISON SYNDROME. This disease is due to loss-of-function of the MEN1 gene, a tumor suppressor gene (GENES, TUMOR SUPPRESSOR) on CHROMOSOME 11 (Locus: 11q13). Year introduced: 1995

Multiple Endocrine Neoplasia - A group of autosomal dominant diseases characterized by the combined occurrence of tumors involving two or more ENDOCRINE GLANDS that secrete PEPTIDE HORMONES or AMINES. These neoplasias are often benign but can be malignant. They are classified by the endocrine glands involved and the degree of aggressiveness. The two

A Glossary of MeSH terms for all types of cancer (neoplasms)

major forms are MEN1 and MEN2 with gene mutations on CHROMOSOME 11 and CHROMO-SOME 10, respectively. Year introduced: 1995

Multiple Endocrine Neoplasia Type 2b - Similar to MEN2A, it is also caused by mutations of the MEN2 gene, also known as the RET proto-oncogene. Its clinical symptoms include medullary carcinoma (CARCINOMA, MEDULLARY) of THYROID GLAND and PHEOCHROMO-CYTOMA of ADRENAL MEDULLA (50%). Unlike MEN2a, MEN2b does not involve PARATHYROID NEOPLASMS. It can be distinguished from MEN2A by its neural abnormalities such as mucosal NEUROMAS on EYELIDS; LIP; and TONGUE, and ganglioneuromatosis of GASTROINTESTINAL TRACT leading to MEGACOLON. It is an autosomal dominant inherited disease. Year introduced: 1995

Multiple Endocrine Neoplasia Type 2a - A form of multiple endocrine neoplasia characterized by the presence of medullary carcinoma (CARCINOMA, MEDULLARY) of the THYROID GLAND, and usually with the co-occurrence of PHEOCHROMOCYTOMA, producing CALCI-TONIN and ADRENALINE, respectively. Less frequently, it can occur with hyperplasia or adenoma of the PARATHYROID GLANDS. This disease is due to gain-of-function mutations of the MEN2 gene on CHROMOSOME 10 (Locus: 10q11.2), also known as the RET proto-oncogene that encodes a RECEPTOR PROTEIN-TYROSINE KINASE. It is an autosomal dominant inherited disease. Year introduced: 1995

Muscle Neoplasms - Tumors or cancer located in muscle tissue or specific muscles. They are differentiated from NEOPLASMS, MUSCLE TISSUE which are neoplasms composed of skeletal, cardiac, or smooth muscle tissue, such as MYOSARCOMA or LEIOMYOMA. Year introduced: 1996

Nasopharyngeal Neoplasms - Tumors or cancer of the NASOPHARYNX.

Neoplasm, Residual - Remnant of a tumor or cancer after primary, potentially curative therapy. (Dr. Daniel Masys, written communication) Year introduced: 1995

Neoplasms by Site - A collective term for precoordinated organ/neoplasm headings locating neoplasms by organ, as BRAIN NEOPLASMS; DUODENAL NEOPLASMS; LIVER NEOPLASMS; etc. Year introduced: 1998

Neoplasms by Histologic Type - A collective term for the various histological types of NEOPLASMS. It is more likely to be used by searchers than by indexers and catalogers. Year introduced: 1998

Neoplasms - New abnormal growth of tissue. Malignant neoplasms show a greater degree of anaplasia and have the properties of invasion and metastasis, compared to benign neoplasms. Year introduced: /diagnosis was NEOPLASM DIAGNOSIS 1964-1965

Neoplasms, Vascular Tissue - Neoplasms composed of vascular tissue. This concept does not refer to neoplasms located in blood vessels.

A Glossary of MeSH terms for all types of cancer (neoplasms)

Neoplasms, Unknown Primary - Metastases in which the tissue of origin is unknown. Year introduced: 1987

Neoplasms, Radiation-Induced - Tumors, cancer or other neoplasms produced by exposure to ionizing or non-ionizing radiation.

Neoplasms, Nerve Tissue - Neoplasms composed of nerve tissue. This concept does not refer to neoplasms located in the nervous system or its component nerves. Year introduced: 1994

Neoplasms, Muscle Tissue - Neoplasms composed of muscle tissue: skeletal, cardiac, or smooth. The concept does not refer to neoplasms located in muscles. Year introduced: MYOBLASTOMA was heading 1963-1993

Neoplasms, Multiple Primary - Two or more abnormal growths of tissue occurring simultaneously and presumed to be of separate origin. The neoplasms may be histologically the same or different, and may be found in the same or different sites. Year introduced: 1965

Neoplasms, Hormone-Dependent - Certain tumors that 1, arise in organs that are normally dependent on specific hormones and 2, are stimulated or caused to regress by manipulation of the endocrine environment. Year introduced: 1979

Neoplasms, Glandular and Epithelial - Neoplasms composed of glandular tissue, an aggregation of epithelial cells that elaborate secretions, and of any type of epithelium itself. The concept does not refer to neoplasms located in the various glands or in epithelial tissue. Year introduced: 1994

Neoplasms, Experimental - Experimentally induced new abnormal growth of TISSUES in animals to provide models for studying human neoplasms.

Neoplasms, Germ Cell and Embryonal - Neoplasms composed of primordial GERM CELLS of embryonic GONADS or of elements of the germ layers of the EMBRYO, MAMMALIAN. The concept does not refer to neoplasms located in the gonads or present in an embryo or FETUS. Year introduced: 1994 (1963)

Neoplasms, Connective Tissue - Neoplasms composed of connective tissue, including elastic, mucous, reticular, osseous, and cartilaginous tissue. The concept does not refer to neoplasms located in connective tissue.

Neoplasms, Plasma Cell - Neoplasms associated with a proliferation of a single clone of PLASMA CELLS and characterized by the secretion of PARAPROTEINS. Year introduced: 2008

Neoplasms, Gonadal Tissue - Neoplasms composed of tissues of the OVARY or the TESTIS, not neoplasms located in the ovaries or testes. Gonadal tissues include GERM CELLS, cells from the sex cord, and gonadal stromal cells. Year introduced: 1994

A Glossary of MeSH terms for all types of cancer (neoplasms)

Neoplasms, Squamous Cell - Neoplasms composed of squamous cells of the epithelium. The concept does not refer to neoplasms located in tissue composed of squamous elements. Year introduced: 1994

Neoplasms, Neuroepithelial - Neoplasms composed of neuroepithelial cells, which have the capacity to differentiate into NEURONS, oligodendrocytes, and ASTROCYTES. The majority of craniospinal tumors are of neuroepithelial origin. (From Dev Biol 1998 Aug 1;200(1):1-5) Year introduced: 1994

Neoplasms, Mesothelial - Neoplasms composed of tissue of the mesothelium, the layer of flat cells, derived from the mesoderm, which lines the body cavity of the embryo. In the adult it forms the simple squamous epithelium which covers all true serous membranes (peritoneum, pericardium, pleura). The concept does not refer to neoplasms located in these organs. (From Dorland, 27th ed) Year introduced: 1994

Neoplasms, Ductal, Lobular, and Medullary - Neoplasms, usually carcinoma, located within the center of an organ or within small lobes, and in the case of the breast, intraductally. The emphasis of the name is on the location of the neoplastic tissue rather than on its histological type. Most cancers of this type are located in the breast. Year introduced: 1998

Neoplasms, Cystic, Mucinous, and Serous - Neoplasms containing cyst-like formations or producing mucin or serum. Year introduced: 1998

Neoplasms, Basal Cell - Neoplasms composed of cells from the deepest layer of the epidermis. The concept does not refer to neoplasms located in the stratum basale. Year introduced: 1994

Neoplasms, Adnexal and Skin Appendage - Neoplasms composed of sebaceous or sweat gland tissue or tissue of other skin appendages. The concept does not refer to neoplasms located in the sebaceous or sweat glands or in the other skin appendages. Year introduced: 1998

Neoplasms, Fibroepithelial - Neoplasms composed of fibrous and epithelial tissue. The concept does not refer to neoplasms located in fibrous tissue or epithelium. Year introduced: 1994

Neoplasms, Fibrous Tissue - Neoplasms composed of fibrous tissue, the ordinary connective tissue of the body, made up largely of yellow or white fibers. The concept does not refer to neoplasms located in fibrous tissue. Year introduced: 1994

Neoplasms, Bone Tissue - Neoplasms composed of bony tissue, whether normal or of a soft tissue which has become ossified. The concept does not refer to neoplasms located in bones. Year introduced: 1994

Neoplasms, Adipose Tissue - Neoplasms composed of fatty tissue or connective tissue made up of fat cells in a meshwork of areolar tissue. The concept does not refer to neoplasms located in adipose tissue. Year introduced: 1994

A Glossary of MeSH terms for all types of cancer (neoplasms)

Neoplasms, Connective and Soft Tissue - Neoplasms developing from some structure of the connective and subcutaneous tissue. The concept does not refer to neoplasms located in connective or soft tissue. Year introduced: 1998

Neoplasms, Complex and Mixed - Neoplasms composed of more than one type of neoplastic tissue. Year introduced: 1998

Neoplasms, Post-Traumatic - Tumors, cancer or other neoplasms caused by or resulting from trauma or other non-radiation injuries. Year introduced: 1993

Neoplasms, Second Primary - Abnormal growths of tissue that follow a previous neoplasm but are not metastases of the latter. The second neoplasm may have the same or different histological type and can occur in the same or different organs as the previous neoplasm but in all cases arises from an independent oncogenic event. The development of the second neoplasm may or may not be related to the treatment for the previous neoplasm since genetic risk or predisposing factors may actually be the cause. Year introduced: 1992

Nerve Sheath Neoplasms - Neoplasms which arise from nerve sheaths formed by SCHWANN CELLS in the PERIPHERAL NERVOUS SYSTEM or by OLIGODENDROCYTES in the CENTRAL NERVOUS SYSTEM. Malignant peripheral nerve sheath tumors, NEUROFI-BROMA, and NEURILEMMOMA are relatively common tumors in this category. Year introduced: 2006 (1994)

Nervous System Neoplasms - Benign and malignant neoplastic processes arising from or involving components of the central, peripheral, and autonomic nervous systems, cranial nerves, and meninges. Included in this category are primary and metastatic nervous system neoplasms. Year introduced: 1980

Neuroectodermal Tumors, Primitive - A group of malignant tumors of the nervous system that feature primitive cells with elements of neuronal and/or glial differentiation. Use of this term is limited by some authors to central nervous system tumors and others include neoplasms of similar origin which arise extracranially (i.e., NEUROECTODERMAL TUMORS, PRIMITIVE, PERIPHERAL). This term is also occasionally used as a synonym for MEDULLOBLASTOMA. In general, these tumors arise in the first decade of life and tend to be highly malignant. (From DeVita et al., Cancer: Principles and Practice of Oncology, 5th ed, p2059) Year introduced: 2000(1994)

Nose Neoplasms - Tumors or cancer of the NOSE.

Odontogenic Tumors - Neoplasms produced from tooth-forming tissues. Year introduced: 1980

Optic Nerve Neoplasms - Benign and malignant neoplasms that arise from the optic nerve or its sheath. OPTIC NERVE GLIOMA is the most common histologic type. Optic nerve neoplasms

143

A Glossary of MeSH terms for all types of cancer (neoplasms)

tend to cause unilateral visual loss and an afferent pupillary defect and may spread via neural pathways to the brain. Year introduced: 1998

Orbital Neoplasms - Neoplasms of the bony orbit and contents except the eyeball.

Oropharyngeal Neoplasms - Tumors or cancer of the OROPHARYNX. Year introduced: 1991(1985)

Otorhinolaryngologic Neoplasms - A general concept for tumors or cancer of any part of the EAR; the NOSE; the THROAT; and the PHARYNX. It is used when there is no specific heading. Year introduced: 1984

Ovarian Neoplasms - Tumors or cancer of the OVARY. These neoplasms can be benign or malignant. They are classified according to the tissue of origin, such as the surface EPITHE-LIUM, the stromal endocrine cells, and the totipotent GERM CELLS.

Palatal Neoplasms - Tumors or cancer of the PALATE, including those of the hard palate, soft palate and UVULA.

Pancreatic Neoplasms - Tumors or cancer of the PANCREAS. Depending on the types of ISLET CELLS present in the tumors, various hormones can be secreted: GLUCAGON from PANCREATIC ALPHA CELLS; INSULIN from PANCREATIC BETA CELLS; and SOMATOSTATIN from the SOMATOSTATIN-SECRETING CELLS. Most are malignant except the insulin-producing tumors (INSULINOMA).

Paranasal Sinus Neoplasms - Tumors or cancer of the PARANASAL SINUSES.

Parathyroid Neoplasms - Tumors or cancer of the PARATHYROID GLANDS.

Parotid Neoplasms - Tumors or cancer of the PAROTID GLAND.

Pelvic Neoplasms - Tumors or cancer of the pelvic region.

Penile Neoplasms - Cancers or tumors of the PENIS or of its component tissues.

Peripheral Nervous System Neoplasms - Neoplasms which arise from peripheral nerve tissue. This includes NEUROFIBROMAS; SCHWANNOMAS; GRANULAR CELL TUMORS; and malignant peripheral NERVE SHEATH NEOPLASMS. (From DeVita Jr et al., Cancer: Principles and Practice of Oncology, 5th ed, pp1750-1) Year introduced: 2000(1966)

Peritoneal Neoplasms - Tumors or cancer of the PERITONEUM.

Perivascular Epithelioid Cell Neoplasms - A family of mesenchymal tumors composed of histologically and immunohistochemically distinctive perivascular epithelioid cells. These cells do not have a normal anatomic homolog. (From Fletcher CDM, et. al., World Health Organization Classification of Tumors: Pathology and Genetics of Tumors of Soft Tissue and Bone, 2002). Year introduced: 2009

A Glossary of MeSH terms for all types of cancer (neoplasms)

Pharyngeal Neoplasms - Tumors or cancer of the PHARYNX.

Pinealoma - Neoplasms which originate from pineal parenchymal cells that tend to enlarge the gland and be locally invasive. The two major forms are pineocytoma and the more malignant pineoblastoma. Pineocytomas have moderate cellularity and tend to form rosette patterns. Pineo-blastomas are highly cellular tumors containing small, poorly differentiated cells. These tumors occasionally seed the neuroaxis or cause obstructive HYDROCEPHALUS or Parinaud's syndrome. GERMINOMA; CARCINOMA, EMBRYONAL; GLIOMA; and other neoplasms may arise in the pineal region with germinoma being the most common pineal region tumor. (From DeVita et al., Cancer: Principles and Practice of Oncology, 5th ed, p2064; Adams et al., Principles of Neurology, 6th ed, p670)

Pituitary Neoplasms - Neoplasms which arise from or metastasize to the PITUITARY GLAND. The majority of pituitary neoplasms are adenomas, which are divided into non-secreting and secreting forms. Hormone producing forms are further classified by the type of hormone they secrete. Pituitary adenomas may also be characterized by their staining properties (see ADENOMA, BASOPHIL; ADENOMA, ACIDOPHIL; and ADENOMA, CHROMOPHOBE). Pituitary tumors may compress adjacent structures, including the HYPOTHALAMUS, several CRANIAL NERVES, and the OPTIC CHIASM. Chiasmal compression may result in bitemporal HEMIANOPSIA.

Pleural Neoplasms - Neoplasms of the thin serous membrane that envelopes the lungs and lines the thoracic cavity. Pleural neoplasms are exceedingly rare and are usually not diagnosed until they are advanced because in the early stages they produce no symptoms.

Prostatic Intraepithelial Neoplasia - A premalignant change arising in the prostatic epithelium, regarded as the most important and most likely precursor of prostatic adenocarcinoma. The neoplasia takes the form of an intra-acinar or ductal proliferation of secretory cells with unequivocal nuclear anaplasia, which corresponds to nuclear grade 2 and 3 invasive prostate cancer. Year introduced: 1996

Prostatic Neoplasms - Tumors or cancer of the PROSTATE.

Prostatic Neoplasms, Castration-Resistant - Tumors or cancer of the PROSTATE which can grow in the presence of low or residual amount of androgen hormones such as TESTOSTER-ONE. Year introduced: 2014

Rectal Neoplasms - Tumors or cancer of the RECTUM.

Respiratory Tract Neoplasms

Retinal Neoplasms - Tumors or cancer of the RETINA. Year introduced: 1998

Retroperitoneal Neoplasms

Salivary Gland Neoplasms - Tumors or cancer of the SALIVARY GLANDS.

A Glossary of MeSH terms for all types of cancer (neoplasms)

Sebaceous Gland Neoplasms - Year introduced: 1968

Sigmoid Neoplasms - Tumors or cancer of the SIGMOID COLON.

Skin Neoplasms - Tumors or cancer of the SKIN.

Skull Base Neoplasms - Neoplasms of the base of the skull specifically, differentiated from neoplasms of unspecified sites or bones of the skull (SKULL NEOPLASMS). Year introduced: 1997

Soft Tissue Neoplasms - Neoplasms of whatever cell type or origin, occurring in the extraskeletal connective tissue framework of the body including the organs of locomotion and their various component structures, such as nerves, blood vessels, lymphatics, etc. Year introduced: 1976

Spinal Neoplasms - Self explicit.

Spinal Cord Neoplasms - Benign and malignant neoplasms which occur within the substance of the spinal cord (intramedullary neoplasms) or in the space between the dura and spinal cord (intradural extramedullary neoplasms). The majority of intramedullary spinal tumors are primary CNS neoplasms including ASTROCYTOMA; EPENDYMOMA; and LIPOMA. Intramedullary neoplasms are often associated with SYRINGOMYELIA. The most frequent histologic types of intradural-extramedullary tumors are MENINGIOMA and NEUROFIBROMA.

Splenic Neoplasms - Tumors or cancer of the SPLEEN.

Stomach Neoplasms - Tumors or cancer of the STOMACH.

Sublingual Gland Neoplasms - Neoplasms of the sublingual glands. Year introduced: 1991(1986)

Submandibular Gland Neoplasms Year introduced: 1991(1981)

Supratentorial Neoplasms - Primary and metastatic (secondary) tumors of the brain located above the tentorium cerebelli, a fold of dura mater separating the CEREBELLUM and BRAIN STEM from the cerebral hemispheres and DIENCEPHALON (i.e., THALAMUS and HYPOTHALAMUS and related structures). In adults, primary neoplasms tend to arise in the supratentorial compartment, whereas in children they occur more frequently in the infratentorial space. Clinical manifestations vary with the location of the lesion, but SEIZURES; APHASIA; HEMIANOPSIA; hemiparesis; and sensory deficits are relatively common features. Metastatic supratentorial neoplasms are frequently multiple at the time of presentation. Year introduced: 1989

Sweat Gland Neoplasms Year introduced: 1968

Testicular Neoplasms - Tumors or cancer of the TESTIS. Germ cell tumors (GERMINOMA) of the testis constitute 95% of all testicular neoplasms. Year introduced: 1963

A Glossary of MeSH terms for all types of cancer (neoplasms)

Thoracic Neoplasms

Thymus Neoplasms - Tumors or cancer of the THYMUS GLAND.

Thyroid Neoplasms - Tumors or cancer of the THYROID GLAND.

Tongue Neoplasms - Tumors or cancer of the TONGUE.

Tonsillar Neoplasms - Tumors or cancer of the PALATINE TONSIL.

Tracheal Neoplasms - Tumors of the Trachea

Triple Negative Breast Neoplasms - Breast neoplasms that do not express ESTROGEN RECEPTORS; PROGESTERONE RECEPTORS; and do not overexpress the NEU RECEPTOR/HER-2 PROTO-ONCOGENE PROTEIN. Year introduced: 2014

Trophoblastic Neoplasms - Trophoblastic growth, which may be gestational or nongestational in origin. Trophoblastic neoplasia resulting from pregnancy is often described as gestational trophoblastic disease to distinguish it from germ cell tumors which frequently show trophoblastic elements, and from the trophoblastic differentiation which sometimes occurs in a wide variety of epithelial cancers. Gestational trophoblastic growth has several forms, including HYDATIDI-FORM MOLE and CHORIOCARCINOMA. (From Holland et al., Cancer Medicine, 3d ed, p1691) Year introduced: 1994

Ureteral Neoplasms - Cancer or tumors of the URETER which may cause obstruction leading to hydroureter, HYDRONEPHROSIS, and PYELONEPHRITIS. HEMATURIA is a common symptom.

Urethral Neoplasms - Cancer or tumors of the URETHRA. Benign epithelial tumors of the urethra usually consist of squamous and transitional cells. Primary urethral carcinomas are rare and typically of squamous cells. Urethral carcinoma is the only urological malignancy that is more common in females than in males.

Urinary Bladder Neoplasms - Tumors or cancer of the URINARY BLADDER. Year introduced: 2007 (1963)

Urogenital Neoplasms - Tumors or cancer of the UROGENITAL SYSTEM in either the male or the female.

Urologic Neoplasms - Tumors or cancer of the URINARY TRACT in either the male or the female. Year introduced: 1978

Uterine Neoplasms - Tumors or cancer of the UTERUS.

Uterine Cervical Neoplasms - Tumors or cancer of the UTERINE CERVIX. Year introduced: 2006 (1963)

A Glossary of MeSH terms for all types of cancer (neoplasms)

Uveal Neoplasms - Tumors or cancer of the UVEA. Year introduced: 1981

Vaginal Neoplasms - Tumors or cancer of the VAGINA.

Vascular Neoplasms - Neoplasms located in the vasculature system, such as ARTERIES and VEINS. They are differentiated from neoplasms of vascular tissue (NEOPLASMS, VASCULAR TISSUE), such as ANGIOFIBROMA or HEMANGIOMA. Year introduced: 1996

Vulvar Neoplasms - Tumors or cancer of the VULVA.

Chapter 9

Clinical Trials

In the previous chapter (the PubMed/MEDLINE database), it was discussed how research progresses to publication. At some point, a commercial company or an agency decides that a line of research is worth developing into a medical application. Before a particular medical procedure is studied in humans, studies on animals will have been done to understand potential toxicity and sometimes efficacy. Then, upon the approval by government agencies, experimental treatments are conducted in four phases.

In Phase I Clinical Trials, studies are performed to evaluate the safety of diagnostic, therapeutic, or prophylactic drugs, devices, or techniques in healthy, human subjects and to determine the safe dosage range. These tests also are used to determine pharmacological and pharmacokinetic properties (toxicity, metabolism, absorption, elimination, and preferred route of administration). They involve a small number of persons and usually last about 1 year.

In Phase II Clinical Trials, studies are performed on several hundred volunteers, including a limited number of patients with the target disease or disorder, and they last about two years.

In Phase III Clinical Trials, studies are done on patients with the target disease or disorder and they are monitored closely by physicians to identify any adverse reactions from long-term use. These studies are performed on groups of patients large enough to identify clinically significant responses and usually last about three years.

In Phase IV Clinical Trials, studies are done, post-marketing, to further evaluate the safety and efficacy of a product.

People are enlisted or can enroll in the Clinical Trials, usually at Phase II and III. The following procedures explain how to see what might be available in your situation.

Expert Summary

❧ *Go to:* http://www.cancer.gov/clinicaltrials/search .

❧ *Select:* The particular cancer of interest in the drop-down menu.

❧ *Select:* Other criteria in the various sections: Stage/Subtype, location, Trial/Treatment Type, etc., if you know them.

❧ *Select:* The "search" button at the bottom.

❧ *Review:* The selected protocols.

Go to the National Cancer Institute site: **http://www.cancer.gov/** .
Select the "**Clinical Trials**" link.

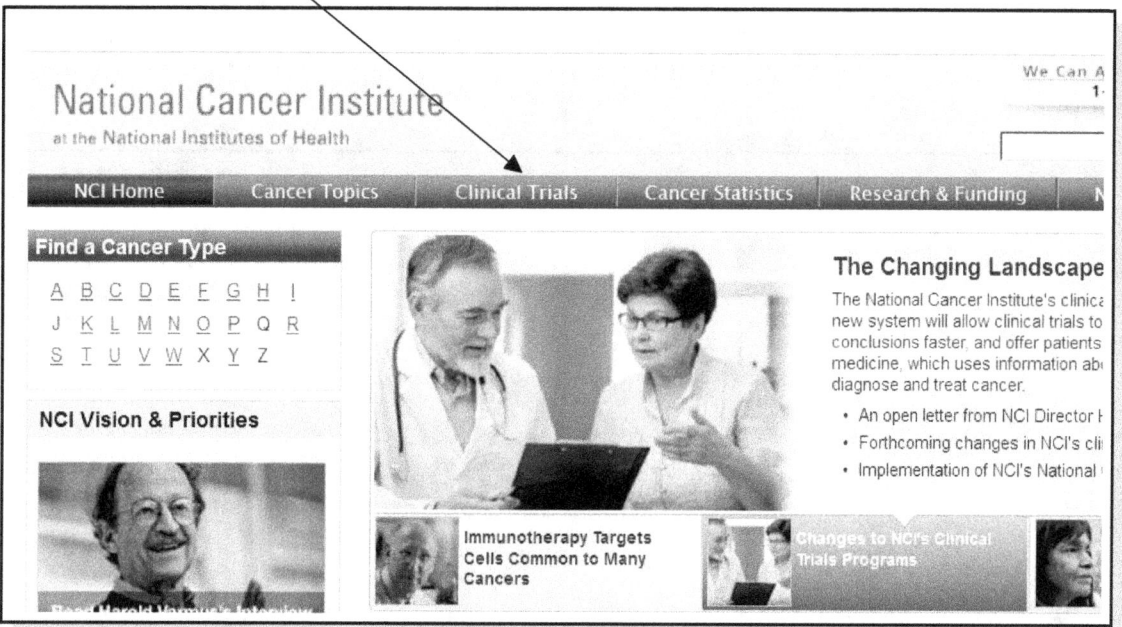

Note the various functions. Select "**Find a Clinical Trial**"

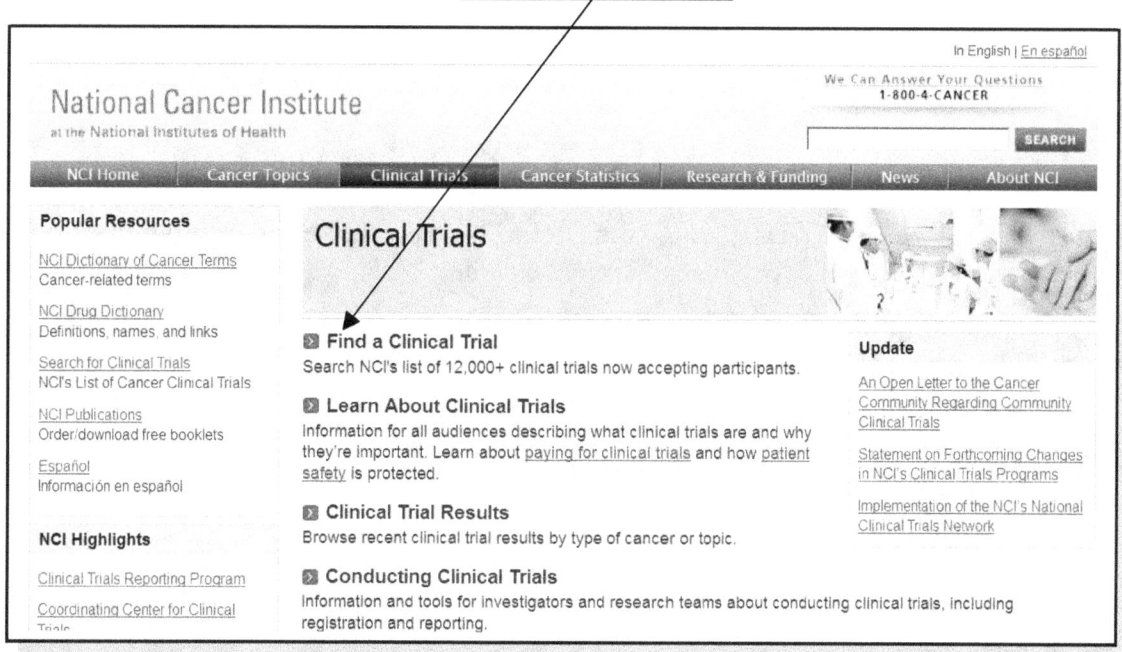

Chapter 9 - Clinical Trials

Select the **Cancer Type/Condition** from the pull-down menu. **A**lso, some conditions which are associated with cancer and are subject to treatment are included in that list. Note also the instructional **Video Guide** and **Popular Resources** in the left-hand column.

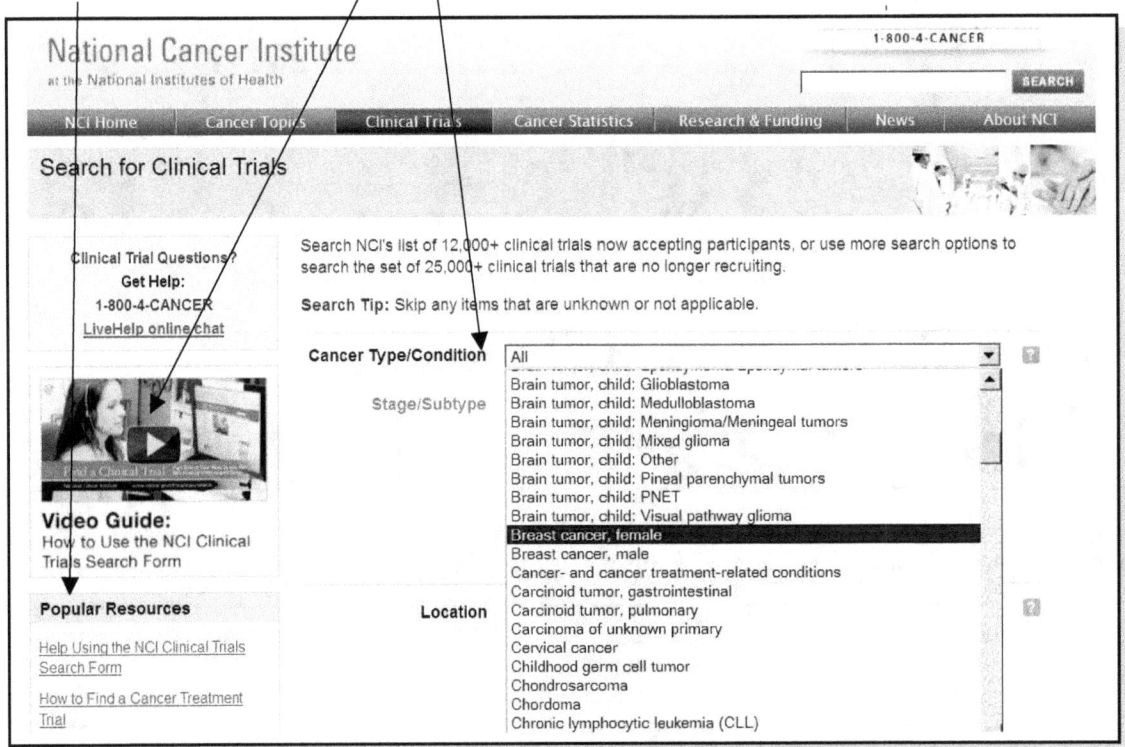

Having selected the Cancer Type, you will be asked to select the **"Stage/Subtype"**. This your physician can tell you. Or you can leave the default "All".

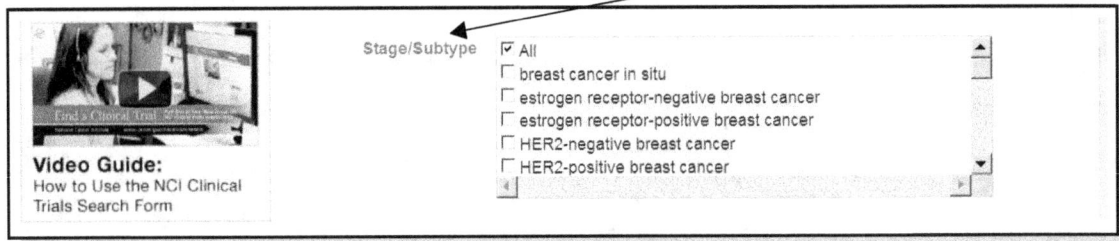

Specify the **Location** that is appropriate - either by Zip Code, Hospital, or City and also the **proximity**. There are other options which can further define the search; but for the first pass, leave it at these basics.

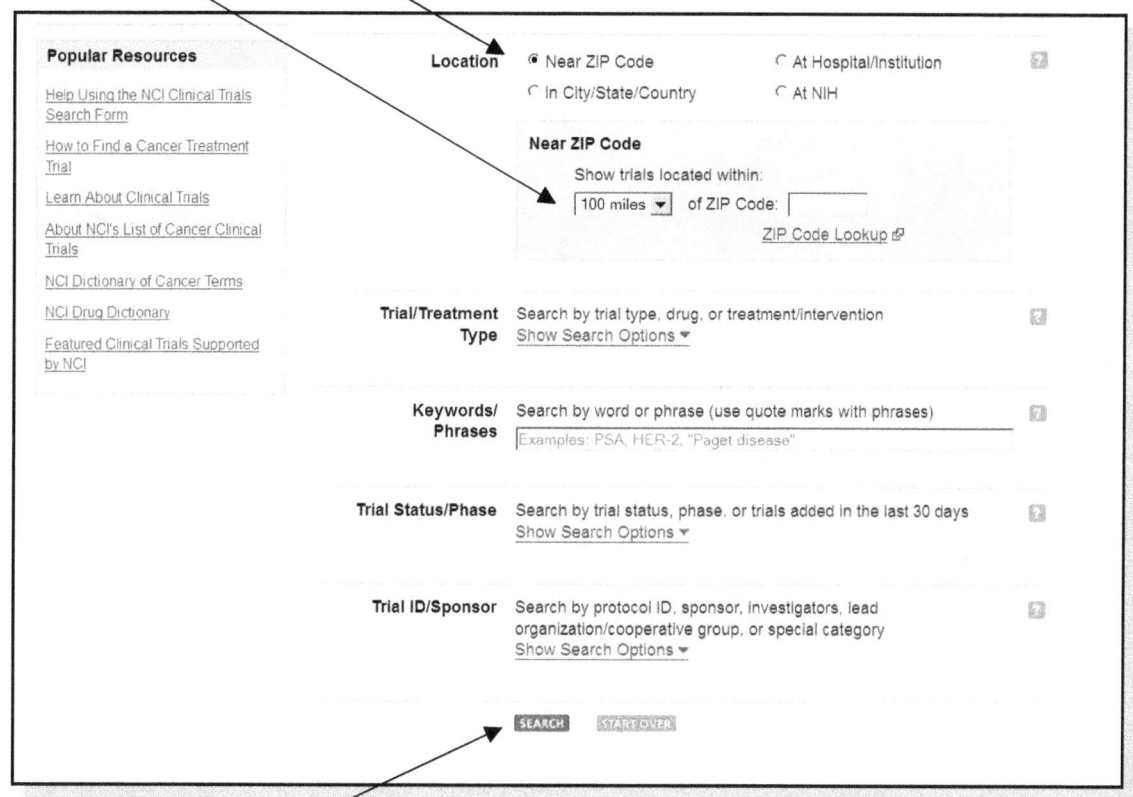

Finally, select the "**search**" button.

Chapter 9 - Clinical Trials

You will then be presented with a listing of the **abstracts** of those Clinical Trials within the **criteria which you specified**.

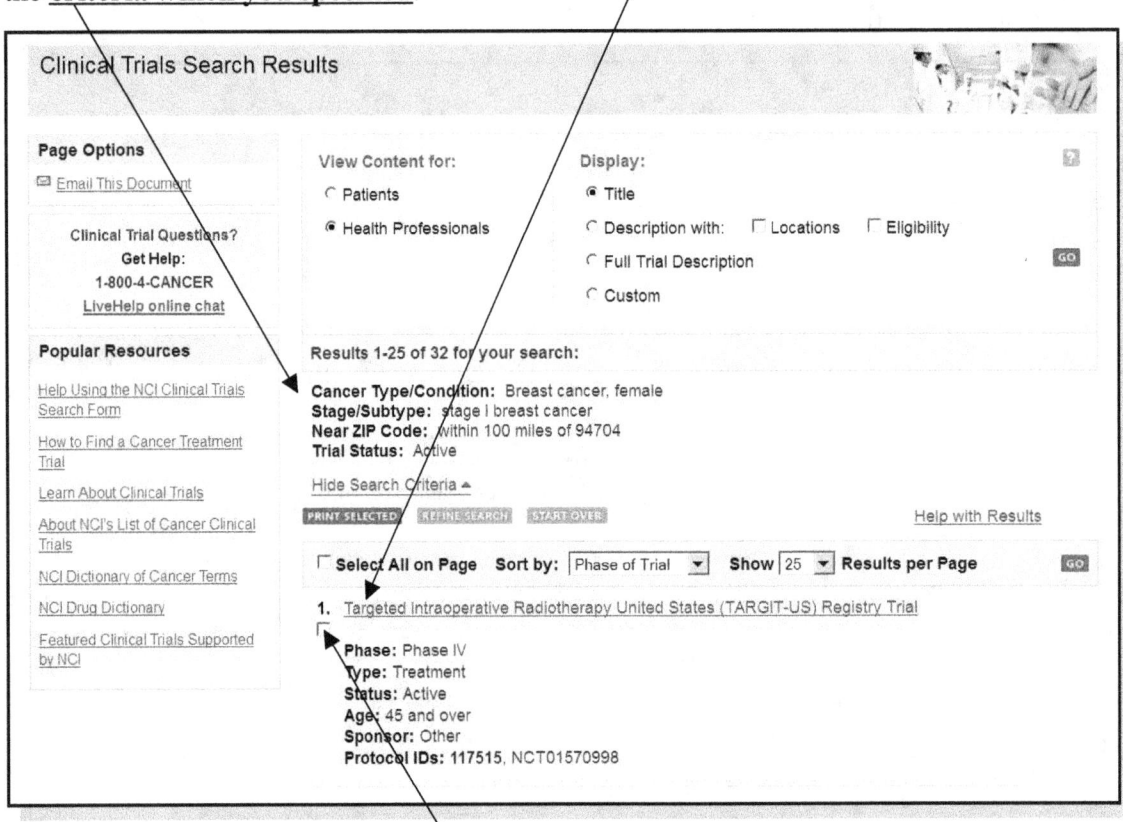

Scroll down through the abstracts; **select** the ones of possible interest; continue on to the additional pages (your prior selections will be preserved); and at the end, use the "print selected" button. **Y**ou will receive a listing of your selections. **T**he numbering between the original index and the final selection will change.

Finally, go back to the index listing which you marked, and select the **link** to the more complete report.

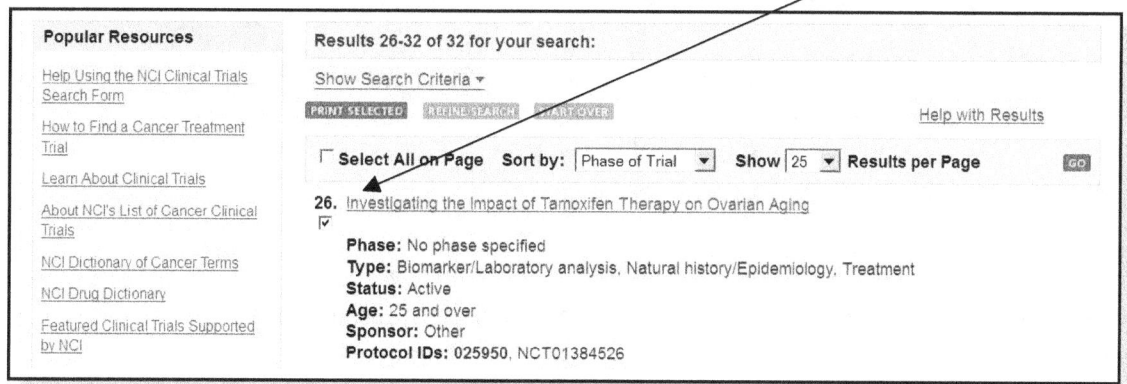

That takes you to the more detailed report which you can "**Print This Page**" or "**Email This Document**". **D**o this routine with each of the studies which you selected.

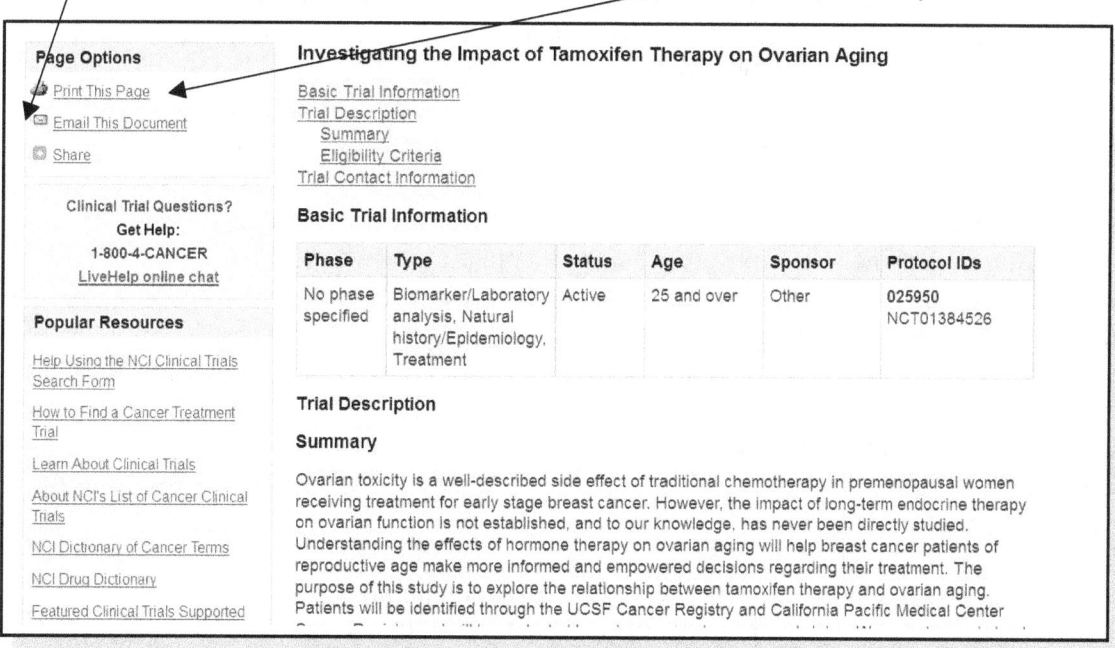

From this point, you will have to have your doctor evaluate the suitability of a clinical trial in your particular case and to advance under that physicians supervision; or, in some instance, you can directly contact the Principal Investigator of the study and apply for entry.

Chapter 10

Phase I - Life-Extension Modalities

"The good physician treats the disease; the great physician
treats the patient who has the disease." - an admonition to
treat the whole person. William Osler (1849 – 1919) one of
the founders of modern, clinical medicine.

In the Introduction to this book, it was briefly mentioned that this work deals with one
component (Curative Medicine) of a more comprehensive approach to long-range health,
one which we call the Life-Extension & Control of Ageing Program. That program
encompasses two sets of modalities or procedures: "Phase I - Life-Extension Modalities"
and "Phase II - Life-Extension Modalities".

Phase I modalities includes those procedures and practices which have been reasonably
demonstrated to help improve and maintain health (i.e., biological vitality) such that a
person has the prospect of living to one's genetically programmed, maximum life-span in a
condition of reasonable functionality. For most people, that would mean 80-90 years of
age. Apart from the extension of quality survival, this also gives a person, who is so
inclined, extended time for the prospect of taking advantage of advances in research as
they become developed - thus, gaining further improvements in vitality and longevity.
Phase II modalities include those procedures and practices which deal with the control of
natural ageing - i.e., slowing those intrinsic, degenerative processes and ultimately revers-
ing them, with the target system being a physical condition which one had at about the age
of 20 ± 5 (i.e., the phase of optimal biological vitality). Phase II modalities are still in the
research and experimental stage; the science in that regard is moving forward rapidly; what
is needed is a well financed, targeted strategy, that is managed properly; and we intend to
be a key player in that movement. In fact, writing this book is one method of supporting
that effort.

Phase I Life-Extension Modalities (those that help to maintain health) include procedures
in the following areas: 1) Nutrition, 2) Physical Conditioning, 3) Toxicology, 4) Preventive
Medicine; 5) Psychological Practices; and 6) Curative Medicine. For each of these categories, in their own respective manner, there is reasonable evidence to show that certain
procedures help to maintain biological vitality and contribute to enabling a person to live
the full genetic potential. Ideally, the recommended practices in all of these categories
should be applied concurrently as part of one's general life-style; however, when a serious
medical condition arises (as will happen at some point to almost everyone) then item #6,

155

Curative Medicine, takes priority with the other modalities acting in a supportive role as Complementary Therapies or, in some instances, Alternative Therapies.

As stated in the beginning, this book assumes that the reader is concerned about the treatment of some form of cancer and wants to establish a treatment strategy that is most appropriate for a particular person. Accordingly, all of the chapters, up to this point, have focused on that objective in category 6) Curative Medicine. In **Chapter 1**, we covered the single most important element - the PDQ (Physician Data Query) database, which is maintained by the National Cancer Institute; and this provides state-of-the-art diagnostic and treatment protocols for all of the major forms of life-threatening cancer. If you do nothing more than follow the instructions in Chapter 1, you will be able to see what the most advanced, "conventional" medicine has to offer you; and this understanding should make a significant contribution to your medical treatment. In **Chapter 2**, a commentary was provided on the subjects of "Conventional Medicine", a "History of Medicine In General" and "Cancer - What Is It?". The purpose there is to give a picture of how the medicine which you may receive is derived - that it is changing, that it is bound by the current state of scientific knowledge as well as economics, cultures, and the how medical doctors are educated. Further, the molecular mechanisms of cancer are beginning to be understood, and this should (with some reservations) lead to a substantially different approach to this disease. **Chapter 3** deals with keeping your medical records and **Chapter 4** with using some of the wider Internet resources. In **Chapter 5**, suggestions are made about secondary opinions, and **Chapter 6** deals with the demographics of particular cancers. Then in **Chapter 7**, a history of the National Library of Medicine is given as an introduction to **Chapter 8**, which is the Library's major database called MEDLINE with its search engine called PubMed and which gives you access to the worlds research literature over the last 100+ years - although only the last 10 years will be relevant to most people. Next, in **Chapter 9**, an introduction is given about how to investigate on-going, clinical trials of new, experimental therapies and methods of diagnosis. In all, these 9 chapters will give you a comprehensive understanding of what constitutes Curative Medicine (one of the 6 areas of Phase I - Life-Extension Modalities) and the tools for evaluating the most appropriate approach to dealing with any type of cancer, whether you may be the Patient, the Facilitator, and even the treating Physician.

Next, we will review the other 5, Phase I - Life-Extension Modalities, which apart from their independent value in terms of maintaining health, also serve as Complimentary therapies to conventional treatments and sometimes as Alternative therapies to such. Because each person is unique in terms of one's biology, psychology, circumstances, and cultural traditions, only general guidelines can be given here, with how they are to be applied, remaining for each person to decide together with one's physician or other consultants.

1- Nutrition

Diet and Nutrition are closely related. "Diet" refers to the foods which we eat and "Nutrition" refers to the substances in food that are the nutrients for building and maintaining one's body and, in a broader sense, the way we digest and use these nutrients. Diet has been used to treat disease since the earliest of human history and was a major modality of the first modern physician, Hippocrates (c. 460 – c. 370 BCE). In contrast, Nutrition has only become understood, in scientific terms, during the last 100 years - so, this is fairly recent knowledge that is becoming increasingly refined.

Incidentally, it is frequently said that cancer did not exist before the modern industrial age - implying that industrial chemicals and industrialize foods are the cause of cancer. This is simply not true. Cancer can be seen in Egyptian mummies, was reported in the earliest medical works, exists in plants and animals, and the same molecular mutations can be seen in the earliest multi-celled organism. It is said that 10% of the cancers have a genetic component, 10% are from infectious agents and toxic chemicals (mostly tobacco and alcohol usage, and some industrial chemicals including, paradoxically, some chemotherapeutic drugs that are used to treat cancer), and the remaining 80% of cancers are mishaps of normal metabolism and, as will be discussed in Chapter 11, the ageing process. The reason that it appears that cancer was of lower incidence in more ancient times is because cancer is a disease that is associated with (caused by) ageing and most people, back then, died early in life and before the age at which most cancers manifest. It has only been in more recent history that most people are now surviving beyond middle age, when most cancer becomes expressed.

In terms of Diet *vis a vis* health and longevity, there are numerous and conflicting recommendations in both the popular media and the scientific community; however basic Nutrition is quite simple. It is important to understand that, fundamentally, your body makes itself from the intake of some 40 different, elemental nutrients which come from various types of foods; and as long as those nutrients are in one's diet, it makes little difference what kind that diet is. These nutrients include: water; glucose (from carbohydrates in plant material); 8 amino acids (from proteins in plants and animals); 2 or more essential fatty acids (from animal and plants); some 13 essential vitamins; and some 14 essential minerals. When you eat food, your digestive processes break down that material to those essential molecules and then your own DNA and metabolic processes re-construct all of your diverse tissues from those building-blocks. If your intake of essential nutrients is periodically low or deficient, your body will conserve or substitute; and if your intake is excessive, it will store. Accordingly, for general health, the following guidelines are recommended.

- **M**aintain a routine diet of "balanced meals" that insure a sufficient intake of the essential 40 nutrients.

- **K**eep the routine diet mostly in whole foods with refined, "junk" foods kept to a minimum to avoid excessive salt and calories from sugar and fat.

- **R**otate the food groups to help insure against deficiency of nutrients as well as to prevent allergic reactions to certain types of food.

- **S**upply ample fiber in the diet for bulk and as an aid to digestion.

- **T**he total caloric intake should be one that reduces and then keeps one's body weight close to what you had at about the age of 25.

- **S**upplement a full-spectrum vitamin/mineral compound (low dosage and United States Pharmacopeia grade) to insure that there are no inadequacies. Mega-dosages of vitamins show no advantage and may add to metabolic stress.

There is no need to be over-meticulous or obsessive about the diet. For example, in controlled, scientific studies on animals with respect to longevity, no special diet or supplementation of nutritional essentials has ever increased the maximum, genetically programmed life-span, with one exception - caloric restriction, which is the minimization of nutrition. Some years ago, in researching this subject, I came across a report which studied diet and longevity (I do not currently have the citation). The diet which they used achieved the greatest longevity in the entire history of life-extension. It was astoundingly unsophisticated. The researchers were studying the effects of restricting the total intake of calories on the life-span of rats. Because it was a long-tern study and they did not have much money, they fed the animals the cheapest possible diet - a diet which had 20% protein (from casein, a milk protein), 30% fat (from lard which is pig fat), 40% carbohydrates (from corn starch), and 10% fiber. They added a full spectrum vitamin/mineral powder to insure against deficiencies. In other words, this was a life-time diet of pellets made from crude protein, pig fat, and corn starch with vitamins and minerals as administered under a regime of restricting the intake of total calories. Of course, this kind diet would be next to impossible for anyone to tolerate as would any long-term, calorie-restricted diet. The point is that the body constructs itself if supplied with basic foods.

In more specific terms of diet as a treatment for cancer, numerous diets have been promoted as therapies either directly for or adjuvant to conventional treatment. Recently, a team of oncologists at the Goethe University in Frankfurt, Germany reported the following. They reviewed the clinical data on 13 cancer diets, including: Alkaline Diet; Bircher-Benner Diet; Breuss cancer cure; Budwig's Diet; Fasting; Gerson's Regime, Kelly/Gonzales Regimen, Ketogenic Diet; Livingston-Wheeler Regimen; Macrobiotics; Moermann Diet; Raw Food; Vegan Diet. Their conclusion was: "Considering the lack of evidence of benefits from cancer diets and potential harm by malnutrition, oncologists should engage more in counseling cancer patients on such diets." [1] In other words, if a patient wants go on a special diet regime, then one should do so under some clinical observation.

Apart from the basic Phase I nutritional recommendations, as reviewed above, various people have recommended such things as: higher Vitamin C intake, a low-dosage aspirin or other non-steroidal anti-inflammatory drug, increased anti-oxidants during radiation diagnosis or therapy; good hydration with plain water (sodas, coffee, alcoholic drinks are not good hydration); and the avoidance of sugar, both *per se* and as an additive in refined foods. However, these and other adjuvants to one's treatment protocol should be discussed with the treating oncologist.

Finally, you can study some of the resources, below, that are related to diet and nutrition.

National Cancer Institute:

http://www.cancer.gov/cancertopics/pdq/supportivecare/nutrition/patient/

http://www.cancer.gov/cancertopics/pdq/supportivecare/nutrition/healthprofessional/

American Institute for Cancer Research:

http://www.aicr.org/patients-survivors/

PubMed/MEDlINE for current research and specialized studies:

Go to: http://www.ncbi.nlm.nih.gov/pubmed and, in the search box, type:

"neoplasms"[MeSH] AND "diet"[MeSH] OR "Nutritional Sciences"[Mesh]

Next, the other categories of Phase I Life-Extension Modalities are reviewed.

---

[1] Huebner J *et alia*; "Counseling patients on cancer diets: a review of the literature and recommendations for clinical practice"; Anticancer Res. 2014 Jan;34(1):39-48.).

2- Physical Conditioning

Like nutrition, there can be many different opinions about the best exercise program; but also like nutrition, the essentials are fairly simple. (Put aside any notion of becoming a body builder or performance athlete - those routines do more damage than good to long range health.) The body was made to **move**, **strain**, and **bend**; and these three elements are the foundation of any exercise program. **Moving** the body (by walking, swimming, jogging, cycling, etc.) increases the blood circulation - thus, helping to distribute the nutrients to cells, eliminate metabolic waste, provide the tissues with oxygen, and stimulate tissue regeneration. **Straining** (weight training) causes the muscles and bones to increase in strength as well as improve the nervous system. And **bending** (stretching or Hatha yoga exercises) increases the flexibility of joints and tissues. All forms of exercise maintain and enhance physical coordination and improve mental faculties; and the basic exercise routines are common knowledge. A personal program will depend on one's present condition, motivation, and access to facilities. The central ideas for all modes of training include: 1) start training from where you are and slowly graduate out-ward from there; 2) give yourself intermittent rest so that the tissues have time to accommodate and build; and 3) make the exercise pleasant so that you feel good during and after the process and, thus, encourage yourself psychologically to want to come back. If you over exercise and cause pain, then your mind will invent a thousand reasons for why you have something else to do. You have to become addicted to physical exercise and that requires reinforcement by pleasure. Modern life-styles frequently do not require adequate physical exercise; thus some deliberate attention needs to be given to this aspect of health maintenance. A structured and reinforcing environment, such as a work-out studio, is helpful - if you can get yourself to the gym then there will be less psychological resistance and the work routine will tend to be more automatic. Again, it is always a good idea to notify any treating physician about one's exercise plan. Record your exercise in your medical records Journal.

For research studies on this subject, review the procedures for PubMed/MEDLINE in Chapter 8. Go to: http://www.ncbi.nlm.nih.gov/pubmed and, in the search box, type: ("Neoplasms"[Mesh]) AND "Exercise"[Mesh] .

3 - Toxicology

The third category of Phase I - Life-Extension Modalities is the minimization or mitigation of exposure to toxic substances. Like Nutrition and Physical Conditioning, there are many common misapprehensions about exposure to toxic substances; and there is no need to become hysterical about toxins, as the media seem inclined to make of it. Smoking and alcohol abuse are the most common toxic substances which contribute to cancer and the other chronic diseases - the former should be eliminated and the latter kept at a minimum. Certainly, we need to make a concerted effort to implement technologies for clean water, waste removal, polluting the atmosphere, develop industrial products that do not contaminate the ecology, and, in general, create a sanitary and sustainable environment. However, even in a completely sterile environment of zero exposure to toxic substances or infectious agents, disease will still occur and the life-span will not exceed our present 80-90 years. Experiments with animals who live in a clean environment show that they do not live much longer than those living in a dirty environment - as long as they have adequate nutritional intake.

Keep in mind the basic principle of biology: you construct yourself from your own DNA plus the ~ 40 essential nutrients from the environment and other life-forms; and anything that is not made by yourself is, in some degree, toxic and is generally dismantled by your normal metabolic processes and converted to useful molecules or eliminated. We exist in a sea of toxic chemicals including infectious agents. That is unavoidable and usually not detrimental to one's health. In this respect, paradoxically, the natural foods which we normally eat are our single biggest exposure to toxic substances; and that, obviously, is unavoidable. Food contains massive amounts of foreign proteins which must be dismantled into their essential amino acids which you can use; and plants, which do not have active immune systems, defend themselves with very toxic chemicals which you neutralize with digestive processes. Certain occupations do have a high exposure to toxins (e.g., farm workers to pesticides and herbicides; industrial workers and people who live close to industrial plants) and special protective measures need to be taken; but the concentration of these toxins to which the consumer is exposed is very small and mostly inconsequential. There is one noteworthy exception and that is therapeutic pharmaceuticals. These are powerful, foreign chemicals that are ingested into the system in high concentrations; and attention needs to be given to their adverse effects and the trade-off between those detriments and their therapeutic effect.

4 - Preventive Medicine

Preventive Medicine means the monitoring of biological parameters in an effort to observe conditions which, if they progress, could lead to disease and would require Curative Medicine. Preventive Medicine then attempts to intervene early so that actual disease can be avoided. With the above practices in Nutrition, Physical Conditioning, and Toxicology, a general life-style can be established that improves and maintains health. Therefore, one's risk to disease can be lowered, and that will go a long way toward disease prevention. With biological monitoring, it takes prevention one step further. There are comprehensive, multi-phasic examinations (physical examination, blood chemistries, physiologic measurements, electro-cardiography, etc.) which are performed at appropriate intervals; and then there are specialized monitorings for specific risk factors, as would be performed during and after cancer therapy. The specifics of these procedures are quite detailed and vary by individual and will not be covered here. One precautionary note warrants mentioning. When doing Preventive Medicine, it is important to take precaution that aggressive medical intervention is not done too early and thereby doing unnecessary treatments and causing adverse effects. "Watchful Waiting" and emphasis on the other Phase I Modalities (i.e., Nutrition, Physical Conditioning, and Toxicology) is advised while the close monitoring of specific risk factors determines if the pre-clinical condition(s) are progressing or remising either by themselves or due to life-style changes.

5 - Psychology

What are the psychological components which facilitate a person in living a fulfilling and healthy life, including a positive coping with adversity? How best to live, to develop a good character, and what kind of a frame-of-mind one should hold in order to adapt to the oscillations of fortune is a very broad subject. This is an ancient discussion, which constitutes much of philosophy and religion. Here, two points warrant consideration with respect to cancer.

First, being confronted with cancer and the prospect of dying is, without any qualification, a major psychological trauma - regardless of how strong one's personality might be. Further, dealing with the consequent therapy is both a physical and psychological trauma. In recent times, the term "Post-Traumatic Stress Disorders" has gained a lot of attention and is relevant, here. Within the general medical category of "Psychiatry and Psychology" and "Mental Disorders", there is a gradation from the more general "Anxiety Disorders" to "Traumatic Stress Disorders". And then there is "Post-Traumatic Stress Disorders" (PTSD) - i.e., the after-effects from a traumatic stress. Usually, it is associated with traumatic events such as war, a hurricane, sexual assault, physical abuse, or a bad accident, all of which makes one feel stressed and afraid after the danger is over. It is a continuing anxiety which disrupts the healing process. It affects your personal life and the lives of people around you. PTSD entered the medical vocabulary in 1981 and is defined, more formally, as follows:

> "Stress Disorders, Post-Traumatic. A class of traumatic stress disorders
> with symptoms that last more than one month. There are various forms of
> post-traumatic stress disorder, depending on the time of onset and the
> duration of these stress symptoms. In the acute form, the duration of the

symptoms is between 1 to 3 months. In the chronic form, symptoms last more than 3 months. With delayed onset, symptoms develop more than 6 months after the traumatic event."

Thus, dealing with cancer is a major cause of psychological stress and anxiety. Numerous studies have proven a relationship between chronic stress and anxiety and cancer progression or recurrence and have shown the positive effects of stress/anxiety management on the quality of life of cancer patients. Practices which help dealing with PTSD include: 1) periodic meditation and learning how to control one's breathing, 2) physical exercise, 3) various yoga practices, 4) letting go of negative thoughts and controlling thinking, 5) taking more involvement in understanding and planning one's treatment strategy. For a more detailed discussions see:

http://www.nlm.nih.gov/medlineplus/posttraumaticstressdisorder.html

Also, go to: http://www.ncbi.nlm.nih.gov/pubmed and type in: "Neoplasms"[Mesh] and "Cognitive Therapy"[Mesh])

The second consideration is the various stages of emotional adjustment that are associated with the prospect of serious illness and death. In the 1960's, a psychiatrist by the name of Elisabeth Kübler-Ross introduced a model of emotional adjustment when faced with dying. This is now being applied more generally to any situation involving a loss and transition. There are 5 stages in this model: 1) denial, 2) anger, 3) bargaining, 4) depression, and 5) acceptance. These can be interwoven and oscillate back and forth. Denial is the first order coping device which we use routinely in all kinds of situations that we do not want. Denial is usually discussed in a negative sense; but in truth it can have positive benefits (some problems actually resolve by themselves without intervention), and it gives one some time to make adjustments. If the situation persists, anger frequently arises and is directed at the situation, the people involved (even people who are helpful), and one's self. This resolves partially in accepting the situation by bargaining for some kind of extension. Depression is usually involved in varying degrees and may need some medication for a brief time. The finaly stage of emotional reconciliation is acceptance of the situation as it is. This can have an emotionally liberating effect and help free a person to make the best of one's circumstances.

For details, see: http://en.wikipedia.org/wiki/K%C3%BCbler_ross

In summary, Phase I Life-Extension Modalities are largely common sense adjustments in life-style and behavior together with a modicum of medical technology. They help to prevent disease and optimize life-span and can be used together with or as alternatives to

163

conventional medical treatment in cancer and other chronic diseases. In principle, they are quite simple; but in practice, they can be complicated and difficult because they involve the modification of personal behavior. They must fit each particular individual. Regardless of how one gets there: bring the body weight down to about that which one had at age 25; have a routine physical exercise program, avoid excessive exposure to toxic substances; learn how to manage chronic psychological stress and anxiety; understand the principles of preventive medicine; find the most appropriate curative medicine for your situation; and stay in touch with research advances.

The real scientific challenge is in the control of ageing, and we will turn to that in the next Chapter.

Chapter 11

Cancer and the Control of Ageing

Previously, the claim has been made that the fundamental cause of cancer is biological ageing and that, until ageing can be cured, it will be impossible to cure or prevent cancer or even improve much upon the conventional therapies that are or will be available to us. Here, that thesis will be explained. Although it is widely recognized that ageing is a "risk factor" for cancer, that does not say anything about the mechanism regarding the cause of cancer *vis-a-vis* ageing. And ageing is not currently viewed as a causative factor by the general public, the medical profession, scientific community, nor government. With this book, it is hoped that we can raise consciousness to this idea and mobilize support for advancing the control of ageing as an approach to cancer.

Let's start with a rather astounding observation from statistical facts. In the National Vital Statistics Reports of May 31, 2013 [1], the calculation is presented for various gains in life-expectancy due to the elimination of specific causes of death. (The latest calculations are for the year 2001.) If we had some miraculously effective treatments and preventive measures and cancer were completely eradicated in the population, then there would be an increase of 2.99 years in average life-expectancy. That is it - only about a 3 year increase, if cancer were eliminated entirely. Further, because the goal of medicine is to cure or prevent all disease, we can ask: what benefit would that have? Below is the table of the specific diseases that are the cause of all morbidity and mortality. If all of the killing diseases were eliminated (again by some impossibly miraculous, medical technologies and environmental measures), then that would yield a gain in life-expectancy by only 11.29 years. This would increase the life-expectancy from about 80 years (as it presently is) out to the maximum human life span of slightly over 90 years (true, there are a small number of people who do live over 100 but not in any kind of desirable condition).

	THE GAIN IN LIFE-EXPECTANCY (AT AGE **50**) DUE TO THE ELIMINATION OF THE COMMON CAUSES OF DEATH.	
	CAUSE OF DEATH:	**YEARS GAINED:**
1	MAJOR CARDIOVASCULAR DISEASES	5.42
2	ALL MALIGNANT NEOPLASMS (CANCERS)	2.99

---

1   Center for Disease Control; National Vital Statistics Reports May 31, 2013; Volume 61, Number 9; Table 22. Gain in expectation of life due to elimination of specified causes of death, by exact age, for the total population: United States, 1999–2001.
http://www.cdc.gov/nchs/data/nvsr/nvsr61/nvsr61_09.pdf

	THE GAIN IN LIFE-EXPECTANCY (AT AGE 50) DUE TO THE ELIMINATION OF THE COMMON CAUSES OF DEATH.	
	CAUSE OF DEATH:	YEARS GAINED:
3	CEREBROVASCULAR DISEASES	0.64
4	CHRONIC LOWER RESPIRATOR DISEASES	0.56
5	DIABETES MELLITUS	0.32
6	ACCIDENTS ALL TYPES	0.23
7	INFLUENZA & PNEUMONIA	0.22
8	ALZHEIMER'S	0.15
9	NEPHRITIS AND KIDNEY DISEASES	0.15
10	SEPTICEMIA	0.13
11	LIVER DISEASE AND CIRRHOSIS	0.13
12	ALCOHOL INDUCED CAUSES	0.08
13	SUICIDE	0.07
14	PNEUMONITIS - SOLIDS AND LIQUIDS	0.06
15	INJURY BY FIREARMS	0.05
16	HUMAN IMMUNO-DEFICIENCY	0.03
17	DRUG INDUCED CAUSES	0.03
18	HOMICIDE	0.02
19	CONGENITAL MALFORMATIONS	0.01
	TOTAL YEARS GAINED	**11.29**

Thus, contrary to the prospect of curing all diseases as being a great blessing, 100% of the population never having a terminal disease and living to 90+ years would be a social and humanitarian catastrophe, with everyone spending their final years in over-crowed geriatric wards and eventually dying of senescence and with much of the younger generation having to spend their careers in tending to them. This prospect was first observed in the 1950's by demographers, who noted the increasing percentage of the population over 60 that was starting to occur at that time and which is now in full sway - they predicted, what they called, a social "gerontocracy". Therefore, curing specific diseases is clearly not the answer. What is required is a radically different approach - one which will focus on whole system, biological regeneration - i.e., the control of ageing.

What Is Ageing?

In humans, the period of optimum biological vitality for every member of our specie is 15-25 years of age (20 ± 5). (It was Bernard Strehler, professor of biochemistry at the University of Southern California and an early advocate of curing ageing, who first used this observation as the ultimate goal of the life-extension sciences.) That period of development (20 ± 5) is the peak of form and function; and there is virtually no morbidity nor mortality in that condition. If this biological condition could be restored and maintained, then disease would be minimal and, if it did occur, easy to treat; functioning would remain optimal and enable the human potential to keep expanding; and life-expectancy would be greatly extended. Under present conditions, after about the age of 30 and regardless of how good one's genetics, environment, behavior, affluence, access to advanced medical technology, standard of living, gender, religion, ethnicity, or any other such factors may be, biological vitality is not maintained and metabolic wear-and-tear (ageing) accumulates. As ageing progresses, tissues deteriorate and there is loss of cell number, metabolic rate, and structure. Functions decline and the risk of the chronic diseases (cancer being one) increases exponentially. In modern society, the ageing process is the underlying cause of most disease and is what limits the human life-expectancy to an average of about 80 years and a maximum life-span of not much more than about 95, the latter portion of which is not very functional. Consider the microscopic photos below of young tissue on the left and old tissue on the right. [2]

VITALITY AT THE CELLULAR LEVEL

---

2   This photograph is from the laboratory of Jaime Miquel at NASA Ames, taken in 1975 of
    Drosophila tissue. I happened to have been in the lab at the time Miquel was preparing
    the tissue samples. He did much of the radiation research for astronauts; and like many early
    gerontologists, it was radiation biology that got him interested in ageing - radiation accelerates ageing.

Chapter 11 - Cancer and the Control of Ageing

Observe, in those slides, the young tissue on the left. All of the cells are like little, pristine robots, rigidly uniform, well positioned in the same direction, densely packed, and clean, and with an intact matrix between them - something which will be emphasized, later, in reviewing the work of Mina Bissell. In contrast, the old cells are disorganized and lack uniformity, are congested with waste material, are mutated, and the extra-cellular matrix or micro-environment is gone. This ageing at the cellular level translates into what we observe as "natural" ageing. In humans, at about the age of 60, the deterioration of tissues looks like this.

Young to Aged   **Regenerated to Young**

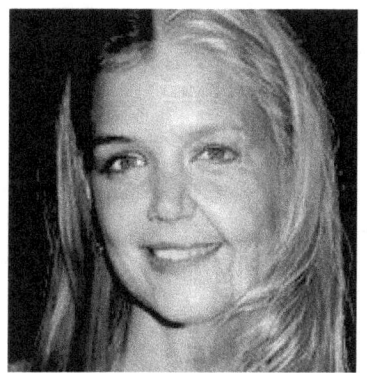 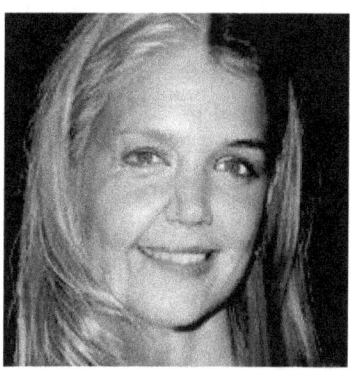

Each specie has a different, fixed maximum life-span. Thus, we say that the life-span is genetically programmed. Below is a listing of the average and maximum life-spans in months for various life-forms. [3]

Common Name	Life-span in months	
	Mean	Maximum
Human	849	1,380
Chimpanzee	210	534
Domestic cattle	276	360
Horse	300	744
Indian elephant	480	840
Cat	180	336
Domestic dog	180	408
Mouse	18	42
House rat	30	56
Houseflies	1	3

---

3   Rockstein M, Chesky JA, Susman ML, 1977; Comparative Biology and Evolution of Aging;

Chapter 11 - Cancer and the Control of Ageing

Consider the adjacent animals. The hummingbird is a small and frail creature. Living in the wild, it works extremely hard, spending a lot of energy in its annual migration of about 2,000 miles and living off of a simple diet of nectar, pollen, and some insects. Yet it can have a maximum life-span of 12 years even under highly arduous conditions. In contrast, the experimental mouse, living in a controlled environment with complete nutrition and good sanitation and virtually no hazards, cannot live longer than 3 years with cancer being a major cause of death. That maximum life-span of 3 years applies to all species of rodents, except the Naked Mole Rat, below, which can live to 35 years and still breeding at that age, with minimal incidence of cancer. Even more remarkable, it lives some 20 feet underground in filthy conditions and in an atmosphere that is highly toxic - it being low in oxygen and extremely high in carbon dioxide from their breathing and ammonium from their urine. So, how can the fragile hummingbird live for 12 years, in arduous migrations, but the well protected mouse for only 3, in protected laboratories, and the naked mole rat for 35, in harsh underground conditions?

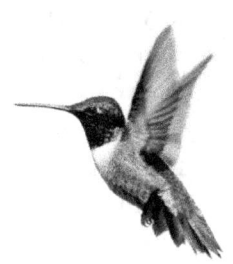

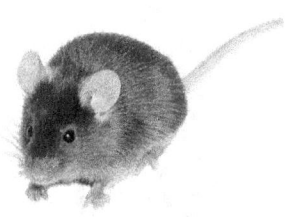

Clearly it is not the form that matters; rather it is **the maintenance of the form** that counts! (There is nothing intrinsic to "Time" that causes ageing or a limited life-span; it is the change in form and function that demarcates time.) Again, if we could regenerate back to and maintain our biological form at its optimal condition (what we had during the age range of 20 ± 5), then our functioning would remain optimal, disease would be low, if disease did occur it would be easy to cure, our potential would be open-ended, and our life-expectancy and span would be greatly extended. This, then, is the ultimate goal of life-extension science.

169

Chapter 11 - Cancer and the Control of Ageing

Ageing as the cause of disease

Aging is characterized by a decline in biological vitality due to loss of cell number, rate, and structure. Below are various graphs of deaths due to specific diseases as juxtaposed to the decline in biological vitality due to ageing. As can be seen by the red curve, **biological vitality peaks between the age range of 15-25**. It observably declines after the age of 30 and, then, begins an exponential decline, thereafter, into senescence. The green bars represent the incidences of **specific diseases as they increase commensurately with biological ageing** - (incidence being defined as the numbers of deaths per 100,000 population).

Here is biological vitality *vis a vis* cancers.

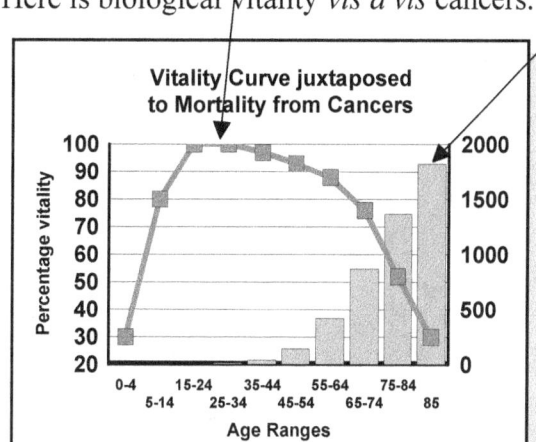

And so it is with heart diseases.

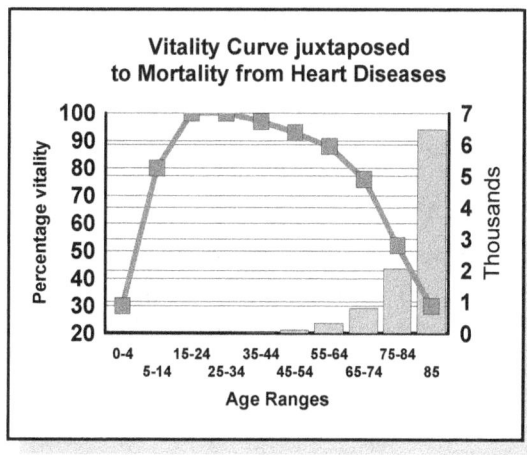

Chapter 11 - Cancer and the Control of Ageing

And the same correlation applies between biological vitality and the other diseases - even such things as accidents that greatly accelerate in the more advanced aged.

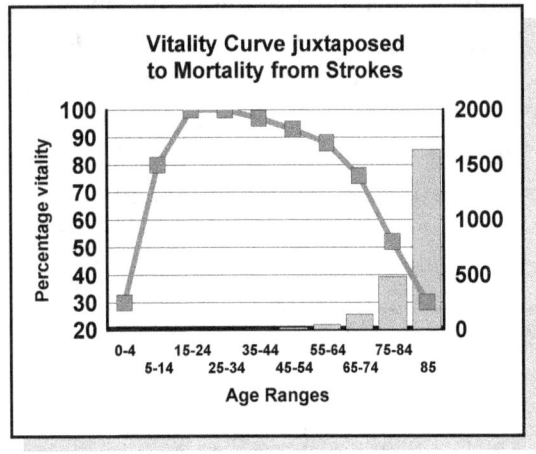

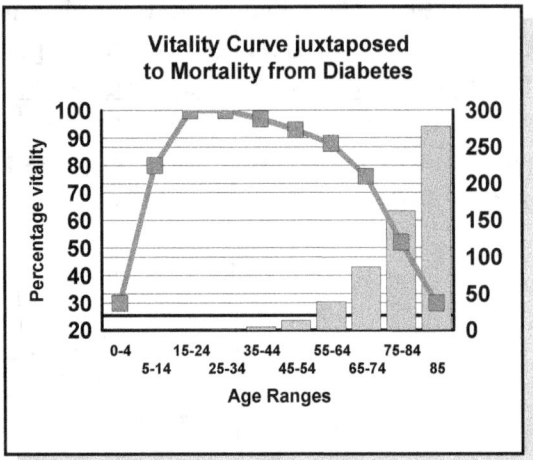

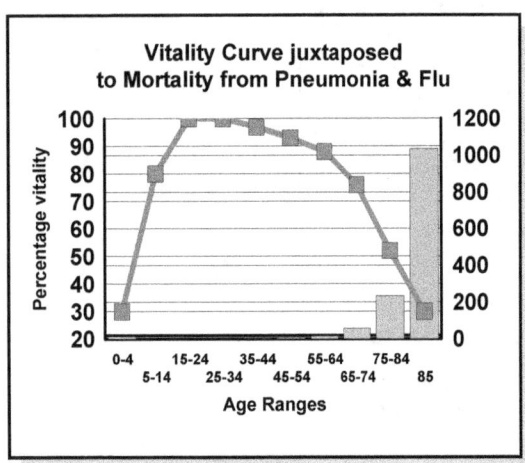

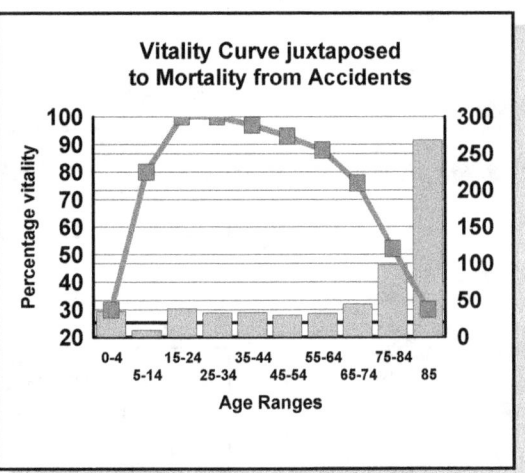

Note in the various graphs, above, there are effectively no deaths from any of the major diseases during the age range of 20 ± 5 - i.e., the zone of optimal vitality in terms of number of cells, their metabolic rate, and their quality of components.

Chapter 11 - Cancer and the Control of Ageing

A Review of Basic Principles

Recall the graphic illustration of developmental biology from Chapter 2. Each of us was created by the union of one sperm and one ovum into a single cell with the capacity to create all of the some 50+ trillion cells that make up the whole body. With the exception of the sperm and ovum, each of which has only 50% of the genetic blue-print (DNA), and red blood cells, which have no nuclear DNA, every cell in your body has a complete copy of the DNA in its nucleus and, under the right circumstances, could make a brand-new copy of you (a clone). We are like a hologram, in which the

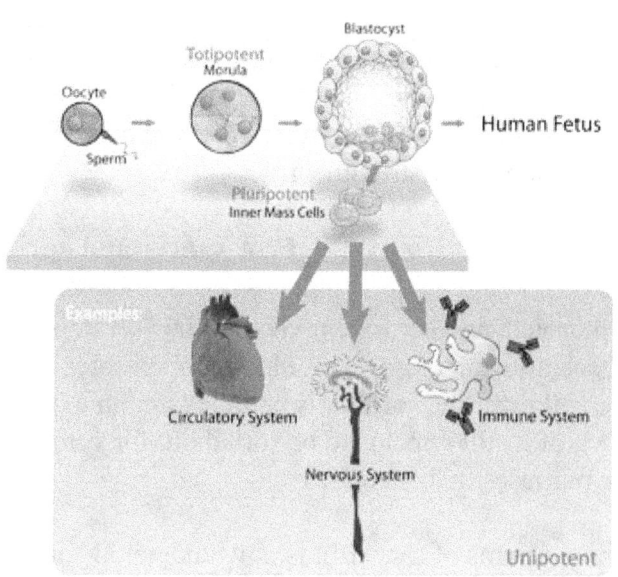

information for the whole is contained in all of the component parts. In the process of development, the original cell (egg) begins its division: first into a cluster of similar, "totipotent" cells, which can make a complete being. Those proliferate into somewhat differentiated cells (pluripotent), which can make only certain cell types, and then into the array of more specialized stem cells and, finally into, fully differentiated cells that create the working structures (tissues and organs) of your body. Some of these differentiated cells last throughout one's life-span. For example, heart muscle cells, soon after birth, stop dividing (cell division or mitosis is a process that causes complete reconstruction of the entire cell). There are stem cells through-out the heart tissue; but they seem to be naturally inactivated. In other words, you have the same heart muscle cells that you had when you were a new born; however, every 90 days or so each heart muscle cell completely reconstructs all of its component parts without renewing its DNA by cell division. The same is true of other cells such as: the neurons in your brain, skeletal muscles, and your eye lens. In contrast, your skin cells, intestine, endocrine tissues wear out and die off and are renewed by their respective stem cells. Both dividing and non-dividing cells eventually accumulate wear and tear; and when not replaced, that is what is called "ageing". During this process of cell division and maintenance, DNA can get damaged and make mistakes in cellular construction and metabolism. Anything that speeds up metabolism (i.e., chronic infection or exposure to toxic chemicals will increase the probability of mistakes). There are certain inherited genetic weaknesses that can make mistakes more likely. Also, there are numerous mechanisms by which such mutations are corrected and cells with mutations to be destroyed. However, if ever a mutation leads to a series of genetic changes that lead to unlimited cell division, then that is cancer. During early development, when growth and metabolism are highest, the number of mutations are greatest, yet the incidence of cancer is almost zero. Biopsies on younger people who have died from accidents show that cancer mutations are common in young people but, obviously, are kept in check and do not manifest. Thus, we are naturally getting cancer all of the time; but normal processes keep them benign or destroy them.

How cancer and ageing converge

A thorough and accurate review of the current state of knowledge with respect to ageing, regeneration, and cancer would be impossible. There is a deluge of on-going research from all over the world; it is complex and in a dynamic and rapid state of change; and much of it still remains to be sorted out for veracity. Let this general over-view suffice for our purposes in this book.

First, in terms of cancer, it is now understood and generally agreed that cancer arises when normal cells experience genetic "instability" (mutation to DNA), which causes a change in their metabolism and structure (phenotype) and that proceed to multiply in an uncontrolled manner. This instability can be caused by infectious and toxic agents (10% of the cases) and/or genetic weaknesses (another 10%); but 80% happen spontaneously by accidents of normal metabolism that are unavoidable. Again, we are getting cancer continuously and have been since birth; but a gauntlet of control mechanisms almost always eliminates the mutated cells, such that the development of cancer is a rare event until ageing ensues. The progression from a normal cell to cancer cells proceeds in the following metabolic "hallmarks". [4]

	Hallmark	Comments
1	Sustaining proliferation signaling.	Cancer cells acquire the capability of stimulating themselves to grow and divide.
2	Evading growth suppressors.	Cancer cells acquire the ability to circumvent normal anti-growth signals from other cells.
3	Resisting cell death.	Cancer cells lose the normal self-destruction mechanisms (apoptosis).

---

4   Hanahan, Douglas and Weinberg, Robert A. (2011). Hallmarks of Cancer: The Next Generation. Cell 144, March 4, 2011.

Chapter 11 - Cancer and the Control of Ageing

	Hallmark	Comments
4	Enabling replicative immortality.	Cancer cells divide indefinitely.
5	Reprogramming of energy metabolism.	Cancer cells modify normal metablism.
6	Evading immune destruction.	They evade being destroyed by the immune system.
7	Inducing angiogenesis.	They recruit a blood supply to themselves.
8	Activating invasion and metastasis.	They can invade surrounding tissue and migrate.

All of these hallmarks of cancer have a basis in DNA mutations and alternations of cellular proteins. Current research is focusing on exactly what particular molecular alterations occur in cancer cells, as a basis for attempting to invent therapies which target one or more such processes. However, the problem with this approach is that these cellular processes are likely to be also involved in the metabolism of normal cells; and while it might be therapeutic to disrupt them in cancer cells, that also might disrupt the metabolism of normal cells and thereby cause serious adverse effects. But we will have to see if and how this line of investigation results in real therapies. And do keep in mind that, as previously discussed, the cure of cancer will not significantly increase life-expectancy nor improve the quality of life.

Again, ageing is a process of irreversible decrease in biological vitality that, in all humans, happens naturally and starts to manifest at about the ages of 30-35. When we talk about young versus old, health versus disease, prevention, longevity, quality of life, performance, we are, fundamentally, talking about "Biological Vitality"; and in terms of therapeutic aims, we mean restoring Biological Vitality and maintaining it. What, then, constitutes Biological Vitality? It is about three, interrelated factors: 1) cell number, 2) the rate of cell functioning, and 3) the quality of cell components. During normal metabolism and under conditions of disease, all three components can be impaired; but normally their condition and functions are restored. However, because of some, as yet not understood genetic defect, the capacity to completely restore is inhibited or limited and the system generally deteriorates over time (i.e., ages), causing chronic diseases, leading to senescence, and limiting the maximum life-span. Cell number, rate, and quality are the criteria for Vitality and the aim of life-extension science and medicine would have to focus on the restoration and maintenance of those three factors. If our theory that ageing is a causative factor of

174

cancer, then what evidence supports that concept? In the previous graphs of age, disease incidences, and biological vitality, it is shown that the decline in biological vitality (ageing) correlates with the increased incidence of cancer and the other chronic diseases. Thus, the decline in Biological Vitality is one factor that correlates with ageing as a possible cause of cancer. For a more definitive correlation, we should look to experimental evidence in which ageing is slowed not only resulting in life-extension but also showing a delaying or decrease in cancer. Experimental, caloric restriction provides an example of such evidence.

In 1935, nutritional scientists (McCay, Crowell, and Maynard) reported their study in which the objective was stated as follows:

> "In a preliminary report, the literature concerning the effect of retarded growth upon the life span was reviewed (McCay and Crowell, '34). In this report was also included a summary in the nature of a progress report dealing with a study employing rats to determine the effect of retarding growth upon the total length of life.

> The present summary represents a complete, final report of this experiment employing white rats and covering a period of nearly 4 years. The object of this study was to determine the effect of retarding growth upon the total length of life and to measure the effects of retarded growth upon the ultimate size of the animal's body. In the present study, growth was retarded by limiting the calories." [5]

In their study, they restricted the total caloric intake of the animals to 60% of what the rats normally eat, attempting to make sure that they still had complete nutrition. In the following graph, their data are represented.

---

[5] McCay CM, Crowell MF, Maynard LA. The effect of retarded growth upon the length of life span and upon the ultimate body size. J Nutr. 1935;10:63–79.

Chapter 11 - Cancer and the Control of Ageing

Apparently, they were still working out the proper diet for caloric restriction because much of the restricted group died early. However, the life-extension effect of caloric restriction is highly discernible in 50% of the population, group **"B"**, over the control animals, group **"A"**.

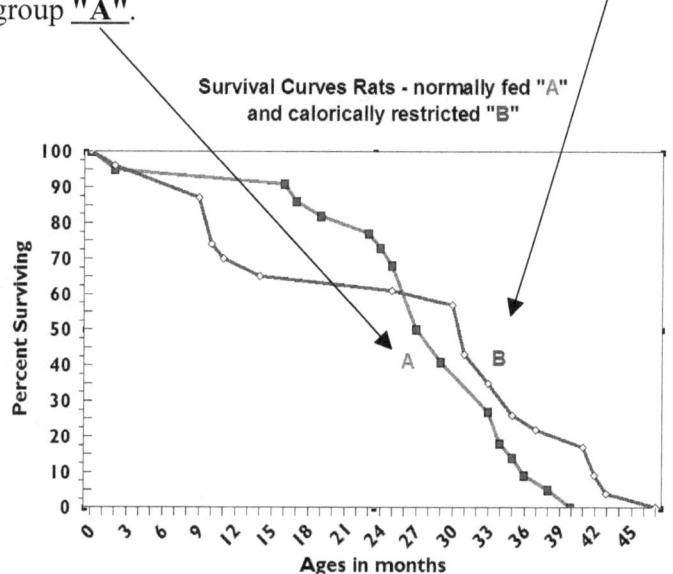

McCay's study of caloric restriction and its effect of slowing ageing were rudimentary and remained essentially ignored by the scientific community for some 50 years - being considered mostly an irrelevant curiosity. **H**owever, in the early 1990's, Roy Walford (a Professor of Pathology at the UCLA School of Medicine and gerontologist) started investigating caloric restriction as a means of life-extension as well as a model for studying the ageing process. **R**egarding the latter, the idea became that, if caloric restriction slows ageing, then how it does so might be a clue for how the natural ageing process happens and, therefore, could elucidate potential therapies. **C**aloric restriction does slows ageing in virtually all life-forms and more recently it has been demonstrated to do so in rhesus monkeys, a primate model similar to humans.

> "Caloric restriction (CR) without malnutrition increases longevity and delays the onset of age-associated disorders in short-lived species, from unicellular organisms to laboratory mice and rats. The value of CR as a tool to understand human ageing relies on translatability of CR's effects in primates. Here we show that CR significantly improves age-related and all-cause survival in monkeys on a long-term ~30% restricted diet since young adulthood.... Our data indicate that the benefits of CR on ageing are conserved in primates. [6]

---

[6]   Caloric restriction reduces age-related and all-cause mortality in rhesus monkeys.

Chapter 11 - Cancer and the Control of Ageing

As a result of Walford's influence, the study of caloric restriction and its effect on ageing flourished, with some 1,400 reports currently being cited in the MEDLINE database on that subject.

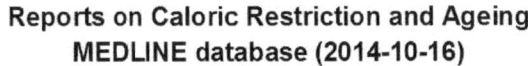

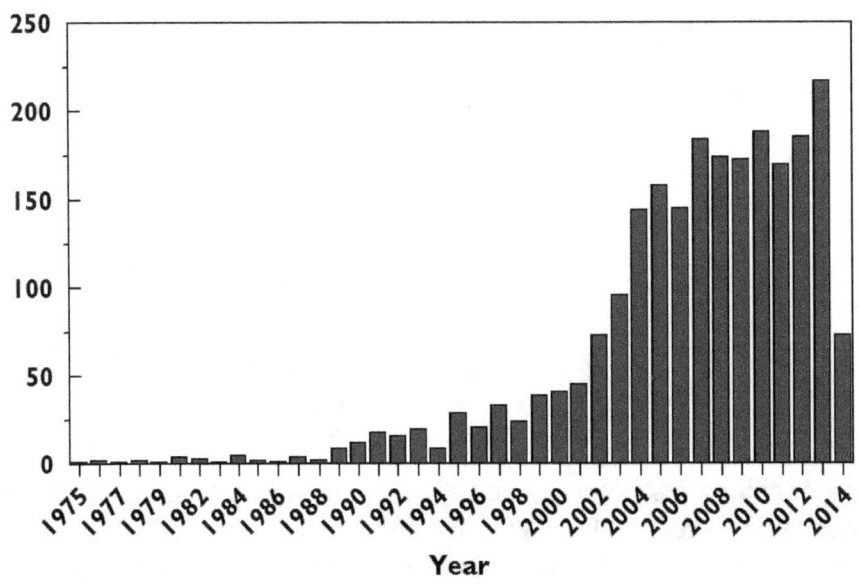

Colman RJ, Beasley TM, Kemnitz JW, Johnson SC, Weindruch R, Anderson RM; Nat Commun. 2014 Apr 1;5:3557.

Chapter 11 - Cancer and the Control of Ageing

In life-extension science and the study of ageing, the "Survival Curve" is the definitive way of determining if a particular therapy affects biological ageing. Below is a stylized graphic representation of the 3 basic Survival Curves. When a group of animals is studied throughout their entire life-span, one sees a normal, control Survival Curve with a standard mortality rate as in "(A)". Then, if you make beneficial modifications in the environment or provide some therapy which improves survival without changing the genetically programmed ageing, one will see a bowing of the Survival Curve where an increasing percentage of the population lives to the full potential life-span as in "(B)". If a therapy were to slow biological ageing, directly, then it will shift the entire Survival Curve to the right, extending not only the average but also the maximum life-span as in "C".

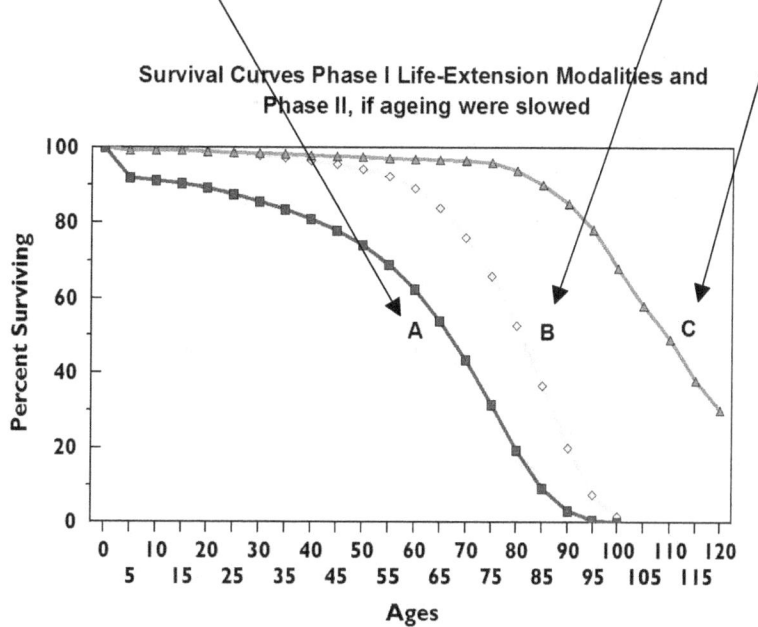

Survival Curves Phase I Life-Extension Modalities and Phase II, if ageing were slowed

Our present human population is experiencing a shift in our Survival Curve as in "B", where improvements in the environment and medicine are causing almost all of the population to live to our maximum life-span. As previously said, this is leading to a catastrophe where more and more people are surviving to a condition of senescence. What are needed are therapies which slow and reverse biological ageing as in Curve "C". And that is a completely new medical paradigm.

If caloric restriction slows ageing, which it does to some degree, and if that general biological deterioration which we call ageing plays a causative role in cancer, then calorically restricted animals should show a decrease in cancer incidence. And so it does. As far back as the 1940's, Albert Tannenbaum reported an experiment using caloric restriction

Chapter 11 - Cancer and the Control of Ageing

to study the incidence of spontaneous tumors in mice. [7] **Below** are the data table and note the following: 1) the **ages** of the animals; 2) the control group **N42** (allowed to eat freely) and the number surviving and their tumors; and 3) the caloric-restricted animals **N45** with their survival and tumors.

TABLE 1

THE EFFECT OF A CALORIE-RESTRICTED DIET ON THE FORMATION OF SPONTANEOUS MAMMARY TUMORS IN DBA VIRGIN FEMALE MICE

Age weeks	N42: *ad-libitum* controls			N45: calorie-restricted		
	Mean weight gm.	Animals alive and tumor-free	Cumu-lative tumor count	Mean weight gm.	Animals alive and tumor-free	Cumu-lative tumor count
10*	20	50	0	21	50	0
40	28	48	0	19	50	0
48	30	47	1	19	50	0
56	30	45	2	20	49	0
64	31	40	6	21	48	0
72	30	35	11	20	46	0
80	29	27	16	20	41	0
88	—	15	23	—	39	0
96	—	8	25	—	31	0
100	—	6	26	—	29	0

* Animals placed on experimental diets at 10 weeks of age.

---

7   Tannenbaum A; Effects of varying caloric intake upon tumor incidence and tumor growth; Annals of the New York Academy of Sciences; Volume 49, Nutrition in Relation to Cancer pages 5–18, September 1947

Chapter 11 - Cancer and the Control of Ageing

Graphing the data from the previous Table of Tannenbaum's experiment, you get the survival curves, below. "**A**" represents the normal survival curve for this specie of mouse, and the experimental, callorically restricted group is "**B**" - clearly indicated a slowing of the ageing process and dramatic increase in life-span

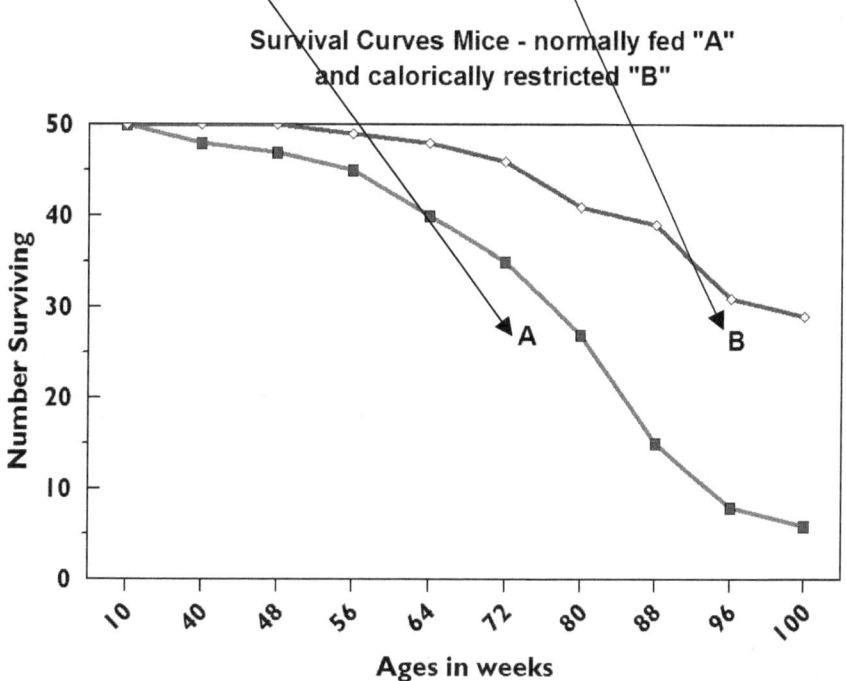

Survival Curves Mice - normally fed "A" and calorically restricted "B"

Further, the rather astounding observation is that in the calorically restricted group, there were zero tumors over their extended life-span. What then is the research related to cancer incidence and caloric restriction? See the following graph of reports in the MEDLINE database since 1947. As of this writing, there are a total of 646 reports. Some are related to mechanism, but all which pertain to the incidence of cancer and caloric restriction show a marked decreased in the incidence of cancers when the ageing process(es) are retarded by a calorically restricted regimen.

Chapter 11 - Cancer and the Control of Ageing

Reports on Caloric Restriction and Cancer
MEDLINE database (2014-10-16)

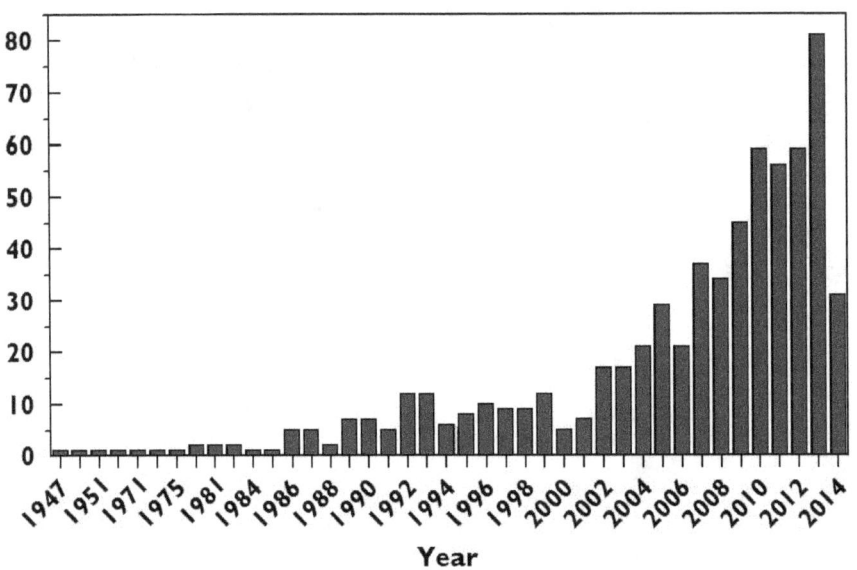

In summary, the prevailing paradigm of dealing with cancer as an independent disease will not yield any significant increase in life-expectancy and quality of life (on a statistical basis) even under ideal conditions of perfect cures. Ageing is a decline in Biological Vitality which is a loss of cell number, metabolic rate, and structure. As ageing progresses, the incidence of virtually all chronic diseases increase; and this is true of cancer. As experimental evidence of the thesis that ageing is a causative agent in cancer, caloric restriction extends life-span by slowing ageing while concurrently lowering cancer incidence. Therefore, a substantive approach to the treatment and prevention of cancer would be the control of ageing by regeneration of tissue back to the optimal condition which one had at about the age of 20 ± 5.

To conclude this final chapter, I want to review the work of one particular investigator, Mina Bissell, who seems particularly relevant to this thesis of approaching cancer by systemic regeneration. There are numerous scientists who are doing relevant work, but one can get a better feel by following a few scientists who have pursued a coherent and consistent line of investigation over a long period of time; and Dr. Bissell's work is exemplary.

Chapter 11 - Cancer and the Control of Ageing

Mina Bissell is a Distinguished, Senior Scientist at the Lawrence Berkeley National Laboratory (LBNL). The term "Distinguished" is reserved for those who "have a sustained history of distinguished scientific and technical achievements and/or have directly contributed to the Laboratory's preeminence," according to the Lab Regulations and Procedures Manual. The incumbents are "seen as nationally or internationally recognized authorities and leaders in their field; their expertise is sought after by professional colleagues."
LBNL is a federal research laboratory that is adjacent to the University of California, Berkeley (UCB) and is administered by that university. She is involved in a variety of projects related to cancer.
Born in Iran, she came to the United States for higher education; and after completing her Master and Doctorate degrees at Harvard in bacteriology, biochemistry, microbiology, and molecular genetics, she received a fellowship at UCB and became a staff scientist at LBNL - advancing since the 1970's to hold various administrative positions in the laboratory as well as faculty positions in four departments at the university while in pursuit of her unique line of research. She has received many awards and honors for her research, has served on national and international

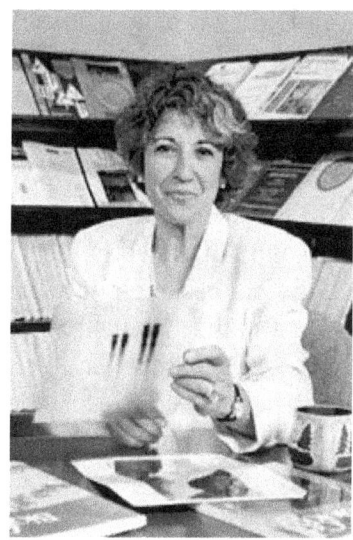

Dr. Mina Bissell

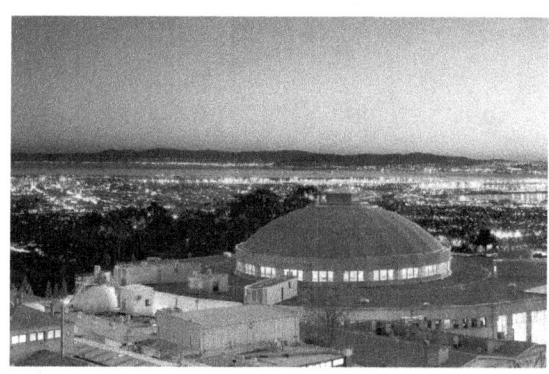

LBNL - Lawrence Berkeley
National Laboratory

scientific committees and review boards, belongs to a host of professional societies, has been an associate editor and on the editorial boards of many different scientific societies, is the holder of various patents, and has published over 300 reports in the scientific literature either by herself or, usually, as the senior investigator. Virtually all of this has been associated with cancer research; and she is internationally recognized for her lifetime contributions to the fields of breast cancer research, the enhanced role of the extra-cellular matrix (ECM) and the nucleus environment *vis-a-vis* to gene expression in normal and malignant tissues. Without reservation, Dr. Bissell is one of the leading scientists in this field.

Chapter 11 - Cancer and the Control of Ageing

A chronological sketch of Bissell's career will illustrate the thesis, as presented here, that cancer must be approached by systemic regeneration or control of ageing. Bissell's line of investigation can be characterized by several interrelated themes, which are reviewed as follows.

Two Enigmas In Biology. First, how it can happen that each and every cell has a complete copy of the entire genetic code that can construct all of the different tissues in an entire body but each cell only expresses certain sections of that code to become differentiated into specialized cells that determine the particular tissues? How do the cells that make the nose stay that way for life and do not make some other organ? In fact cancer can be seen as being derived from a cell that has de-differentiated into some anomalous type of tissue that is growing on its own? Further, given that the human body has some 50 trillion cells (it is estimated) and during normal metabolism there are a large number of mutations that occur constantly, of which a considerable number of such mutations are cancerous, why does so little cancer occur and at such a late stage in life - particularly given that the metabolic rate and number of mutations are so much higher during early development, when the incidence of cancer is essentially zero? As Bissell says in her lectures, pondering, exploring, and trying to answer these enigmas has bracketed her entire career.

The Rous Sarcoma Virus and Cancer. In 1911, Peyton Rous, was investigating the cause of a particular type of cancer in chickens. Taking a cell-free extract of the tumor, he discovered that by injecting the fluid into healthy chickens the cancer could be reproduced. The causative agent, it was discovered subsequently, was a virus. Later, other cancer-causing viruses were discovered; and this led to great interest in the possibility that cancer might be a result of infection that could be prevented by vaccination. Eventually, only a small number of viruses could be linked to cancer but using this model has been highly informative in understanding the genetic basis of cancer cells. (This was the generative force behind the National Cancer Act of 1971 which expanded the National Cancer Institute and which has become the world's largest organization that is dedicated solely to cancer research.) The Institute's resources have been used in the book in Chapter 1 (Physicians Data Query), Chapter 6 (Cancer Statistics), and Chapter 9 (Clinical Trials).) Bissell's early scientific carrier involved investigating the Rous Sarcoma Virus model. From 1976 to 1994, she published some 19 reports in this area. She found that the initiation of a cancer by this virus was generated by the trauma at the site of the injection. Although, from the injection, the virus was distributed throughout the cells of the entire body, it was only at the injection site where the tumor developed. The conclusion was that damage to the tissue structure at the site of the injection was what enabled the virus to become active as a cancer causing agent. She also found that the Rous Sarcoma Virus, when injected into a chicken embryo, would not develop into a tumor and thus something in the embryonic

Chapter 11 - Cancer and the Control of Ageing

environment inhibited the cancer-causing potential of the virus. This started her thinking along the lines that expression of cancer causing genes depended on extra-cellular environment.

3-Dimensional Cell Culture Medium. Much of the study of cellular biology is conducted in culture (*in vitro*) where the cells are transferred to an artificial medium in a plate. The cells can survive and reproduce in that environment; and it is much easier than studying them in the living system. Until recently, all such experiments were done on a two-dimensional surface, however, the problem has been that when cells are transferred from their normal, living (*in vivo*) environment to the artificial one, they radically change form and functions to adapt to that artificial environment; and accordingly, one cannot be sure that what is being studied is representative of living tissue. In 1989, Bissell became one of the early investigators using a three-dimensional matrix for culturing cells using a reconstituted basement membrane to simulate natural conditions. Further, she demonstrated that the cultured mammary cell line regained much of their natural form and also secreted milk proteins when grown on a more natural culture medium. This is seen in the adjacent microscopic

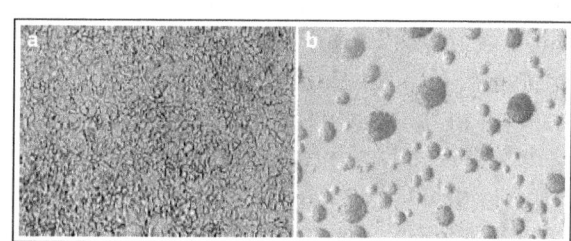

Mammary gland epithelial cells cultured on 2D plastic gel (a) where form and function are lost and on 3D matrix gel (b) where natural form and function are retained. [8]

photo from another investigator, where cells plated on the usual plastic base become unnaturally disorganized and differently shaped versus one plated on a three-dimensional environment that retain and recover their natural shape and functions. In a 1997 report, Bissell states:

"In a recently developed human breast cancer model, treatment of **tumor cells** in a 3-dimensional culture ... led to a striking morphological and functional reversion [of the tumor cells] to a normal phenotype [or form].... Our results illustrate that the extracellular matrix and its receptors dictate

---

8   2009; M. Kozlowski, et al.; Differences in growth and transcriptomic profile of bovine mammary epithelial monolayer and three-dimensional cell cultures; J Physiol Pharmacol. 2009 May;60 Suppl 1:5-14.

the phenotype of mammary epithelial cells, and thus in this model system the tissue phenotype is dominant over the cellular genotype." [9]

Bissell has continued to develop and refine this 3D experimental model for better understanding the interaction between the cellular extra-cellular matrix and micro-environment in relationship to the interactions of cells between each other, with their individual expression of DNA and the making of cellular components and those relevant to cancer.

Using the Mammary Gland as a Model System. In the 1980's Bissell began working with the mammary epithelial cells as an experimental model for the study of normal and malignant cells in culture. She has worked with both mouse and human mammary tissues. This gland has unique features for studying a complex biological system. Until puberty, it is developmentally quiescent, resting in the breast tissue as rudimentary nodes. Then upon pregnancy, those nodes blossom into "acini" as in the microscopic photo, adjacent. The word "acinus" is Latin for a cluster of cells that resemble a berry shape, containing multiple alveolar glands, as in the graphic representation. The "Luminal Epithelial Cells" (**1**) secrete milk that is exuded into the "Lumen" (**2**) and delivered to the nipple through a network of ducts. Then there are "Myoepithelia Cells" (**3**) that are muscle cells, interlaced around the Lumen Epithelial Cells which contract to work those cells into secreting milk. And around this acinus is an "Extracellular Matrix" (**4**) which is produced by resident cells and secreted into a molecular fabric that provides structural and biochemical

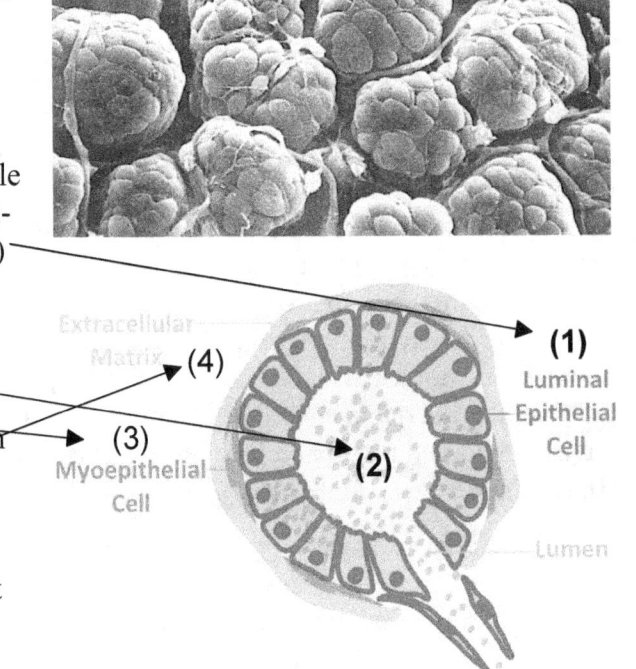

---

9   1997; Bissell MJ et al.; Reversion of the malignant phenotype of human breast cells in three-dimensional culture and in vivo by integrin blocking antibodies. J Cell Biol. 1997 Apr 7;137(1):231-45.

support to the surrounding cells, allowing adhesion of the cells to each other, cell-to-cell molecular communication, maintain differentiation, and probably many other functions that are still under investigation. The Luminal Epithelial Cells are the major site for breast carcer.

The above review does not properly convey the large amount of detailed work over decades by Bissell and the many people associated with her and the larger scientific community. For a better feel of that, see one of her recent lectues:

http://www.youtube.com/watch?v=xukDIWFMU9Y

The Over-arching Theme. The culmination of Bissell's work is, thus far, that although the mutation of genes (nuclear DNA) is essential for cells to transform into cancer, it is the structure of the Extra-cellular Matrix and the Micro-environment that governs the expression of the DNA and determines structure and function of the tissue. In a recent paper, she summarizes:

> "The study of biological form and how it arises is the domain of the developmental biologists; but once the form is achieved, the organ poses a fascinating conundrum for all the life scientists: how are form and function maintained in adult organs throughout most of the life of the organism? That they do appears to contradict the inherently plastic nature of organogenesis during development. How do cells with the same genetic information arrive at, and maintain such different architectures and functions, and how do they keep remembering that they are different from each other? It is now clear that narratives based solely on genes and an irreversible regulatory dynamics cannot answer these questions satisfactorily, and the concept of microenvironmental signaling needs to be added to the equation. During development, cells rearrange and differentiate in response to diffusive morphogens, juxtacrine signals, and the extracellular matrix (ECM). These components, which constitute the modular microenvironment, are sensitive to cues from other tissues and organs of the developing embryo as well as from the external macroenvironment. On the other hand, once the organ is formed, these modular constituents integrate and constrain the organ architecture, which ensures structural and functional homeostasis and therefore, organ specificity. We argue here that a corollary of the above is that once the organ architecture is compromised in adults by mutations or by changes in the microenvironment such as **aging** or inflammation, that organ becomes subjected to the developmental and embryonic circuits in search of a new identity. But since the microenvironment is no longer embryonic, the

Chapter 11 - Cancer and the Control of Ageing

confusion leads to cancer: hence as we have argued, tumors become new evolutionary organs perhaps in search of an elusive homeostasis." [10]

Recall what has been said previously. Biological vitality is a function of cell number, rate of metabolism, and structural quality. The peak of each human's biological vitality is between the ages of 20 ± 5 years of age. If that condition could be regenerated and maintained, then functioning would remain optimal; disease minimal and, if it does occur, easy to treat; and the potential life-expectancy greatly extended. The development of a medical technology which enables such regeneration should be the ultimate aim of both medicine and the life-extension sciences. Bissell's work points the way for such a fundamentally new approach toward that aim, showing that the biological vitality of cells is, in large measure, a function of the quality of their Extra-Cellular Matrix and Micro-Environment. She is poised to take her work to the next logical step - methods to regeneration the Extra-Cellular Matrix and Micro-Environment and evaluate the consequence of that on medical cures, health maintenance, and longevity.

---

10   Bhat Rl, Bissell MJ. Of plasticity and specificity: dialectics of the microenvironment and macroenvironment and the organ phenotype. Wiley Interdiscip Rev Dev Biol. 2014 Mar-Apr;3(2):147-63. 2013 Nov 18.

Chapter 11 - Cancer and the Control of Ageing

Epilog & Follow-up

We opened this work with the following statement:

> "The claim is made that there is one and, really, only one rational approach to cancer, as is explained in this book. Within about 30 minutes, using the easy to follow routines here, you can obtain the state-of-the-art protocols for the diagnosis and treatment of any type of cancer.
>
> Then, advance to the information on Alternative and Supportive care and how Experimental Trials and "Phase I" Life-Extension Applications might apply to your interests.
>
> The conventional approach to cancer is not really working; and we are in a rapid transition to a new order of medical science. However, it will require the involvement of a large number of people to advance it. And the eventual conquest of cancer requires a fundamentally different direction - one which we call the "Life-Extension & Control of Ageing Approach".
>
> This book is relevant at any stage (i.e., newly diagnosed, in treatment, in remission, or recurrent) as well as for prevention. If you are dealing with cancer - this book is an essential tool."

We believe that the material in this book supports those assertions - as bold as they may appear. If you are dealing with cancer, then the first objective is to evaluate what conventional medicine has to offer and to plan a therapeutic strategy that is appropriate to the individual person. In tandem with that, a personal program of Phase I Life-Extension Applications should be implemented to improve biological vitality and over-all health. Next, become informed about cancer in general and the specific type of concern. Evaluate what experimental therapies might be of value; and, if possible, become skilled at reviewing the scientific literature. Many of the procedures which we explain should also be of value to the treating Physician(s). Further, we have also interjected the new perspective that the control of ageing is critical to the eventual solution to cancer as well as to the other chronic diseases and to health in general.

We encourage you to register with us for supporting and follow-up information:

http://www.doctorinternet.com/cancer

The current medical paradigm is poised to make a radical change from treating only specific pathology with the traditional techniques of surgery, chemotherapy, and radiation toward personalized medicine based on the particular genetics of the individual and toward regeneration medicine.

Your involvement is appreciated and important in making this happen.

CAE

www.ingramcontent.com/pod-product-compliance
Lightning Source LLC
Chambersburg PA
CBHW080807180526

45168CB00006B/2350